Y0-AQW-522

Pediatric Cancer

Pediatric Cancer: Volume 3

Diagnosis, Therapy, and Prognosis

For further volumes:
http://www.springer.com/series/10167

Pediatric Cancer
Volume 3

Diagnosis, Therapy, and Prognosis

Pediatric Cancer

Diagnosis, Therapy, and Prognosis

Edited by

M.A. Hayat
Distinguished Professor
Department of Biological Sciences,
Kean University, Union, NJ, USA

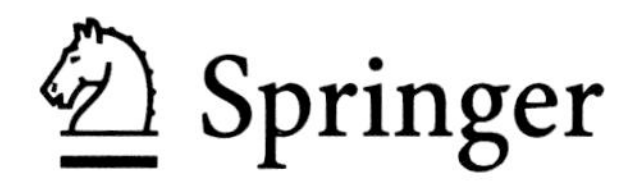

Editor
M.A. Hayat
Department of Biological Sciences
Kean University
Room 213, Library building
Morris Avenue 1000
Union, NJ 07083
USA

ISSN 2211-7997 ISSN 2211-8004 (electronic)
ISBN 978-94-007-4527-8 ISBN 978-94-007-4528-5 (eBook)
DOI 10.1007/978-94-007-4528-5
Springer Dordrecht Heidelberg New York London

Library of Congress Control Number: 2012942469

Printed on acid-free paper

Springer is part of Springer Science+Business Media (www.springer.com)

Although touched by technology, surgical pathology always has been, and remains, an art. Surgical pathologists, like all artists, depict in their artwork (surgical pathology reports) their interactions with nature: emotions, observations, and knowledge are all integrated. The resulting artwork is a poor record of complex phenomena.

Richard J. Reed, M.D.

One Point of View

All small tumors do not always keep growing, especially small breast tumors, testicular tumors, and prostate tumors. Some small tumors may even disappear without a treatment. Indeed, because prostate tumor grows slowly, it is not unusual that a patient may die at an advanced age of some other causes, but prostate tumor is discovered in an autopsy study. In some cases of prostate tumors, the patient should be offered the option of active surveillance followed by PSA test or biopsies. Similarly, every small kidney tumor may not change or may even regress. Another example of cancer or precancer reversal is cervical cancer. Precancerous cervical cells found with Pap test may revert to normal cells. Tumor shrinkage, regression, dormancy, senescence, reversal, or stabilization is not impossible. Can prosenescence therapy be an efficient alternative strategy to standard therapies for cancer prevention and treatment?

Another known example of cancer regression is found in pediatric neuroblastoma patients. Neuroblastoma shows one of the highest rates of spontaneous regression among malignant tumors. In addition to the well-known spontaneous regression in stage 4S disease, the high incidence of neuroblastoma remnants found during autopsy of newborns suggests that localized lesions may undergo a similar regression (Guin et al. 1969). Later studies also indicate that spontaneous regression is regularly seen in infants with localized neuroblastoma and is not limited to the first year of life (Hero et al. 2008). These and other studies justify the "wait and see" strategy, avoiding chemotherapy and radiotherapy in infants with localized neuroblastoma, unless MYCN gene is amplified. Infants with nonamplified MYCN and hyperdiploidy can be effectively treated with less intensive therapy. Infants with disseminated disease without MYCN have excellent survival with minimal or no treatment. Another example of spontaneous shrinkage and loss of tumors without any treatment is an intradural lipoma (Endoh et al. 1998).

Although cancers grow progressively, various lesions such as cysts and thyroid adenomas show self-limiting growth. Probably, cellular senescence occurs in many organ types following initial mutations. Cellular senescence, the growth arrest seen in normal mammalian cells after a limited number of divisions, is controlled by tumor suppressors, including p53 and p16, and so this phenomenon is believed to be a crucial barrier to tumor development. It is well-established that cell proliferation and transformation induced by oncogene activation are restrained by cellular senescence.

Metastasis is the main cause of death from cancer. Fortunately, metastasis is an inefficient process. Only a few of the many cancer cells detached from the primary tumor succeed in forming secondary tumors. Metastatic inefficiency varies depending on the location within an organ, but the malignancy may continue to grow preferentially in a specific tissue environment. Some of the cancer cells shed from the primary tumor are lost in the circulation due to hemodynamic forces or the immune system, macrophages, and natural killer cells.

Periodic rejection of a drug by FDA, which was previously approved by the FDA, is not uncommon. Most recently, the FDA ruled that Avastin should not be used to treat advanced breast cancer, although it remains on the market to treat certain other cancers, including colon and lung malignancies. Side effects of Avastin include high blood pressure, massive bleeding, heart attack, and damage to the stomach and intestines.

Unwanted side effects of some drug excipients (e.g., propylene glycol and menthol) may also pose safety concerns in some patients. Excipients are defined as the constituents of the pharmaceutical formulation used to guarantee stability, and physicochemical, organoleptic, and biopharmaceutical properties. Excipients frequently make up the majority of the volume of oral and parenteral drugs. Not all excipients are inert from the biological point of view. Although adverse drug reactions caused by the excipients are a minority of all adverse effects of medicinal products, the lack of awareness of the possible risk from excipients should be a concern for regulatory agencies, physicians, and patients (Ursino et al. 2011). Knowledge of the potential side effects of excipients is important in clinical practice.

It is known that chemotherapy can cause very serious side effects. One most recent example of such side effects was reported by Rubsam et al. (2011). Advanced hepatocellular carcinoma (HCC) induced by hepatitis C virus was treated with Sorafenib. It is an oral multikinase inhibitor that interferes with the serine/threonine kinases RAF-1 and B-Raf and the receptor tyrosine kinases of the vascular endothelial growth factor receptors and the platelet-derived growth factor receptor-beta. Although sorafenib is effective in regressing HCC, it shows serious side effects including increasingly pruritic and painful skin changes (cutaneous eruption).

An example of unnecessary surgery is the removal of all the armpit lymph nodes after a biopsy when a sentinel node shows early stage breast cancer; removal of only the sentinel node may be needed. Limiting the surgery to the sentinel node avoids painful surgery of the armpit lymph nodes, which can have complications such as swelling and infection (such limited surgery is already being practiced at the Memorial Sloan-Kettering Cancer Research Center). Radiation-induced second cerebral tumors constitute a significant risk for persons undergoing radiotherapy for the management of cerebral neoplasms. High-grade gliomas are the most common radiation-induced tumors in children (Pettorini et al. 2008). The actual incidence of this complication is not known, although it is thought to be generally low.

Medical Radiation

Chromosome aberrations induced by ionizing radiation are well known. Medical radiation-induced tumors are well documented. For example, several types of tumors (sarcomas, meningiomas) can develop in the CNS after irradiation of the head and neck region (Parent 1990). Tumorigenic mechanisms underlying the radiation therapy of the CNS are discussed by Amirjamshidi and Abbassioun (2000).

Women treated with therapeutic chest radiation may develop cancer. This possibility becomes exceedingly serious considering that 50,000–55,000 women in the United States have been treated with moderate to high-dose chest radiation (~20 Gy). This possibility is much more serious for pediatric or young adult cancer patients, because these women are at a significantly increased risk of breast cancer and breast cancer mortality following cure of their primary malignancy (Mertens et al. 2008). A recent study also indicates that such young women develop breast cancer at a young age, which does not appear to plateau (Henderson et al. 2010). In this high-risk population, ironically there is a benefit associated with early detection. In other words, young women with early stage breast cancer following chest radiation have a high likelihood for favorable outcome, although a life-long surveillance is needed.

Presently, although approximately 80% of the children with cancer are cured, the curative therapy could damage a child's developing organ system; for example, cognitive deficits following cranial radiotherapy are well known. Childhood survivors of malignant diseases are also at an increased risk of primary thyroid cancer (Sigurdson et al. 2005). The risk of this cancer increases with radiation doses up to 20–29 Gy. In fact, exposure to radiation therapy is the most important risk factor for the development of a new CNS tumor in survivors of childhood cancer, including leukemia and brain tumors. The higher risk of subsequent glioma in children subjected to medical radiation at a very young age reflects greater susceptibility of the developing brain to radiation. The details of the dose–response relationships, the expression of excess risk over time, and the modifying effects of other host and treatment factors have not been well defined (Neglia et al. 2006).

A recent study indicates that childhood brain tumor survivors are at an increased risk of late endocrine effects, particularly the patients treated with cranial radiation and diagnosed at a younger age (Shalitin et al. 2011). Among children with cancer, the application of radiotherapy, therefore, should not be taken lightly, and it should be administered only when absolutely necessary to successfully treat the primary tumor. When radiotherapy is administered, use of the minimum effective dose tends to minimize the risk of second CNS neoplasms (late effect). Prolonged follow-up of childhood cancer survivors (particularly those treated with radiation) is necessary because of the long period between treatment and the development of malignancy. This practice should be a part of the effective therapy of the primary disease.

It is well established that radiation doses are related to risk for subsequent malignant neoplasms in children with Hodgkin's disease. It has been reported that increasing radiation dose was associated with increasing standardized incidence ratio (p=0.0085) in survivors of childhood Hodgkin's disease (Constine et al. 2008). Approximately 75% of subsequent malignancies occurred within the radiation field. Although subsequent malignancies occur, for example, in breast cancer survivors in the absence of radiotherapy, the rise increases with radiation dose.

The pertinent question is: Is it always necessary to practice tumor surgery, radiotherapy, chemotherapy or hormonal therapy or a combination of these therapies? Although the conventional belief is that cancer represents an "arrow that advances unidirectionally," it is becoming clear that for cancer to progress it requires cooperative microenvironment (niche), including immune system and hormone levels. However, it is emphasized that advanced (malignant) cancers do not show regression and require therapy. In the light of the inadequacy of standard treatments of malignancy, clinical applications of the stem cell technology need to be expedited.

Prostate Cancer

There were an estimated 217,730 new cases of prostate cancer in the United States in 2010 with 32,050 deaths, making it the second leading cause of cancer deaths in men. Currently, there are more than 2,000,000 men in the United States who have had radical or partial prostate surgery performed. Considering this huge number of prostate surgeries and the absence of a cumulative outcome data, it seems appropriate to carefully examine the benefits of radical surgery, especially in younger men.

Clinical prostate cancer is very rare in men of the ages younger than 40 years. In this age group, the frequency of prostate malignancy is 1 in 10,000 individuals. Unfortunately, the incidence of malignancy increases over the ensuing decades, that is, the chance of prostate malignancy may reach to 1 in 7 in men between the ages of 60 and 79 years. Reactive or aging-related alterations in the tumor microenvironment provide sufficient influence, promoting tumor cell invasion and metastasis. It has been shown that nontumorigenic prostate epithelial cells can become tumorigenic when cocultured with fibroblasts obtained from regions near tumors (Olumi et al. 1999).

Prostate cancer treatment is one of the worst examples of overtreatment. Serum prostate specific antigen (PSA) testing for the early detection of prostate cancer is in wide use. However, the benefit of this testing has become controversial. The normal cut-off for serum levels of PSA is 4 ng/ml, so any man presenting a PSA above this level is likely to require rectal biopsy, but only in 25% of men with serum levels of PSA between 4 ng and 10 ng/ml have cancer (Masters 2007). The PSA threshold being used for biopsy ranges between 2.5 and 3.4 ng/ml. Up to 50% of men presenting with prostate cancer have PSA levels within the normal range. It is apparent that screening of prostate cancer using PSA has a low specificity, resulting in many unnecessary biopsies, particularly for gray zone values (4 ng–10 ng/ml). According to one point of view, the risks of prostate cancer overdetection are substantial. In this context, overdetection means treating a cancer that otherwise would not progress to clinically significant disease during the lifetime of the individual. Overdetection results in overtreatment. The advantages and limitations of PSA test in diagnosing prostate cancer were reviewed by Hayat (2005, 2008).

Androgen deprivation therapy (ADT) is an important treatment for patients with advanced stage prostate cancer. This therapy is carried out by blocking androgen receptor or medical or surgical castration. Although ADT is initially very effective, treated tumors inevitably progress to androgen-independent prostate cancer (AIPC), which is incurable. One possible mechanism responsible for the development of AIPC is modulation of the tissue microenvironment by neuroendocrine-like cancer cells, which emerge after ADT (Nelson et al. 2007).

Recently, Pernicova et al. (2011) have further clarified the role of androgen deprivation in promoting the clonal expansion of androgen-independent prostate cancer. They reported a novel linkage between the inhibition of the androgen receptor activity, down-regulation of S-phase kinase-associated protein 2, and the formation of secretory, senescent cells in prostate tumor cells. It is known that several components of the SASP secretome, such as IL-6, IL-8, KGH, and epidermal growth factor, are capable of transactivating androgen receptor under androgen-depleted conditions (Seaton et al. 2008). It needs to be pointed out that androgen deprivation therapy, used in high-risk patients with prostate cancer, may cause reduced libido, erectile dysfunction, fatigue, and muscle loss; osteoporosis is also a late complication. Therefore, periodic bone density scanning needs to be considered.

Recently, the FDA cleared the use of NADiA (nucleic acid detection immunoassay) ProsVue prognostic cancer test. This proprietary nucleic acid detection immunoassay technology identifies extremely low concentrations of proteins that have not been routinely used as a diagnostic or prognostic aid. It is an in vitro diagnostic assay for determining the rate of change of serum total PSA over a period of time. The assay can quantitate PSA at levels <1 ng/ml. This technique can be used as a prognostic marker in conjunction with clinical evaluation as an aid in identifying the patients at reduced risk for recurrence of prostate cancer for years following prostatectomy. It targets the early detection of proteins associated with cancer and infectious diseases. This technique combines immunoassay and real-time PCR methodologies with the potential to detect proteins with femtogram/ml sensitivity (10–15 g/ml). Additional clinical information is needed regarding its usefulness in predicting the recurrence.

A significant decrease in the risk of prostate cancer-specific mortality is observed in men with few or no comorbidities. Indeed, active surveillance in lieu of immediate treatment (surgery or radiation, or both) is gaining acceptance. Most men with prostate cancer, even those with high-risk disease, ultimately die as a result of other causes (Lu-Yao et al. 2009). Debate on this controversy is welcome, but narrow opinions and facile guidelines will not lead to facts and new information; men worldwide deserve it (Carroll et al. 2011). Automatic linking positive diagnosis with treatment, unfortunately, is a common clinical practice. Unfortunately, even men who are excellent candidates for active surveillance in the United States often undergo some treatment. Deferment of treatment is advised in men with low-risk disease, especially of a younger age.

Active surveillance is proposed for patients with low-risk prostate cancer in order to reduce the undesirable effects of overdiagnosis. Prostate-specific antigen serum level lower than 10 ng/L and Gleason score lower than 7 are the main criteria to select patients for active surveillance. The correct use of these two criteria is essential to differentiate between aggressive and nonaggressive prostate cancer. Autopsy studies indicate that approximately one out of three men older than 50 years show histological evidence of prostate cancer (Klotz 2008). Thus, a large proportion of prostate cancers are latent, never destined to progress, and affect the life of the patient. It is estimated that the percentage of low-risk prostate cancer is between 50% and 60% of newly diagnosed cases. A large number of patients die having prostate cancer, but not because of this cancer (Filella et al. 2011).

First whole genome sequences of prostate tumors were recently published online in Nature journal (vol. 470: 214–220, 2011). This study revealed that rather than single spelling errors the tumor has long "paragraphs" of DNA that seem to have broken off and moved to another part of the genome (rearrangement of genes), where they are most active. These portions of DNA contain genes that help drive cancer progression. The mutated genes involved include PTEN, CADM2, MAG12, SPOP, and SPTA1. This information may lead to the development of more efficient, less invasive ways to diagnose and treat this cancer. Such information, in addition, should lead to personalized therapeutics according to sequencing results of different gene mutations or chromosomal rearrangements. The urgent need of such studies becomes apparent considering the huge number of new cases of prostate problem reported every year.

In contrast to prostate cancer, cardiovascular disorders take the heavier toll of life. In other words, the risk of death for men in the United States between the ages of 55 and 74 years due to cardiovascular disease surpasses that of prostate cancer. Cardiovascular disease is the most common of the chronic non-communicable diseases that impact global mortality. Approximately 30% of all deaths worldwide and 10% of all healthy life lost to disease are accounted for by cardiovascular disease alone.

In conclusion, initial treatment with standard surgery, irradiation, chemotherapy, or hormonal therapy, or combination of these protocols can result in both local and systemic sequelae. Therefore, surveillance for late recurrence and secondary primary malignancies is recommended for most cancer patients. Patients with breast, lung, prostate, colorectal, and head and neck cancers constitute the largest groups requiring long-term monitoring and follow-up care.

Eric M.A. Hayat

References

Amirjamshidi A, Abbassioun K (2000) Radiation-induced tumors of the central nervous system occurring in childhood and adolescence. Childs Nerv Syst 16:390–397

Carroll PR, Whitson JH, Cooperberg MR (2011) Serum prostate-specific antigen for the early detection of prostate cancer; always, never, or only sometimes? J Clin Oncol 29:345–346

Constine LS, Tarbell N, Hudson MM et al (2008) Subsequent malignancies in children treated for Hodgkin's disease: associations with gender and radiation dose. Int J Radiat Oncol Biol Physol 72:24–33

Endoh M, Iwasaki Y, Koyanagi I, Hida K, Abe H (1998) Spontaneous shrinkage of lumbosacral lipoma in conjunction with a general decrease in body fat: case report. Neurosurgery 43(1):150–151; discussion 151–152

Filella X, Alcover J, Molina R (2011) Active surveillance in prostate cancer: the need to standardize. Tumor Biol 32:839–843

Guin P, Gilbert E, Jones B (1969) Incidental neuroblastoma in infants. Am J Clin Pathol 51:126–136

Hayat MA (2005) Prostate carcinoma: an introduction. In: Immunohistochemistry and in situ hybridization of human carcinomas, vol 2. Elsevier, San Francisco, pp 279–297

Hayat MA (2008) Prostate carcinoma. In: Methods of cancer diagnosis, therapy, and prognosis, vol 2. Springer Science, New York, pp 391–396

Henderson TO, Amsterdam A et al. (2010) Surveillance for breast cancer in women treated with chest radiation for a childhood, adolescent or young adult cancer: a report from Children's Oncology Group. Ann Intern Med 152:1–22

Hero S, Simon T, Spitz R, Ernestus K, Gnekow A, Scheel-Walter H, Schwabe D, Schilling F, Benz-Bohm G, Berthold F (2008) Localized infant neuroblastomas often show spontaneuous regression: results of the prospective trials NB95-S and NB 97. J Clin Oncol 26:1504–1510

Klotz L (2008) Low-risk prostate cancer can and should often be managed with active surveillance and selective delayed intervention. Nat Clin Pract Urol 5:2–3

Lu-Yao GL, Albertsen PC, Moore DF et al (2009) Outcomes of localized prostate cancer following conservative management. JAMA 302:1202–1209

Masters JR (2007) Clinical applications of expression profiling and proteomics in prostate cancer. Anticancer Res 27:1273–1276

Mertens AC, Liu Q, Neglia JP et al (2008) Cause-specific late mortality among 5-year survivors of childhood cancer: the Childhood Cancer Survivor Study. J Natl Cancer Inst 100:1368–1379

Neglia JP, Robison LL, Stovall M, Liu Y, Packer RJ et al (2006) New primary neoplasms of the central nervous system in survivors of childhood cancer: a report from the childhood cancer survivor study. J Natl Cancer Inst 98:1528–1537

Nelson EC, Cambio AJ, Ok JH, Lara PN Jr, Evans CP (2007) Clinical implications of nueroendocrine differentiation in prostate cancer. Prostate Cancer Prostatic Dis 10:6–14

Olumi AF, Grossfeld GD, Hayward SW, Carroll PR, Tlsty TD, Cunha GR (1999) Carcinoma-associated fibroblasts direct tumor progression of initiated human prostatic epithelium. Cancer Res 59:5002–5011

Parent AD (1990) Late complications of radiation-induced neoplasms. Neurosurgery 26:1090–1091

Pernicova Z, Slabakova E, Kharaishvill G, Bouchal J, Kral M, Kunicka Z, Machalam M, Kozubik A, Soucek K (2011) Androgen depletion induces senescence in prostate cancer cells through down-regulation of SKp2. Neoplasia 13:526–536

Pettorini BL, Park Y-S, Caldarelli M, Massimi L, Tamburrini G, DiRocco C (2008) Radiation induced brain tumors after central nervous system irradiation in childhood: a review. Childs Nerv Syst 24:793–805

Rubsam K, Flaig MJ, Ruzicka T, Prinz JC (2011) Erythema marginatum hemorrhagicum: a unique cutaneous side effect of sorafenib. J Am Acad Dermatol 64:1194–1196

Seaton A, Scullin P, Maxwell PJ, Wilson C, Pettigrew J, Gallagher R, O'Sullivan JM, Johnston PG, Waugh DJ (2008) Interleukin-8 signaling promotes androgen-independent proliferation of prostate cancer cells via induction of androgen receptor expression and activation. Carcinogenesis 6:1148–1156

Shalitin S, Gal M, Goshen Y, Cohen I, Yaniv I, Philip M (2011) Endocrine outcome in long-term survivors of childhood brain tumors. Horm Res Paediatr 76:113–122

Sigurdson AJ, Ronckers CM, Mertens AC et al (2005) Primary thyroid cancer after a first tumor in childhood (the childhood cancer survivor study): a nested case-control study. Lancet 365:2014–2023

Ursino MG, Poluzzi E, Caramella C, DePonti F (2011) Excipients in medicinal products used in gastroenterology as a possible cause of side effects. Regul Toxicol 60:93–105

Preface and Introduction

It is recognized that scientific journals and books not only provide current information but also facilitate exchange of information, resulting in rapid progress in the medical field. In this endeavor, the main role of scientific books is to present current information in more detail after careful additional evaluation of the investigational results, especially those of new or relatively new diagnostic approaches and therapeutic methods and their potential toxic side effects.

Although subjects of diagnosis, cancer recurrence including brain tumors, resistance to chemotherapy, assessment of treatment effectiveness, including cell therapy and side effects of a treatment are scattered in a vast number of journals and books, there is need of combining these subjects in single volumes. An attempt is made to accomplish this goal in the projected multi-volume series of handbooks.

In the era of cost-effectiveness, my opinion may be minority perspective, but it needs to be recognized that the potential for false-positive or false-negative interpretation on the basis of a single laboratory test in clinical pathology does exist. Interobserver or intraobserver variability in the interpretation of results in pathology is not uncommon. Interpretative differences often are related to the relative importance of the criteria being used.

Generally, no test always performs perfectly. Although there is no perfect remedy to this problem, standardized classifications with written definitions and guidelines will help. Standardization of methods to achieve objectivity is imperative in this effort. The validity of a test should be based on the careful, objective interpretation of the tomographic images, photo-micrographs, and other tests. The interpretation of the results should be explicit rather than implicit. To achieve accurate diagnosis and correct prognosis, the use of molecular criteria and targeted medicine is important. Equally important are the translation of molecular genetics into clinical practice and evidence-based therapy. Translation of medicine from the laboratory to clinical application needs to be carefully expedited. Indeed, molecular medicine has arrived.

There are many differences between adult and pediatric brain tumors beyond simple nomenclature; for example, pediatric tumors are often more sensitive to adjuvant irradiation and chemotherapy. Some pediatric tumors may only need complete resection to achieve a cure. It is pointed out that an experienced neurosurgeon should be aware of the difference between the adult tumors and pediatric tumors. It is emphasized, for example, that pediatric low-grade gliomas need lower doses of anticancer drugs such as cisplatin/etoposide. Refinements in clinical and molecular stratification for many types of childhood brain tumors to achieve risk-adapted treatment planning are discussed.

This is the third volume in the series, PEDIATRIC CANCER. Brain tumors are the most common solid tumors of childhood and remain the leading cause of cancer-related mortality in children. A general introduction to the principles of diagnosis, treatment, and prognosis of children with brain tumors is presented in this volume. Molecular characterization of solid tumors is important for providing novel biomarkers of disease and identifying molecular pathways, which may provide putative targets for new therapies. Specifically, this volume discusses in detail molecular genetics, diagnosis, prognosis, and therapy of atypical teratoid/rhabdoid tumor (AT/RT). AT/RT is a highly aggressive embryonal CNS tumor, which is mainly found in children, with a peak incidence in infants younger than 3 years of age. In fact, these tumors are among the most common malignant neoplasms in children. Similarities of the AT/RT with some other CNS tumors (PNET and medulloblastoma) tend to misclassify this tumor, which is pointed out in this volume. Although AT/RT has overlapping histological features with some other tumors, one feature unique to most AT/RTs is the genetic abnormality in the INI1 gene on chromosome 22q11. The presence of this gene and SMARCB1 gene in this tumor is discussed here. Present and future therapies for children with this tumor are presented. Historically, outcomes for patients with the atypical AT/RT have been poor despite surgery and chemotherapy, but new strategies, including intensive multimodel therapy and high-dose chemotherapy with autologous stem cell transplantation, have improved outcomes. Diagnosis of AT/RT type using imaging technology is included in this volume. Various therapies, including total resection followed by aggressive chemotherapy and radiation, for patients with this tumor are presented. Dissemination of this malignancy to the cerebral fluid is explained.

A number of other pediatric tumors are described in this volume. The role of cytogenetic markers in intracranial pediatric ependymoma is explained using comparative genomic hybridization and fluorescent in situ hybridization. Prognostic role of cyclin A and B proteins in pediatric embryonal tumors is pointed out. Treatment of pineal region tumors in childhood is included, so is the complete surgery and ultrasound monitoring of pediatric hepatoblastoma. This volume also contains the details of testicular preserving surgery.

Molecular mechanisms, including hepatocyte growth factor, underlying the initiation and progression of medulloblastoma are discussed. The involvement of MYCN gene amplification, heterozygous germ-line mutations, and hedgehog signaling in medulloblastoma is explained. Immunohistochemical analysis and ultrastructural details of medulloblastoma are also included in this volume. Prognostic factors for this malignancy are described. The importance of Gamma Knife radiosurgery during multimodality management of medulloblastoma/PNET tumors is explained. This volume also describes the diagnosis of retinoblastoma using magnetic resonance imaging and treatment of this malignancy. The role of microsatellite instability in pediatric high grade is deciphered. Effects of radiotherapy in low-grade glioma in children are also included in this volume. Combined therapeutical strategies for pediatric multiple primary cranio-spinal tumors associated with neurofibromatosis type 2 are described in detail. Laminectomy and duraplasty of pediatric intradural lipoma of the cervicothorasic spinal cord are presented.

Many tumor suppressor genes and oncogenes directly participate in or regulate signal transduction pathways. Alterations of these and other cell cycle regulators play a crucial role in the development and progression of human malignancies, including those in children. Although pediatric optic-hypothalamic gliomas have a favorable prognosis with regard to the long-term survival, such children may suffer from neurological deficits. Pediatric patients with high-grade gliomas have a very poor prognosis despite a variety of aggressive therapies. An overview, including epidemiology, etiology, treatment, and prognostic factors, of these high-grade gliomas is presented. Endoscopic neurosurgical techniques for treating pediatric intraventricular brain tumors are explained. The efficacy of using scheduled non-narcotic analgesic regimens following cranial and spine neurosurgery is explained. The use of scheduled doses of alternating acetaminophen and ibuprofen following craniotomy for tumor biopsy or resection is recommended. Neurosurgical management of pediatric low-grade glioma, high-grade glioma, medulloblastoma, retinaoblastoma, teratoid/rhabdoid tumors, spinal tumors, and some other tumor types is explained in detail.

By bringing together a large number of experts (oncologists, neurosurgeons, physicians, research scientists, and pathologists) in various aspects of this medical field, it is my hope that substantial progress will be made against this terrible disease. It would be difficult for a single author to discuss effectively the complexity of diagnosis, therapy, and prognosis of any type of tumor in one volume. Another advantage of involving more than one author is to present different points of view on a specific controversial aspect of the pediatric cancer. I hope these goals will be fulfilled in this and other volumes of this series. This volume was written by 72 contributors representing 16 countries. I am grateful to them for their promptness in accepting my suggestions. Their practical experience highlights their writings, which should build and further the endeavors of the reader in this important area of disease. I respect and appreciate the hard work and exceptional insight into the nature of brain tumors provided by these contributors. The contents of this volume are divided into six subheadings, Teratoid/Rhabdoid, Medulloblastoma, Retinoblastoma, Glioma, Spinal Tumors, and Miscellaneous Tumors, for the convenience of the reader.

It is my hope that the current volume will join the future volumes of the series for assisting in the more complete understanding and cure of globally relevant brain malignancy in children. There exists a tremendous, urgent demand by the public and the scientific community to address to cancer, diagnosis, treatment, cure, and hopefully prevention. In the light of existing cancer calamity, government funding must give priority to eradicating this deadly children's malignancy over military superiority.

I am thankful to Jennifer Russo for assisting in completing this volume.

Eric M.A. Hayat

Contents

Part IV Glioma

Part V Spinal Tumors

Part VI Miscellaneous Tumors

Contents of Volume 1

Contents of Volume 2

Contributors

Nejat Akalan Department of Neurosurgery, Faculty of Medicine, Hacettepe University, Ankara, Turkey

George A. Alexiou Department of Neurosurgery, Children's Hospital "Agia Sofia", Athens, Greece

Atilla Arslanoglu Imaging Center, Beytepe Military Hospital, Ankara, Turkey

Saurabh Aurora Department of Pediatric Retina and Ocular Oncology, Aravind Eye Hospital, Coimbatore, Tamil Nadu, India

Rachel Beddow Central and Southern Genetic Services, Wellington Hospital, Wellington, New Zealand

Lipa Bodner Department of Oral and Maxillofacial Surgery, Soroka University Medical Center, Ben Gurion University of the Negev, Beer Sheva, Israel

Jinbiao Chen Centenary Institute of Cancer Medicine and Cell Biology, Camperdown, NSW, Australia

Junjeong Choi Department of Pediatrics, Yonsei University College of Medicine, 162 Ilsadong Wonju, 220–701, Wonju, Republic of Korea

Krystyna H. Chrzanowska Department of Medical Genetics, The Children's Memorial Health Institute, Warsaw, Poland

Elżbieta Ciara Department of Medical Genetics, The Children's Memorial Health Institute, Warsaw, Poland

Mariela Carolina Coccé Cytogenetics Laboratory, Genetics Department, Garrahan Pediatrics Hospital, Buenos Aires, Argentina

Joseph R. Cohen Semel Institute, Department of Psychiatry and Biobehavioural Sciences, David Geffen School of Medicine, University of California, Los Angeles, CA, USA

Uygur Er Neurosurgery Clinic, TOBB ETU Hospital, The Union of Chambers and Commodity Exchanges of Turkey, Economics and Technology University, Sogutozu C., Fourth Sk., No. 22/7, 06510 Cankaya, Ankara, Turkey

Thomas Flannery Departments of Neurological Surgery and Radiation Oncology, University of Pittsburgh Medical Center, Pittsburgh, PA, USA Department of Neurosurgery, Royal Hospitals Trust, Belfast, and Leeds Gamma Knife Center, St. James's Institute of Oncology, Leeds, UK

Otilia Fufezan Third Pediatric Clinic, University of Medicine and Pharmacy, Cluj Napoca, Romania

Daniel W. Fults University of Utah School of Medicine, Salt Lake City, UT, USA

Marta Susana Gallego Cytogenetics Laboratory, Genetics Department, Garrahan Pediatrics Hospital, Buenos Aires, Argentina

Bora Gürer Department of First Neurosurgery, Dışkapı Yıldırım Beyazıt Research and Education Hospital, Ankara, Turkey

Reiji Haba Department of Pathology and Host Defense, Faculty of Medicine, Kagawa University, Miki-cho, Kita-gun, Kagawa, Japan

Christine Haberler Institute of Neurology, Medical University of Vienna, Vienna, Austria

Murigendra Hiremath Department of Pediatric Urology, KLE University's J N Medical College, KLES Kidney Foundation, KLES Dr. Prabhakar Kore Hospital and MRC, Belgaum, India

Daniela Iacob Third Pediatric Clinic, University of Medicine and Pharmacy, Cluj Napoca, Romania

Eric M. Jackson Department of Neurosurgery, Nationwide Children's Hospital, Columbus, OH, USA

Chris Jones Section of Paediatric Oncology, Institute of Cancer Research, Sutton, Surrey, UK

Elżbieta Jurkiewicz Department of Radiology, MR Unit, The Children's Memorial Hospital Health Institute, Warsaw, Poland

N. Kalpana Department of Pediatric Retina and Ocular Oncology, Aravind Eye Hospital, Coimbatore, Tamil Nadu, India

Hayri Kertmen Department of First Neurosurgery, Dışkapı Yıldırım Beyazıt Research and Education Hospital, Ankara, Turkey

Hyosun Kim Department of Pediatrics, Yonsei University College of Medicine, 50 Yonsei-ro Seodaemun-gu, Seoul, 120–752, Republic of Korea

Se Hoon Kim Department of Pathology, Yonsei University College of Medicine, 50 Yonsei-ro Seodaemun-gu, Seoul, 120–752, Republic of Korea

Douglas Kondziolka Departments of Neurological Surgery and Radiation Oncology, University of Pittsburgh Medical Center, Pittsburgh, PA, USA

Michael J. Kramarz Department of Neurosurgery, Children's Hospital of Philadelphia, University of Pennsylvania Medical Center, Philadelphia, PA, USA

Takashi Kusaka Maternal Perinatal Center, Faculty of Medicine, Kagawa University, Miki-cho, Kita-gun, Kagawa, Japan

Linda M. Liau Jonsson Comprehensive Cancer Center, David Geffen School of Medicine, University of California, Los Angeles, CA, USA

Rishi R. Lulla Hematology, Oncology and Stem Cell Transplantation, Ann & Robert H. Lurie Children's Hospital of Chicago and Northwestern University Feinberg School of Medicine, 225 East Chicago Avenue, Box #30, IL 60611, Chicago

L. Dade Lunsford Departments of Neurological Surgery and Radiation Oncology, University of Pittsburgh Medical Center, Pittsburgh, PA, USA

Esther Manor Genetics, Laboratory, Institute of Human Genetics, Soroka University Medical Center, Ben Gurion University of the Negev, Beer Sheva, Israel

Thomas E. Merchant Division of Radiation Oncology, St. Jude Children's Research Hospital, Memphis, TN, USA

Erin S. Murphy Department of Radiation Oncology, Taussig Cancer Institute, Cleveland Clinic, Cleveland, OH, USA

V. Narendran Department of Pediatric Retina and Ocular Oncology, Aravind Eye Hospital, Coimbatore, Tamil Nadu, India

Rajendra Nerli Department of Pediatric Urology, KLE University's J N Medical College, KLES Kidney Foundation, KLES Dr. Prabhakar Kore Hospital and MRC, Belgaum, India

Masayuki Onodera Department of Pathology and Host Defense, Faculty of Medicine, Kagawa University, Miki-cho, Kita-gun, Kagawa, Japan

Amalia Patereli Department of Pathology, Children's Hospital "Agia Sofia", Athens, Greece

Danuta Perek Department of Radiology, MR Unit, The Children's Memorial Hospital Health Institute, Warsaw, Poland

Annalisa Pezzolo Laboratory of Oncology, Department of Laboratory and Experimental Medicine, Instituto Giannina Gaslini, Genoa, Italy

Neofytos Prodromou Department of Neurosurgery, Children's Hospital "Agia Sofia", Athens, Greece

Rui Manuel Reis Molecular Oncology Research Center, Barretos Cancer Hospital, Rua Antenor Duarte Villela, Paulo, Brazil

Adam C. Resnick Department of Neurosurgery, Children's Hospital of Philadelphia, University of Pennsylvania Medical Center, Philadelphia, PA, USA

Stefan Rutkowski Department of Pediatric Hematology and Oncology, University Medical Center Hamburg-Eppendorf, Hamburg, Germany

Olga Rutynowska Department of Radiology, MR Unit, The Children's Memorial Hospital Health Institute, Warsaw, Poland

Haruhiko Sakamoto Department of Pathology and Host Defense, Faculty of Medicine, Kagawa University, Miki-cho, Kita-gun, Kagawa, Japan

Ahmet Metin Şanlı Department of First Neurosurgery, Dı kapı Yıldırım Beyazıt Research and Education Hospital, Ankara, Turkey

Alexandru Serban Third Pediatric Clinic, University of Medicine and Pharmacy, Cluj Napoca, Romania

Parag K. Shah Department of Pediatric Retina and Ocular Oncology, Aravind Eye Hospital, Coimbatore, Tamil Nadu, India

Aseem Shukla Department of Urologic Surgery, Pediatric Division, University of Minnesota, Minneapolis, MN, USA

Irene Slavc Department of Pediatrics, Medical University of Vienna, Vienna, Austria

Simone Treiger Sredni Neurosurgery Research Program, Children's Hospital of Chicago Research Center and Northwestern University Feinberg School of Medicine, 225 East Chicago Avenue, Box #28, IL 60611, Chicago

Stella Stabouli Pediatric Intensive Care Unit, Hippokration General Hospital, Thessaloniki, Greece

Teresa Stachowicz-Stencel Departments of Pediatrics, Haematology, Oncology, and Endocrinology, Medical University of Gdansk, Gdansk, Poland

Kalliopi Stefanaki Department of Neurosurgery, Children's Hospital "Agia Sofia", Athens, Greece

Phillip B. Storm Department of Neurosurgery, Children's Hospital of Philadelphia, University of Pennsylvania Medical Center, Philadelphia, PA, USA

Cecilia Surace Cytogenetics and Molecular Genetics, Children's Hospital "Bambino Gesú", Rome, Italy

Takashi Tamiya Department of Neurological Surgery, Faculty of Medicine, Kagawa University, Miki-cho, Kita-gun, Kagawa, Japan

Wayne D. Thomas Cell-Innovations Pty Limited, Liverpool, NSW, Australia

Joanna Trubicka Department of Medical Genetics, The Children's Memorial Health Institute, Warsaw, Poland

Masaki Ueno Department of Pathology and Host Defense, Faculty of Medicine, Kagawa University, Miki-cho, Kita-gun, Kagawa, Japan

Ali Varan Department of Pediatric Oncology, Institute of Oncology, Hacettepe University, Ankara, Turkey

Marta Viana-Pereira Life and Health Sciences Research Institute (ICVS), School of Health Sciences, University of Minho, Braga, Portugal

André O.vonBueren Department of Pediatric Hematology and Oncology, University Medical Center Hamburg-Eppendorf, Hamburg, Germany

Gerhard Franz Walter Department of Neuropathology, Klinikum Kassel, Kassel, Germany

James A. Waschek Semel Institute, Department of Psychiatry and Biobehavioural Sciences, David Geffen School of Medicine, University of California, Los Angeles, CA, USA

Douglas A. Weeks Department of Pathology, Oregon Health and Science University, Portland, OR, USA

Faruk Zorlu Department of Radiation Oncology, Faculty of Medicine, Hacettepe University, Ankara, Turkey

Part I

Teratoid/Rhabdoid

1 Early Childhood Atypical Teratoid/Rhabdoid Tumors

Christine Haberler and Irene Slavc

Contents

C. Haberler (✉)
Department of Pediatrics, Medical University of Vienna, Waehringer Guertel 18-20, A-1097 Vienna, Austria
e-mail: christine.haberler@meduniwien.ac.at

I. Slavc
Institute of Neurology, Medical University of Vienna, Waehringer Guertel 18-20, A-1097 Vienna, Austria
e-mail: irene.slavc@meduniwien.ac.at

Abstract

Atypical teratoid rhabdoid tumor (AT/RT) is a highly malignant embryonal tumor of the central nervous system (CNS), which occurs sporadically or in the setting of a rhabdoid predisposition syndrome. A peak incidence of AT/RTs is found in children aged less than 3 years at diagnosis. In this age group ATRT occurs as frequently as medulloblastoma, the most common malignant pediatric CNS tumor.

The characteristic morphological feature of AT/RT is the presence of rhabdoid tumor cells and varying amounts of small -undifferentiated PNET-like, mesenchymal, and/or epithelial differentiated tumor cells. The morphological and imaging similarities with supratentorial PNETs and medulloblastomas may result in misclassification. The vast majority of AT/RTs are characterized by alterations of the *SMARCB1* (*hSNF5*/*INI1*) gene that encodes a ubiquitously expressed protein. Alterations of *SMARCB1* lead to loss of nuclear protein expression, which can be detected by an immunohistochemical staining.

Currently, no definitive guidelines for optimal treatment have been established. Most recent treatment strategies recommend maximal safe surgery followed by multimodal therapy, including intensive chemotherapy often augmented with intrathecal therapy with or without high-dose chemotherapy (HDC), and focal or craniospinal irradiation. With this

M.A. Hayat (ed.), *Pediatric Cancer, Volume 3: Diagnosis, Therapy, and Prognosis*, Pediatric Cancer 3,
DOI 10.1007/978-94-007-4528-5_1,

approach prolonged survival can be achieved in a proportion of patients.

Introduction

Atypical teratoid/rhabdoid tumor (AT/RT) is a rare, highly aggressive embryonal CNS tumour. It may occur sporadically or in the setting of a rhabdoid predisposition syndrome. AT/RTs are mainly encountered in children, with a peak incidence in infants aged less than 3 years.

Rhabdoid tumours were originally described as aggressive variant of Wilms tumours with rhabdomyosarcomatous features (Beckwith and Palmer 1978). Subsequently, non-renal rhabdoid tumours were observed particularly in the CNS and referred to as AT/RT. This term was coined by Rorke in 1987 and defined as an entity in 1996 (Rorke et al. 1996). In 2000, AT/RTs were introduced to the World Health Organization (WHO) brain tumor classification.

The designation AT/RT reflects the complex histological features of this tumour including rhabdoid tumor cells and variable areas of primitive neuroectodermal-like, mesenchymal and/or epithelial differentiated tumour cells. The morphological and imaging similarities with supratentorial PNETs and medulloblastomas may result in misclassification (Haberler et al. 2006; Warmuth-Metz et al. 2008; Woehrer et al. 2010). The characteristic genomic aberration of AT/RTs is the inactivation of the *SMARCB1* (*hSNF5/INI1*) gene located in chromosome band 22q11.2, which is present in the vast majority of AT/RTs and peripheral rhabdoid tumors and can be detected by an immunohistochemical staining.

Epidemiology

AT/RTs occur predominantly in children; only single cases have been reported in adults (Raisanen et al. 2005). Large hospital-based series established the incidence of AT/RT at 1–2% of all pediatric CNS tumors (Rickert and Paulus 2001; Wong et al. 2005; Kaderali et al. 2009). In a population-based study of histopathologically confirmed pediatric brain tumors the age-standarized incidence rate of AT/RTs is 1.38 per 1,000,000 person-years (Woehrer et al. 2010).

Reported median ages at diagnosis are between 16.5 and 24 months (Rorke et al. 1996; Hilden et al. 2004; Woehrer et al. 2010; von Hoff et al. 2011). A peak incidence is observed in children younger than 3 years. In this age group AT/RT occurs as frequently as medulloblastoma, the most common malignant pediatric brain tumor, whereas it is rare in other age groups (Woehrer et al. 2010). In most large series a male predominance is reported (Rorke et al. 1996; Burger et al. 1998; Hilden et al. 2004; Haberler et al. 2006; von Hoff et al. 2011).

Localization and Clinical Features

AT/RTs may occur at any site of the CNS. Most larger hospital-based and one population-based series report AT/RTs to occur more frequently infra- than supratentorially (Rorke et al. 1996; Burger et al. 1998; Woehrer et al. 2010), whereas tumors registered in the German Hit database were found to be equally distributed between the supra- and infratentorial compartment (von Hoff et al. 2011). Few tumors extend supra- and infratentorially. Children with infratentorial tumors are significantly younger than children with supratentorial tumors (Rorke et al. 1996; Tekautz et al. 2005; von Hoff et al. 2011).

Supratentorial tumors are most commonly observed in the cerebral hemispheres and less frequently in the pineal gland or suprasellar region (Rorke et al. 1996; Burger et al. 1998; Woehrer et al. 2010). Infratentorial tumors are most commonly located in the cerebellum, but may occur also in the brainstem and cerebellopontine angle (Rorke et al. 1996; Burger et al. 1998; Woehrer et al. 2010). Infrequently, AT/RTs occur in the spinal cord (Rorke et al. 1996; Burger et al. 1998; Woehrer et al. 2010). A single case of a primary diffuse, cerebral leptomeningeal tumor growth has been reported (El-Nabbout et al. 2010).

Metastatic disease at diagnosis is frequent and may be present in up to 30–40% of the patients

(Rorke et al. 1996; Hilden et al. 2004; Tekautz et al. 2005; Woehrer et al. 2010; Lafay-Cousin et al. 2011; von Hoff et al. 2011). Patients presenting with multiple primary tumors (e.g. CNS and kidney or soft tissue) should be checked for a germline mutation of the *SMARCB1* gene (see rhabdoid predisposition syndrome). The clinical symptoms of AT/RT patients largely depend on the localization and size of the tumor and include signs of increased intracranial pressure (headaches, vomiting, irritability), hemi-or paraplegia, impaired cerebellar function (ataxia), cranial nerve palsies, macrocephaly, head tilt or failure to thrive.

Imaging

The radiological features of AT/RT are nonspecific and resemble those of supratentorial PNETs and medulloblastomas (Rorke et al. 1996; Meyers et al. 2006; Koral et al. 2008; Warmuth-Metz et al. 2008). In the so far largest study on imaging features in AT/RTs, published by Warmuth-Metz et al. (2008), signal intensities values varied widely on T1- and T2-weighted images. In T1 and T2 images homogeneous as well as mixed signal intensities were encountered (Fig. 1.1). Signs of bleeding mainly with a diffuse pattern, and surrounding edema were found in 45% and 52% of the AT/RTs, respectively. Most tumors showed a contrast enhancement of medium to strong intensity. Cystic or necrotic parts were observed in the majority of AT/RTs. In 38% of AT/RTs an unusual pattern consisting of a band-like wavy rim of strong and quite uniform enhancement completely or only partly surrounding a central cystic or necrotic area has been reported (Warmuth-Metz et al. 2008).

In infratentorial tumors, involvement of the cerebellopontine angle is significantly more common in AT/RTs than in medulloblastomas and posterior fossa tumors are significantly smaller at diagnosis than supratentorial tumors (Warmuth-Metz et al. 2008). Large supratentorial tumors with signs of bleeding or infratentorial tumors with involvement of the cerebellopontine angle should raise the suspicion of AT/RT.

Histopathology

Histopathologically, AT/RTs correspond to WHO grade IV. They frequently display a heterogeneous architecture. The characteristic feature is the presence of rhabdoid tumor cells with eccentric vesicular nuclei, prominent nucleoli, and globular eosinophilic cytoplasmic inclusions (Fig. 1.2a). Additionally, varying amounts of small -undifferentiated PNET-like, mesenchymal and/or epithelial differentiated tumor cells may be present (Fig. 1.2b–c). Abundant mitotic figures, nuclear atypia and necrosis are usually detectable, reflecting the malignant nature of this tumor. The diagnosis of AT/RT may be difficult if characteristic rhabdoid tumor cells are not prominent or, especially in small biopsies, lacking due to a sampling error. Such tumors may be misdiagnosed as supratentorial primitive neuroectodermal tumors (sPNET), medulloblastomas, anaplastic ependymomas, choroid plexus carcinomas, glioblastomas, malignant teratomas or sarcomas (Haberler et al. 2006).

Immunohistochemically, rhabdoid tumor cells express typically, but not absolutely specifically vimentin, EMA (epithelial membrane antigen) and less frequently SMA (smooth muscle actin). Expression of NFP (neurofilament protein), synaptopysin, GFAP (glial fibrillary acidic protein) and cytokeratin is also frequently detectable (Fig. 1.2d–g). Germ cell markers are not expressed. An antibody directed against the SMARCB1/INI1 protein has proven as useful marker for AT/RTs and peripheral rhabdoid tumors (Judkins et al. 2004; Haberler et al. 2006) and has considerably facilitated the diagnosis of AT/RT.

SMARCB1/INI1 protein is a ubiquitously expressed nuclear protein, which reflects the status of the *SMARCB1/INI1* gene. Consequently to the inactivation of *SMARCB1/INI1*, nuclear SMARCB1/INI1 expression is characteristically lacking in AT/RTs and peripheral rhabdoid tumors (Fig. 1.2h), but is expressed in normal tissues and the majority of other pediatric CNS tumors (Haberler et al. 2006). Endothelial cells of intratumoral blood vessels in AT/RTs serve as

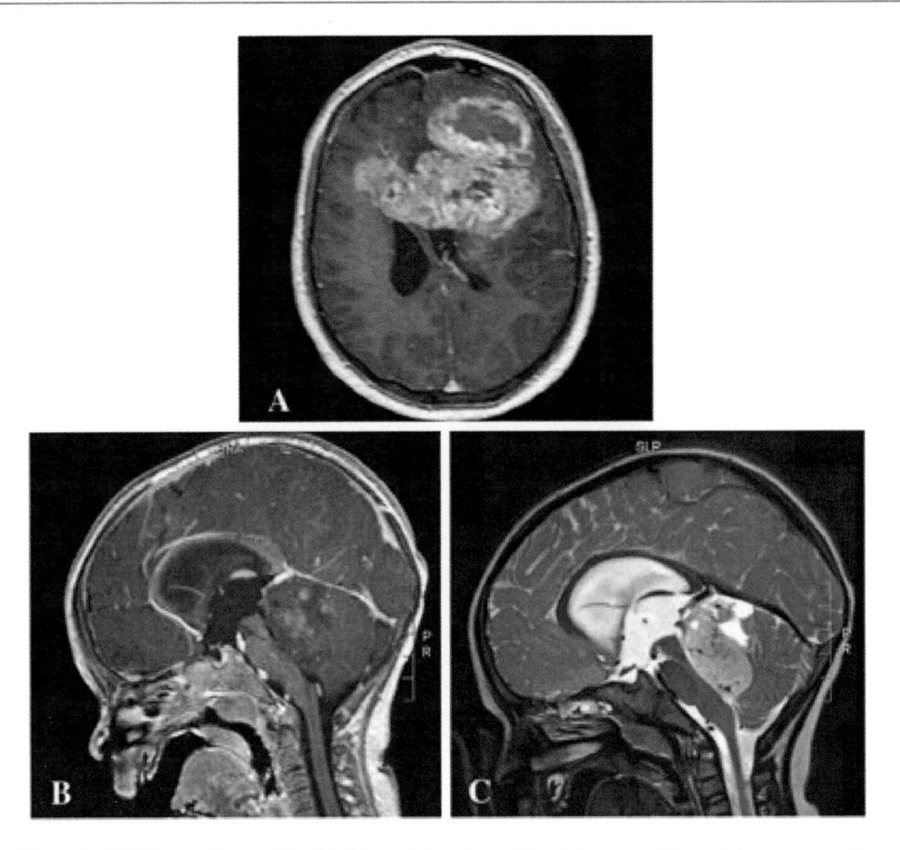

Fig. 1.1 Bifrontal *ATRT* in a 14-year-old girl (**a**). Axial Gd-enhanced T1-weighted image. Inhomogeneously enhancing tumor with a cystic-necrotic part (**a**). *ATRT* tectal region-4th ventricle in a 1-year-old boy (**b**–**c**). Sagittal Gd-enhanced T1-weighted image with an inhomogeneously enhancing tumor (**b**). Sagittal T2-weighted image with tumor-associated cysts, hypointense intratumoral spots (calcification resp. hemorrhage), and occlusive hydrocephalus (**c**)

internal quality control for the staining. Using this antibody, SMARCB1/INI1 immunonegative tumors in the posterior fossa displaying only small undifferentiated PNET-like, but no rhabdoid tumor cells could be detected (Haberler et al. 2006). Postmortem analyses of some of these tumors revealed focally characteristic rhabdoid tumor cells, thus corroborating the diagnosis of AT/RT and highlighting the possibility of misdiagnosis due to a sampling error. Therefore, it is recommended to perform immunohistochemical analysis of SMARCB1/INI1 protein on a routinely basis in malignant pediatric CNS tumors. Yet, SMARCB1/INI1 immunonegative tumors should be diagnosed cautiously, because also other tumor entities in the CNS may be SMARCB1/INI1 immunonegative. These tumors comprise epithelioid sarcomas in the spinal cord, schwannomas occurring in the setting of schwannomatosis, and single recently reported cases of cribriform neuroepithelial tumors (Modena et al. 2005; Hulsebos et al. 2007; Hasselblatt et al. 2009). Therefore, when diagnosing an AT/RT both, morphological features of the tumor and SMARCB1/INI1 immunoreactivity should be considered.

Choroid plexus carcinomas have been also reported to be SMARCB1/INI1 immunonegative. However, most of these reports date from the first years after the definition of AT/RT, when experience with the morphological features of this tumor was still limited. As it could be shown that choroid plexus carcinomas are in general SMARCB1/INI1 immunopositive (Judkins et al. 2005; Haberler

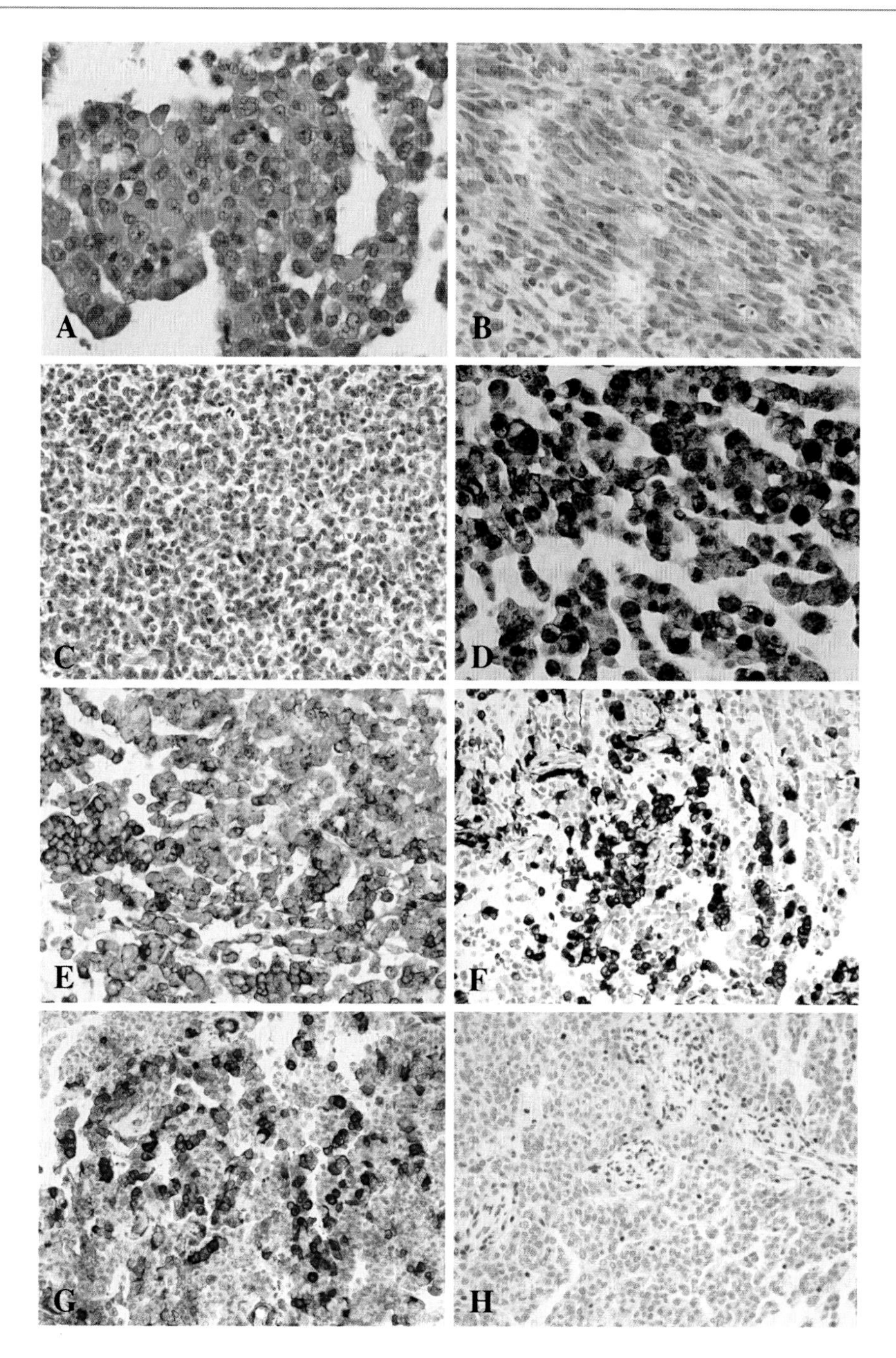

Fig. 1.2 Rhabdoid tumor cells (**a**); mesenchymal differentiated tumor areas (**b**); small PNET-like tumor cells (**c**). Tumor cells expressing Vimentin (**d**), Cytokeratin (**e**), GFAP (**f**), Smooth muscle actin (**g**); Tumor cells lack nuclear SMARCB1 (INI1/BAF47) expression, whereas it is retained in vascular endothelial cells (**h**)

et al. 2006) those tumors most likely represent AT/RTs with extensive epithelial differentiation. Few rhabdoid tumors including AT/RTs have been reported to be SMARCB1/INI1 immunopositive. In single of these tumors inactivation of the *SMARCA4* gene, and loss of SMARCA4 protein could be demonstrated (Schneppenheim et al. 2010; Hasselblatt et al. 2011).

Molecular Genetics

Inactivation of the *SMARCB1* (*hSNF5/INI1*) gene located in chromosome band 22q11.2 is the genetic hallmark in the vast majority of rhabdoid tumors including AT/RTs (Jackson et al. 2009; Kordes et al. 2010; Bourdeaut et al. 2011). SMARCB1 (SWI/SNF related, Matrix associated, Actin dependent Regulator of Chromatin, subfamily B, member 1) has 9 exons and is a core member of the evolutionarily conserved multi-subunit SWI/SNF chromatin remodeling complex, which mobilizes nucleosomes by utilizing the energy of ATP hydrolysis and thereby regulates expression of target genes involved in a broad range of cellular functions including proliferation, cell cycle regulation, DNA repair, mitosis and differentiation (Wilson and Roberts 2011).

Consistent with the role of a tumor suppressor gene biallelic inactivation of *SMARCB1* is present in rhabdoid tumors. To date, the function of *SMARCB1* in the development of rhabdoid tumors is not fully understood. The functions of the SMARCB1 protein and other members of the SWI/SNF chromatin remodeling complex in cancer have been reviewed by Wilson and Roberts (2011). SMARCB1 has been implicated in the Retinoblastoma pathway. Its loss causes cell cycle progression via downregulation of $p16^{INK4a}$ and upregulation of *E2Fs* and *CyclinD1*. SMARCB1 also interacts with *MYC*, a number of nuclear hormone receptors, which control cell proliferation and differentiation, the Hedgehog-Gli pathway and embryonic stem cell programs. Furthermore, *SMARCB1* loss stimulates migration via increase of RhoA activity, which potentially contributes to the invasive and metastatic nature of rhabdoid tumors.

As most of the rhabdoid tumors are diploid and only few recurrent regions of copy number changes other than chromosome 22 are detectable, it is not likely that a second locus is involved in the development of rhabdoid tumors in addition to *SMARCB1* (Jackson et al. 2009). Moreover, it could be shown that disruption of the chromatin remodeling complex SWI/SNF and the resulting epigenetic alterations can largely substitute for genomic instability, usually present in other types of cancer (McKenna et al. 2008). Recently, *SMARCA4* another member of the SWI/SNF complex, has been reported to be mutated in two siblings with rhabdoid tumors and single sporadic AT/RTs (Schneppenheim et al. 2010; Hasselblatt et al. 2011). It remains to be seen whether other members of the SWI/SNF complex are involved in the development of rhabdoid tumors.

Using a combination of sequencing, MLPA (multiplex dependent probe amplification), FISH (fluorescence in situ hybridization) and high-resolution SNP (single nucleotide polymorphism) arrays, a wide spectrum of *SMARCB1* abnormalities, comprising deletions, mutations, and duplications could been identified (Jackson et al. 2009; Kordes et al. 2010; Bourdeaut et al. 2011; Eaton et al. 2011). Deletions comprise small intragenic deletions, larger deletions of 22q11.2 and monosomy of chromosome 22. In more than one third of the patients with sporadic tumors a homozygous *SMARCB1* deletion is present and frequently copy neutral LOH is detectable (Jackson et al. 2009). In patients with a heterozygous deletion the second allele is usually mutated, whereas two coding sequence mutations are rarely encountered.

As constitutional aberrations of *SMARCB1* (see rhabdoid predisposition syndrome) have been detected in up to 42.5% of patients with AT/RT, including also patients with apparently sporadic tumors (Bourdeaut et al. 2011; Eaton et al. 2011), molecular testing of *SMARCB1* should be performed in all newly diagnosed AT/RTs.

Rhabdoid Predisposition Syndrome

The rhabdoid predisposition syndrome is a disorder characterized by an increased risk to develop rhabdoid tumors in the CNS, kidney and soft tissues due to the constitutional inactivation of one allele of the *SMARCB1* gene. Germline aberrations of *SMARCB1* have been described in up to 42.5% of patients with AT/RT (Bourdeaut et al. 2011; Eaton et al. 2011). This incidence of germline mutations in AT/RTs is high compared to renal and soft tissue rhabdoid tumors (Eaton et al. 2011).

Patients with *SMARCB1* germline mutation are most often diagnosed within the first year of life. Almost 60% of rhabdoid tumors in children younger than 6 months occur in the setting of a germline mutation (Bourdeaut et al. 2011). The median age at diagnosis of patients with germline mutation is 5–6 months (Bourdeaut et al. 2011; Eaton et al. 2011) whereas it is 18 months in children with sporadic tumors (Bourdeaut et al. 2011; Eaton et al. 2011). However, there is an overlap in the age ranges and germline mutations can be also found in older children. Children presenting with multiple tumors, affected siblings, or an affected child with a family history of malignant CNS tumors with an autosomal dominant inheritance pattern, are almost surely to have a germline mutation.

The most common *SMARCB1* germline alterations are point or frameshift mutations, resulting in a premature truncation of the protein, followed by heterozygous loss of *SMARCB1*, intragenic deletions and rare duplications (Kordes et al. 2010; Bourdeaut et al. 2011; Eaton et al. 2011). The majority of germline mutations arise de novo. However, analyses in affected children and their parents revealed families with genetic findings consistent with gonadal mosaicism, and asymptomatic germline mutation carrier parents (Ammerlaan et al. 2008; Bourdeaut et al. 2011; Eaton et al. 2011). Interestingly, the same germline mutation may lead to rhabdoid tumors at different ages and sites within a family (Bourdeaut et al. 2011).

It could be shown that constitutional mutations in *SMARCB1* predispose also to schwannomatosis (Hulsebos et al. 2007), a disorder characterized by multiple benign schwannomas. In the majority of to date reported families, *SMARBC1* germline mutations predispose either to malignant rhabdoid tumors or to multiple benign schwannomas. However, recently two families with both rhabdoid tumor and schwannomatosis have been reported (Swensen et al. 2009; Eaton et al. 2011). Thus, unaffected carriers are at risk to develop both malignant and benign tumors including rhabdoid tumors and schwannomas. However, to date the correlation between genotype and phenotype, the expressivity and penetrance of germline *SMARCB1* mutations and thus, the risk to develop a malignant rhabdoid tumor or schwannomatosis are not known.

Treatment

Although substantial progress has been made elucidating the biology of ATRTs no definitive guidelines for optimal treatment have been established. Due to the relatively new introduction of ATRTs into the WHO classification as a distinct entity, the rarity of the disease and the lack of large formal clinical trials affected patients have been treated in a heterogeneous manner. Most patients with an AT/RT of the CNS reported in the literature have undergone attempted radical surgery, followed by chemo- and/or radiotherapy according to protocols used in other high-grade CNS malignancies. In spite of this, most patients have suffered rapid disease recurrence and death due to progression. Given the particularly poor prognosis of young children some centers also tended to direct younger children towards palliative care rather than attempt curative therapy (Rorke et al. 1996; Burger et al. 1998). Therefore, the variability in therapy is large and objective comparison of treatment efficacy between patient groups reported in the literature is problematic. However, long-term survivors including patients with recurrent and disseminated disease have been reported using various intensive treatment protocols (Zimmerman et al. 2005).

Von Hoff et al. (2011) reported on 56 patients diagnosed with an ATRT at a median age of 1.2 years between 1988 and 2004 and registered to the HIT database and trials within the German Society for Paediatric Oncology and Haematology (GPOH). Chemotherapy was based on different HIT protocols in 39 patients. Seventeen patients were treated according to protocols used for extracranial rhabdoid tumors or on the basis of individual decisions of the local physicians. Intraventricular methotrexate was administered to 40 of 54 children. Analysis of the influence of specific chemotherapeutic agents was not performed due to incomplete documentation. Radiotherapy, either local or craniospinal, was administered to 29 patients following primary chemotherapy, or at relapse or progression. The median survival of all patients was 1.2 years. Forty-three children (77%) died and 13 patients were alive with a median follow-up of 3.3 years, 8 of these without tumor progression or relapse. Less than complete resection was associated with a trend for worse EFS. Although it was not possible to evaluate the general impact of radiotherapy on outcome, delay of radiotherapy appeared possible in young children. The authors concluded that a subset of patients with favorable clinical risk factors profits from intensive multimodal therapy.

Lafay-Cousin et al. (2011) reported on a retrospective study conducted through the Canadian Paediatric Brain Tumor Consortium of children ≤18 years diagnosed with an ATRT between 1995 and 2007. There were 50 patients with a median age at diagnosis of 16.7 months. Ten patients (20%) underwent palliation. Among the 40 actively treated patients, 22 received conventional chemotherapy and 18 received high-dose chemotherapy regimens. Nine received intrathecal therapy and 15 received adjuvant radiation. The median survival time was 13.5 months. Thirty of the 40 treated patients relapsed/progressed at a median time of 5.5 months. The chemotherapy regimens of eight of the ten patients surviving without relapse consisted of cisplatin, cyclophospamide, etoposide, and vincristine augmented with MTX in three patients and temozolomide in one and followed by a carboplatin and thiotepa based high dose chemotherapy (HDC). Two further patients surviving without relapse were irradiated but did not receive high-dose chemotherapy. Gross total resection was associated with improved survival. The authors concluded that the use of HDC provides encouraging results. Similarly, all eight long-term survivors of the 19 patients (17 actively treated) in the Austrian registry received combined multimodality therapy, including HDC in seven, intrathecal therapy in six and all received focal irradiation (Woehrer et al. 2010).

Chi et al. (2009) reported on 20 patients enrolled in a disease specific prospective multi-institutional phase II clinical trial based on a protocol for children with rhabdomyosarcoma with parameningeal extension. The median age at diagnosis was 26 months. While this intensive multimodality regimen was rather toxic it resulted in a significant improvement for this poor prognosis disease with 2-year progression-free and overall survival rates of 53% ± 13% and 70% ± 10%.

In conclusion, it appears that a more aggressive therapy has prolonged the survival in a subset of children. Based on the data available from several larger series reported in the literature (Hilden et al. 2004; Tekautz et al. 2005; Chen et al. 2006) conclusions are as follows:

1. The degree of surgical resection appears to be a major factor in predicting prognosis and maximal safe resection is recommended.
2. Quick proper diagnosis is essential (INI1 immunostaining) for immediate start of appropriate therapy because most conventional infant brain tumor protocols are inadequate for AT/RT.
3. AT/RT are chemosensitive tumors when protocols including a combination of platin derivatives, alkylating agents, methotrexate, vincristine, etoposide and possibly doxorubicin are used.
4. High-dose chemotherapy with autologous stem cell rescue appears to improve survival.
5. Radiotherapy seems to be an important component in most reports and has been associated with prolonged survival of older children and adults with AT/RT. Focal radiotherapy is therefore recommended also in young children. However, a proportion of long-term survivors never received radiotherapy.
6. Intrathecal chemotherapy possibly using several agents is recommended particularly in young children in whom craniospinal irradiation is not an option.

Children with multifocal and congenital AT/RT may represent a distinct subgroup of patients requiring specific therapeutic guidelines and genetic counseling.

Pilot studies are currently conducted in pediatric oncology groups around the world.

Outcome and Prognostic Factors

The overall survival of AT/RT patients treated according to conventional treatment protocols, used for other high-grade CNS tumors like medulloblastoma or CNS PNET, is poor. First studies describing the clinical and pathological features of AT/RTs reported a mean/median postoperative survival time of 6 and 11 months, respectively (Rorke et al. 1996; Burger et al. 1998). Recent studies provide evidence that patients benefit from intensified multi- modal therapies, and 2-year overall survival rates of up to 70% have been reported (Chi et al. 2009).

Young age at diagnosis, incomplete tumor resection, and metastatic disease (Chi et al. 2009; von Hoff et al. 2011) are adverse prognostic factors. The reported negative impact of germline mutations may reflect the young patient age rather than being a prognostic factor per se. Interestingly, two long-term survivors (>15 years) with confirmed AT/RTs at the age of 4.5 and 0.6 years have been reported in a family with rhabdoid predisposition syndrome (Ammerlaan et al. 2008). However, to date correlations between genotype and phenotype including age at diagnosis, tumor location, as well as patient outcome, are still unknown.

Acknowledgements All MRIs courtesy of Daniela Prayer, Department of Radiology, Medical University of Vienna, Austria.

References

Ammerlaan AC, Ararou A, Houben MP, Baas F, Tijssen CC, Teepen JL, Wesseling P, Hulsebos TJ (2008) Long-term survival and transmission of INI1-mutation via nonpenetrant males in a family with rhabdoid tumour predisposition syndrome. Br J Cancer 98:474–479

Beckwith JB, Palmer NF (1978) Histopathology and prognosis of Wilms tumors: results from the First National Wilms' Tumor Study. Cancer 41:1937–1948

Bourdeaut F, Lequin D, Brugieres L, Reynaud S, Dufour C, Doz F, Andre N, Stephan JL, Perel Y, Oberlin O, Orbach D, Bergeron C, Rialland X, Freneaux P, Ranchere D, Figarella-Branger D, Audry G, Puget S, Evans DG, Pinas JC, Capra V, Mosseri V, Coupier I, Gauthier-Villars M, Pierron G, Delattre O (2011) Frequent hSNF5/INI1 germline mutations in patients with rhabdoid tumor. Clin Cancer Res 17:31–38

Burger PC, Yu IT, Tihan T, Friedman HS, Strother DR, Kepner JL, Duffner PK, Kun LE, Perlman EJ (1998) Atypical teratoid/rhabdoid tumor of the central nervous system: a highly malignant tumor of infancy and childhood frequently mistaken for medulloblastoma: a Pediatric Oncology Group study. Am J Surg Pathol 22:1083–1092

Chen YW, Wong TT, Ho DM, Huang PI, Chang KP, Shiau CY, Yen SH (2006) Impact of radiotherapy for pediatric CNS atypical teratoid/rhabdoid tumor (single institute experience). Int J Radiat Oncol Biol Phys 64:1038–1043

Chi SN, Zimmerman MA, Yao X, Cohen KJ, Burger P, Biegel JA, Rorke-Adams LB, Fisher MJ, Janss A, Mazewski C, Goldman S, Manley PE, Bowers DC, Bendel A, Rubin J, Turner CD, Marcus KJ, Goumnerova L, Ullrich NJ, Kieran MW (2009) Intensive multimodality treatment for children with newly diagnosed CNS atypical teratoid rhabdoid tumor. J Clin Oncol 27:385–389

Eaton KW, Tooke LS, Wainwright LM, Judkins AR, Biegel JA (2011) Spectrum of SMARCB1/INI1 mutations in familial and sporadic rhabdoid tumors. Pediatr Blood Cancer 56:7–15

El-Nabbout B, Shbarou R, Glasier CM, Saad AG (2010) Primary diffuse cerebral leptomeningeal atypical teratoid rhabdoid tumor: report of the first case. J Neurooncol 98:431–434

Haberler C, Laggner U, Slavc I, Czech T, Ambros IM, Ambros PF, Budka H, Hainfellner JA (2006) Immunohistochemical analysis of INI1 protein in malignant pediatric CNS tumors: lack of INI1 in atypical teratoid/rhabdoid tumors and in a fraction of primitive neuroectodermal tumors without rhabdoid phenotype. Am J Surg Pathol 30:1462–1468

Hasselblatt M, Oyen F, Gesk S, Kordes U, Wrede B, Bergmann M, Schmid H, Fruhwald MC, Schneppenheim R, Siebert R, Paulus W (2009) Cribriform neuroepithelial tumor (CRINET): a nonrhabdoid ventricular tumor with INI1 loss and relatively favorable prognosis. J Neuropathol Exp Neurol 68:1249–1255

Hasselblatt M, Gesk S, Oyen F, Rossi S, Viscardi E, Giangaspero F, Giannini C, Judkins AR, Fruhwald MC, Obser T, Schneppenheim R, Siebert R, Paulus W (2011) Nonsense mutation and inactivation of SMARCA4 (BRG1) in an atypical teratoid/rhabdoid tumor showing retained SMARCB1 (INI1) expression. Am J Surg Pathol 35:933–935

Hilden JM, Meerbaum S, Burger P, Finlay J, Janss A, Scheithauer BW, Walter AW, Rorke LB, Biegel JA (2004) Central nervous system atypical teratoid/rhabdoid tumor: results of therapy in children enrolled in a registry. J Clin Oncol 22:2877–2884

Hulsebos TJ, Plomp AS, Wolterman RA, Robanus-Maandag EC, Baas F, Wesseling P (2007) Germline mutation of INI1/SMARCB1 in familial schwannomatosis. Am J Hum Genet 80:805–810

Jackson EM, Sievert AJ, Gai X, Hakonarson H, Judkins AR, Tooke L, Perin JC, Xie H, Shaikh TH, Biegel JA (2009) Genomic analysis using high-density single nucleotide polymorphism-based oligonucleotide arrays and multiplex ligation-dependent probe amplification provides a comprehensive analysis of INI1/SMARCB1 in malignant rhabdoid tumors. Clin Cancer Res 15:1923–1930

Judkins AR, Mauger J, Ht A, Rorke LB, Biegel JA (2004) Immunohistochemical analysis of hSNF5/INI1 in pediatric CNS neoplasms. Am J Surg Pathol 28:644–650

Judkins AR, Burger PC, Hamilton RL, Kleinschmidt-DeMasters B, Perry A, Pomeroy SL, Rosenblum MK, Yachnis AT, Zhou H, Rorke LB, Biegel JA (2005) INI1 protein expression distinguishes atypical teratoid/rhabdoid tumor from choroid plexus carcinoma. J Neuropathol Exp Neurol 64:391–397

Kaderali Z, Lamberti-Pasculli M, Rutka JT (2009) The changing epidemiology of paediatric brain tumours: a review from the hospital for sick children. Childs Nerv Syst 25:787–793

Koral K, Gargan L, Bowers DC, Gimi B, Timmons CF, Weprin B, Rollins NK (2008) Imaging characteristics of atypical teratoid-rhabdoid tumor in children compared with medulloblastoma. AJR Am J Roentgenol 190:809–814

Kordes U, Gesk S, Fruhwald MC, Graf N, Leuschner I, Hasselblatt M, Jeibmann A, Oyen F, Peters O, Pietsch T, Siebert R, Schneppenheim R (2010) Clinical and molecular features in patients with atypical teratoid rhabdoid tumor or malignant rhabdoid tumor. Genes Chromosomes Cancer 49:176–181

Lafay-Cousin L, Hawkins C, Carret AS, Johnston D, Zelcer S, Wilson B, Jabado N, Scheinemann K, Eisenstat D, Fryer C, Fleming A, Mpofu C, Larouche V, Strother D, Bouffet E, Huang A (2011) Central nervous system atypical teratoid rhabdoid tumours: the Canadian paediatric brain tumour consortium experience. Eur J Cancer 48(3):353–359

McKenna ES, Sansam CG, Cho YJ, Greulich H, Evans JA, Thom CS, Moreau LA, Biegel JA, Pomeroy SL, Roberts CW (2008) Loss of the epigenetic tumor suppressor SNF5 leads to cancer without genomic instability. Mol Cell Biol 28:6223–6233

Meyers SP, Khademian ZP, Biegel JA, Chuang SH, Korones DN, Zimmerman RA (2006) Primary intracranial atypical teratoid/rhabdoid tumors of infancy and childhood: MRI features and patient outcomes. AJNR Am J Neuroradiol 27:962–971

Modena P, Lualdi E, Facchinetti F, Galli L, Teixeira MR, Pilotti S, Sozzi G (2005) SMARCB1/INI1 tumor suppressor gene is frequently inactivated in epithelioid sarcomas. Cancer Res 65:4012–4019

Raisanen J, Biegel JA, Hatanpaa KJ, Judkins A, White CL, Perry A (2005) Chromosome 22q deletions in atypical teratoid/rhabdoid tumors in adults. Brain Pathol 15:23–28

Rickert CH, Paulus W (2001) Epidemiology of central nervous system tumors in childhood and adolescence based on the new WHO classification. Childs Nerv Syst 17:503–511

Rorke LB, Packer RJ, Biegel JA (1996) Central nervous system atypical teratoid/rhabdoid tumors of infancy and childhood: definition of an entity. J Neurosurg 85:56–65

Schneppenheim R, Fruhwald MC, Gesk S, Hasselblatt M, Jeibmann A, Kordes U, Kreuz M, Leuschner I, Martin Subero JI, Obser T, Oyen F, Vater I, Siebert R (2010) Germline nonsense mutation and somatic inactivation of SMARCA4/BRG1 in a family with rhabdoid tumor predisposition syndrome. Am J Hum Genet 86:279–284

Swensen JJ, Keyser J, Coffin CM, Biegel JA, Viskochil DH, Williams MS (2009) Familial occurrence of schwannomas and malignant rhabdoid tumour associated with a duplication in SMARCB1. J Med Genet 46:68–72

Tekautz TM, Fuller CE, Blaney S, Fouladi M, Broniscer A, Merchant TE, Krasin M, Dalton J, Hale G, Kun LE, Wallace D, Gilbertson RJ, Gajjar A (2005) Atypical teratoid/rhabdoid tumors (ATRT): improved survival in children 3 years of age and older with radiation therapy and high-dose alkylator-based chemotherapy. J Clin Oncol 23:1491–1499

von Hoff K, Hinkes B, Dannenmann-Stern E, von Bueren AO, Warmuth-Metz M, Soerensen N, Emser A, Zwiener I, Schlegel PG, Kuehl J, Fruhwald MC, Kortmann RD, Pietsch T, Rutkowski S (2011) Frequency, risk-factors and survival of children with atypical teratoid rhabdoid tumors (AT/RT) of the CNS diagnosed between 1988 and 2004, and registered to the German HIT database. Pediatr Blood Cancer 57:978–985

Warmuth-Metz M, Bison B, Dannemann-Stern E, Kortmann R, Rutkowski S, Pietsch T (2008) CT and MR imaging in atypical teratoid/rhabdoid tumors of the central nervous system. Neuroradiology 50:447–452

Wilson BG, Roberts CW (2011) SWI/SNF nucleosome remodellers and cancer. Nat Rev Cancer 11:481–492

Woehrer A, Slavc I, Waldhoer T, Heinzl H, Zielonke N, Czech T, Benesch M, Hainfellner JA, Haberler C (2010) Incidence of atypical teratoid/rhabdoid tumors in children: a population-based study by the Austrian Brain Tumor Registry, 1996–2006. Cancer 116: 5725–5732

Wong TT, Ho DM, Chang KP, Yen SH, Guo WY, Chang FC, Liang ML, Pan HC, Chung WY (2005) Primary pediatric brain tumors: statistics of Taipei VGH, Taiwan (1975–2004). Cancer 104:2156–2167

Zimmerman MA, Goumnerova LC, Proctor M, Scott RM, Marcus K, Pomeroy SL, Turner CD, Chi SN, Chordas C, Kieran MW (2005) Continuous remission of newly diagnosed and relapsed central nervous system atypical teratoid/rhabdoid tumor. J Neurooncol 72:77–84

Atypical Teratoid/Rhabdoid Tumors

2

Simone Treiger Sredni and Rishi R. Lulla

Contents

S.T. Sredni (✉)
Neurosurgery Research Program, Children's Hospital of Chicago Research Center and Northwestern University Feinberg School of Medicine, 225 East Chicago Avenue, Box #28, IL 60611, Chicago
e-mail: ssredni@luriechildrens.org; ssredni@northwestern.edu

R.R. Lulla
Hematology, Oncology and Stem Cell Transplantation, Ann & Robert H. Lurie Children's Hospital of Chicago and Northwestern University Feinberg School of Medicine, 225 East Chicago Avenue, Box #30, IL 60611, Chicago
e-mail: rlulla@luriechildrens.org

Abstract

Atypical teratoid/rhabdoid tumor is a rare aggressive malignant central nervous system tumor that most often occurs in young children. Though these tumors may have overlapping histological features with other Central Nervous System (CNS) tumors, one feature unique to most atypical teratoid/rhabdoid tumors is a genetic abnormality in the *INI-1* gene on chromosome 22q11. Loss of the INI-1 protein staining is important for distinguishing atypical teratoid/rhabdoid tumors from other tumors. Historically, outcomes for patients with atypical teratoid/rhabdoid tumors have been poor despite surgery and chemotherapy. Promising new strategies, including intensive multimodal therapy and high dose chemotherapy with autologous stem cell transplantation, have significantly improved outcomes. In this chapter, we present a comprehensive overview of atypical teratoid/rhabdoid tumors. We focus upon their epidemiology, molecular genetics, pathologic diagnosis and clinical presentation. In addition, we discuss treatment approaches, prognostic factors, outcomes and future research directions.

Introduction

Atypical teratoid/rhabdoid tumor (AT/RT) is a rare, highly malignant tumor of the central nervous system (CNS) that usually affects very young children. Rhabdoid tumors were first

M.A. Hayat (ed.), *Pediatric Cancer, Volume 3: Diagnosis, Therapy, and Prognosis*, Pediatric Cancer 3,
DOI 10.1007/978-94-007-4528-5_2,

described in the kidney by Beckwith and Palmer in 1978 as part of the National Wilm's Tumor Study, as an aggressive variant of Wilm's tumor (Beckwith and Palmer 1978). The term "rhabdoid" was used because the tumor is morphologically similar to rhabdomyosarcoma under the light microscope but lacks the characteristic skeletal muscle markers by electron microscopy, immunohistochemistry or cytogenetic studies. The rhabdoid phenotype was subsequently noted in extra-renal sites including the liver, soft tissue and the CNS. Rhabdoid tumors of the CNS express multiple cell lineages and morphologically may resemble teratomas. For this reason they were named atypical teratoid-rhabdoid tumors (AT/RT). Due to the presence of overlapping histological features, complex immunophenotypes and co-expression of epithelial, primitive neuroepithelial and mesenchymal markers, AT/RT has been commonly misdiagnosed as medulloblastoma, primitive neuroectodermal tumor (PNET) or choroid plexus carcinoma. Rhabdoid tumors from all locations have a common genetic abnormality, the mutation or deletion of the *INI-1* gene located at the chromosome 22q11 (Versteege et al. 1998; Biegel et al. 1999, 2002a).

Historically, AT/RT was associated with extremely poor outcomes despite surgery, chemotherapy and radiation therapy. Recent reports of improving overall survival (OS) using intensive multimodal therapy are promising (Chi et al. 2009), however, neurocognitive sequelae of this therapy have yet to be fully investigated. Future treatment for AT/RT is dependent on investigators obtaining a better understanding of tumor biology and active molecular pathways in this tumor. Exploration of currently available treatments (including the utility of high dose chemotherapy and autologous stem cell transplantation) and new agents is underway with the goal of increasing survival and minimizing treatment related toxicity.

History and Epidemiology

Rhabdoid Tumors have only recently been recognized as a pathologic entity. Biggs and colleagues described the occurrence of a rhabdoid tumor in the CNS for the first time in 1987 (Biggs et al. 1987). AT/RT was broadly recognized as a distinct entity about 10 years later (Rorke et al. 1996) In 1993, AT/RT was included in the World Health Organization (WHO) classification as a grade IV embryonal neoplasm (Kleihues et al. 2002).

The median age at presentation is approximately 20 months with a slight male predominance (1.6:1) (Rorke et al. 1996). In the United States, 3 children per 1,000,000 or approximately 30 new AT/RT cases are diagnosed each year. According to the WHO, AT/RT represents approximately 1.3% of pediatric tumors of CNS in the general pediatric population and 6.6% in children younger than 2 years of age (Biswas et al. 2009). While most AT/RTs occur in children less than 2 years of age, some new diagnoses are made in older children and adolescents. AT/RT can occur anywhere in the CNS; 50% are located in the posterior fossa and 40% are supratentorial lesions. The remaining 10% occur in other sites in the CNS including the spinal cord. Dissemination via cerebrospinal fluid (CSF) is relatively frequent, occurring in nearly 25% of the patients at the time of diagnosis (Biegel et al. 2002b).

Most cases of AT/RT are sporadic although rare familial cases have been described in rhabdoid tumor predisposition syndrome. In this condition, patients inherit germline mutations in the *INI-1* tumor suppressor gene and are predisposed to the development of rhabdoid tumors of the CNS, kidney and soft tissue and may present with more than one primary tumor. (Biegel et al. 1999). Patients with rhabdoid tumor predisposition syndrome are often diagnosed within the first year of life and tend to have the least favorable prognosis (Janson et al. 2006). Routine testing for germline mutations in *INI*-1 for patients or their unaffected family members without a suggestive family history is not usually recommended. However, this may change as more information about genetic predisposition to AT/RT is understood.

Molecular Genetics

Cytogenetic analysis of AT/RT specimens shows a high frequency of abnormalities involving the long arm of chromosome 22. Over 80% of rhabdoid tumors in the brain, kidney and other sites will have loss of chromosome 22q as a result of either deletion and/or translocation (Biegel et al. 1999). The common area of deletion on chromosome 22q11.2 has been mapped to the *INI-1* gene also known as *SMARCB-1*, *hSNF5* or *BAF47*. Almost every rhabdoid tumor will have an abnormality in the *INI-1* gene. This can be manifested by homozygous deletion, loss of heterozygosity with a coding-sequence mutation in the remaining allele or two independent mutations in the *INI-1* gene (Biegel et al. 2002b).

The *INI-1* gene is the human homologue of the yeast *SNF5* gene and its product is 1 of the 12 proteins of the SWI/SNF complex that is thought to function in an ATP-dependent manner to cause a conformational change in the nucleosome which alters histone-DNA binding facilitating transcription factor access (Kalpana et al. 1994). *INI-1* was recognized as a tumor suppressor gene by Versteege et al. (1998) after mapping the most frequently deleted part of chromosome 22q11.2 from a panel of 13 malignant rhabdoid tumor cell lines. The authors observed homozygous deletions, frameshift or nonsense mutations in the *INI-1* gene (Versteege et al. 1998). Shortly thereafter, Biegel et al. (1999) analyzed 18 AT/RT, 7 renal and 4 extra-renal rhabdoid tumors for mutations in the *INI-1* gene and detected homozygous deletions of 1 or more exons in 15 tumors and other mutations in the additional 14 tumors. Germ-line mutations of *INI-1* were also identified in four children, one with an AT/RT and three with renal rhabdoid tumors (Biegel et al. 1999). The identification of germline mutations of the *INI-1* gene in children with one or more primary tumors as well as the fact that the majority of tumors had evidence of inactivation of both alleles reinforced the hypothesis that *INI-1* functions as a classic tumor suppressor gene (Biegel et al. 2002a). It is known that mutation or deletion of the *INI-1* gene may result in altered transcriptional regulation of genes involved in cell death, cell growth and/or cell differentiation. Nevertheless, the direct tumor suppressor functions of the *INI-1* gene or the functional mechanism of the INI-1 protein loss and tumorigenesis of rhabdoid tumors are yet unknown.

Rhabdoid tumors originating in different anatomical sites are assumed to be the same entity, as they share the same clinical, epidemiological and molecular characteristics. However, Biegel et al. (2002a) characterized chromosome 22 deletions and *INI-1* mutations among 100 primary rhabdoid tumors from diverse anatomical sites and concluded that the deletions and/or mutations of the *INI-1* gene were non-randomly associated with the anatomical site of origin. The authors described two potential "hot-spot" mutations for AT/RT specifically C-to-T transition in codon 201 in exon 5 and a cytosine deletion in exon 9 of the *INI-1* gene. No differences in outcome, however, have been reported in patients with various types of *INI-1* alterations (Biegel et al. 2002a).

Up to 15% of all rhabdoid tumors including AT/RT show no alteration in the *INI-1* gene at the DNA, RNA or protein level (Biegel et al. 2002b). Moreover, the expression of the INI-1 protein can be lost or decreased in the absence of gene mutations or deletions. In an attempt to describe this phenomenon, methylation status of the 5' promoter region of the *INI-1* gene and of the CpG dinucleotides in a GC-rich repeat region within the first intron of the gene were investigated. This phenomenon is yet to be explained as hypermethylation does not account for decreased expression of *INI-1* in tumors without coding sequences mutation (Zhang et al. 2002).

The histogenesis of AT/RT is unknown but it has been suggested that rhabdoid tumors originate from either pluripotent fetal cells or stem cells. Recently Gadd et al. (2010) investigated the *INI-1* mediated pathogenesis of rhabdoid tumors by analyzing the global gene expression of 10 rhabdoid tumors compared with 42 non-rhabdoid kidney tumors. The authors found that 28 of the 114 top differentially expressed genes were involved with neural or neural-crest development and were all sharply down-regulated. This suggests that rhabdoid tumors arise within early progenitor cells during a critical developmental window in which loss of the *INI-1* gene directly results in repression of neural development, loss of cyclin-dependent kinase inhibition, and trithorax/polycomb dysregulation (Gadd et al. 2010). Similarly, Ma et al. (2010) compared the differential gene expression profiling between AT/RT and medulloblastoma and observed embryonic stem-like gene recapitulation in AT/RT also pointing towards the neural-stem cell origin of rhabdoid tumors (Ma et al. 2010).

Pathologic Diagnosis

Histopathology

As with other CNS tumors, an accurate diagnosis is important to determine appropriate treatment for patients with AT/RT. The gross appearance is generally similar to medulloblastoma or PNET although large areas of necrosis and hemorrhage are more common in AT/RT. Microscopically, AT/RT is a heterogeneous lesion. It may consist of large areas of small blue cells that are indistinguishable from medulloblastoma or PNET. Alternatively, it may consist purely of characteristic rhabdoid cells or areas of rhabdoid cells adjacent to mesechymal and epithelial tissue. Rhabdoid cells are the histological hallmark of rhabdoid tumor. They are medium-sized, round to oval shaped cells often clearly identified in cytological preparations (Fig. 2.1a). Cells have eccentrically placed vesicular nuclei, a prominent nucleolus and abundant cytoplasm with occasional pale eosinophilic inclusions (Fig. 2.1b). Rhabdoid cells are usually intermixed with variable components of primitive neuroectodermal, mesenchymal and epithelial cells. Necrosis, frequently with dystrophic calcifications, is a common finding.

Immunohistochemistry and Electron Microscopy

AT/RT is characterized by a polyphenotypic immunoreactive pattern. Unlike medulloblastoma or PNET, AT/RT displays a wide range of immunohistochemical reactivity because of the divergent differentiation of the tumor cells. Cells often show variable immunoreactivity for different epithelial markers, neuronal markers and smooth muscle actin. Clusters of cells intensively positive for vimentin (Fig. 2.1c) and epithelial membrane antigen (EMA) (Fig. 2.1d) are frequently observed. Additionally, AT/RT is usually reactive for other common antigens, including glial fibrillary acidic protein (GFAP), neurofilament proteins, smooth muscle actin (SMA), S-100 protein, cytokeratin, and CD99. Characteristically, AT/RT is not reactive for phenotypic markers specific of skeletal muscle differentiation, including MyoD and desmin. The presence of gland-like structures in AT/RT reflects the epithelial origin of some of the tumor's cells. These can be used to differentiate the lesion from medulloblastoma or PNET which do not contain cells of epithelial origin.

In addition to these markers, the absence of immunostain to the INI-1 protein is useful in differentiating AT/RT from medulloblastoma, PNET, choroid plexus carcinoma and other brain tumors that can mimic AT/RT. The INI-1 protein is constitutively expressed in the nuclei of most of cells. However, the expression is decreased or lost in most AT/RT specimens due to deletion or mutation of its encoding gene *INI-1*. The absence of immunohistochemical staining with an INI-1 antibody in the nucleus of tumor cells correlates with molecular findings of *INI-1* inactivation in AT/RT and is extremely useful to confirm the histological diagnosis (Judkins et al. 2004).

Though electron microscopy is not routine in the evaluation of CNS tumors, AT/RT does have some characteristic findings using this technique. The eosinophilic cytoplasmic inclusions seen on hematoxylin and eosin stained tissue sections of rhabdoid cells typically appears as intracytoplasmic, paranuclear whorls of intermediate filaments at the ultra structural level. Neurosecretory granules are observed in some cases (Parwani et al. 2005).

Differential Diagnoses

Medulloblastoma, PNET and AT/RT can be clinically, radiologically and histopathologically indistinguishable. In these entities, most of the tumor consists of undifferentiated small round cells and the characteristic rhabdoid cells may not be present in every AT/RT specimen. It is important to make this distinction as

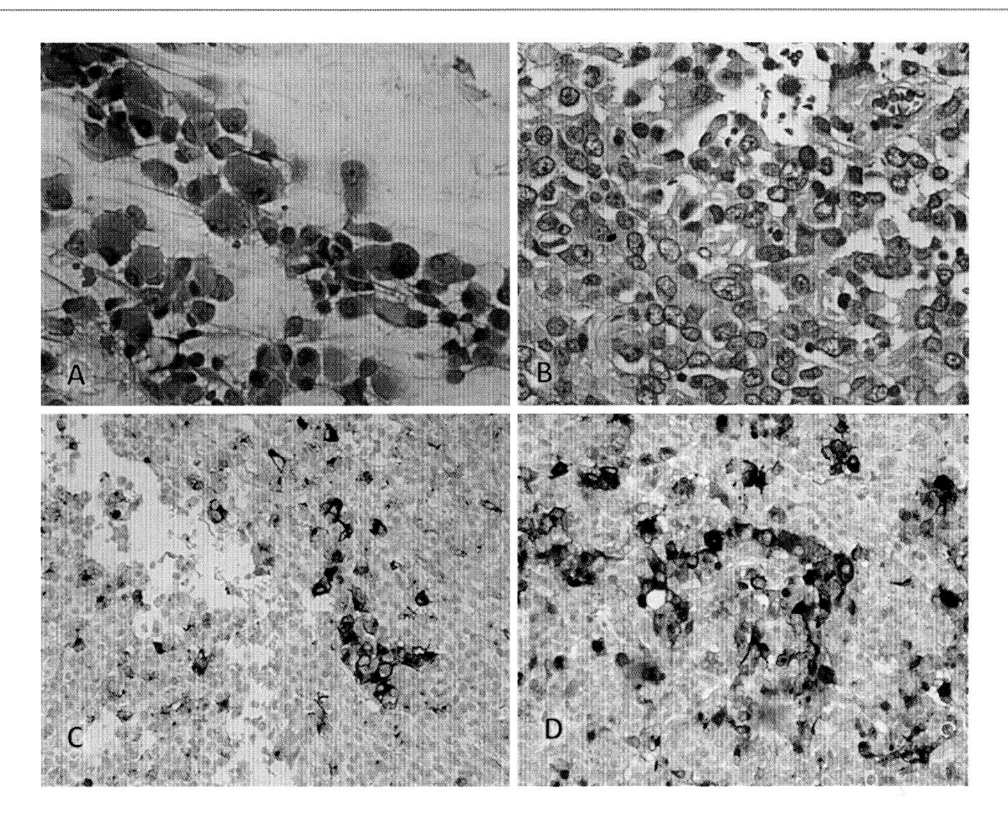

Fig. 2.1 This photomicrograph shows cytology (**a**) and histology (**b**) of *AT/RT*. Rhabdoid tumor cells with large, vesicular nuclei, prominent nucleoli and abundant eosinophilic cytoplasm are present. Many cells have distinct cytoplasmic inclusions (hematoxylin and eosin stain, original magnification ×400). Immunohistochemical staining shows clusters of cells intensely positive for epithelial membrane antigen (*EMA*) (**c**) and Vimentin (**d**) (original magnification ×200). Specimens courtesy of Pauline M. Chou, MD

treatment approaches, prognosis and survival vary significantly. Utsuki et al. (2003) reported on the importance of re-examination of pathologic specimens from patients with non-responsive medulloblastomas. The authors re-examined 15 cases of medulloblastomas and observed that 2 of the 15 cases were immunoreactive for EMA, cytokeratin, vimentin and smooth muscle actin. And although none of them presented with characteristic rhabdoid cells, these cases were reclassified as AT/RT. Both patients were infants and had a significantly shorter OS when compared to the 13 other medulloblastoma patients (6.5 months vs. 86 months) (Utsuki et al. 2003). Negative staining for INI-1 would also be critical in making this distinction.

Another entity which can resemble AT/RT in both clinical and histopathologically features is choroid plexus carcinoma. Histology, ultra structure, routine immunophenotyping or cytogenetic analysis may not distinguish between these two diagnoses. Although loss of INI-1 immunoreactivity has been reported in rare cases of choroid plexus carcinomas, INI-1 expression is still critical to distinguishing choroid plexus carcinoma from AT/RT. Though primary rhabdomyosarcoma of the CNS is extremely rare, metastatic lesions to the CNS can resemble AT/RT. The clinical history and immunoreactivity for striate muscle markers such as MyoD and desmin can clarify this distinction. Finally, many tumors of the CNS including meningioma, glioblastoma and metastatic carcinoma can exhibit a rhabdoid phenotype. In such cases, the diagnosis of primary AT/RT should be considered and ruled out.

Clinical Presentation and Treatment

Clinical Presentation and Radiographic Findings

Atypical teratoid-rhabdoid tumors usually present early in life, however, they have been reported throughout childhood, into adolescence and in adulthood. In general, children with AT/RT have clinical presentations similar to other patients with CNS tumors. Signs and symptoms typically vary by age and tumor location. Initial presenting signs such as vomiting and irritability may be as a result of ventricular dilation and increased intracranial pressure (ICP) from tumor obstruction of cerebrospinal fluid (CSF) flow. An inability to elevate the eyes, otherwise known as the "sun-setting" sign, may also be present. Infants often have more non-specific signs and symptoms such as increasing head circumference, failure to thrive and lethargy (MacDonald 2008). Children older than 3 years of age may report headache and those with supratentorial tumors may present with hemiplegia or other focal motor deficits. Seizures are a relatively uncommon presentation of AT/RT, but have been previously described in the literature (Chen et al. 2005).

Once the signs and symptoms of a brain tumor have been identified, patients are usually referred for diagnostic imaging. Computerized tomography (CT) of the head is typically done first and may demonstrate a mass lesion, enlarged ventricles and/or hemorrhage into the tumor or adjacent brain parenchyma. If a tumor is identified on the CT scan, it usually appears hyperdense compared to adjacent gray matter and may have fine calcifications (Warmuth-Metz et al. 2008). Magnetic resonance imaging (MRI) is the preferred study to characterize CNS AT/RT. As with other brain tumors, it provides the best resolution images of the tumor and its effect on the adjacent normal brain parenchyma. Further, MRI imaging is critical for surgical and radiation therapy planning. There are no specific MRI findings unique to AT/RTs when compared to other malignant lesions in the CNS (Fig. 2.2). The tumors are typically large with cystic and necrotic components and may contain calcifications or hemorrhage (MacDonald 2008). AT/RTs exert mass effect onto adjacent tissues but may not be associated with a significant amount of surrounding edema. In AT/RTs, the predominant MRI signal pattern isointensity on T1-weighted images and T2 shortening with heterogeneity on T2-weighted images (Parmar et al. 2006). Many tumors will also have hyperintense foci on T1-weighted imaging reflecting small intra-tumoral hemorrhages. Tumor enhancement after contrast administration in AT/RTs is variable. Though most tumors will take up gadolinium, in one large series, 16% of tumors demonstrated no contrast enhancement. Further, a characteristic "band-like" wavy enhancing rim which surrounds the central cystic and necrotic component of the tumor may be identified (Warmuth-Metz et al. 2008). If diffusion weighted images are performed, AT/RTs will have a heterogeneous restricted diffusion pattern. Experience with magnetic resonance spectroscopy is limited only to a single case report and revealed a high peak of choline, with decreased creatine and a low N-acetyl-aspartate peak within the tumor (Bing et al. 2009). At the present time, there is no known role for positive emission tomography (PET) in AT/RT.

Treatment

The first step in treatment of a patient with an AT/RT is stabilization, particularly for patients with increased ICP. Often neurosurgical intervention is required, including surgery for obstructive hydrocephalus and placement of either an external ventricular drain or a ventriculo-peritoneal shunt. The use of corticosteroids for tumor related cerebral edema in infants and young children with AT/RT is variable and practitioner dependent. Dexamethasone is the preferred corticosteroid in this setting given its potent anti-inflammatory effect, excellent penetration in the CNS and relatively low mineralocorticoid effect. Patients with minimal peri-tumoral edema may be safely managed without the use of steroids. If they are used, steroids should be rapidly weaned to avoid deleterious side

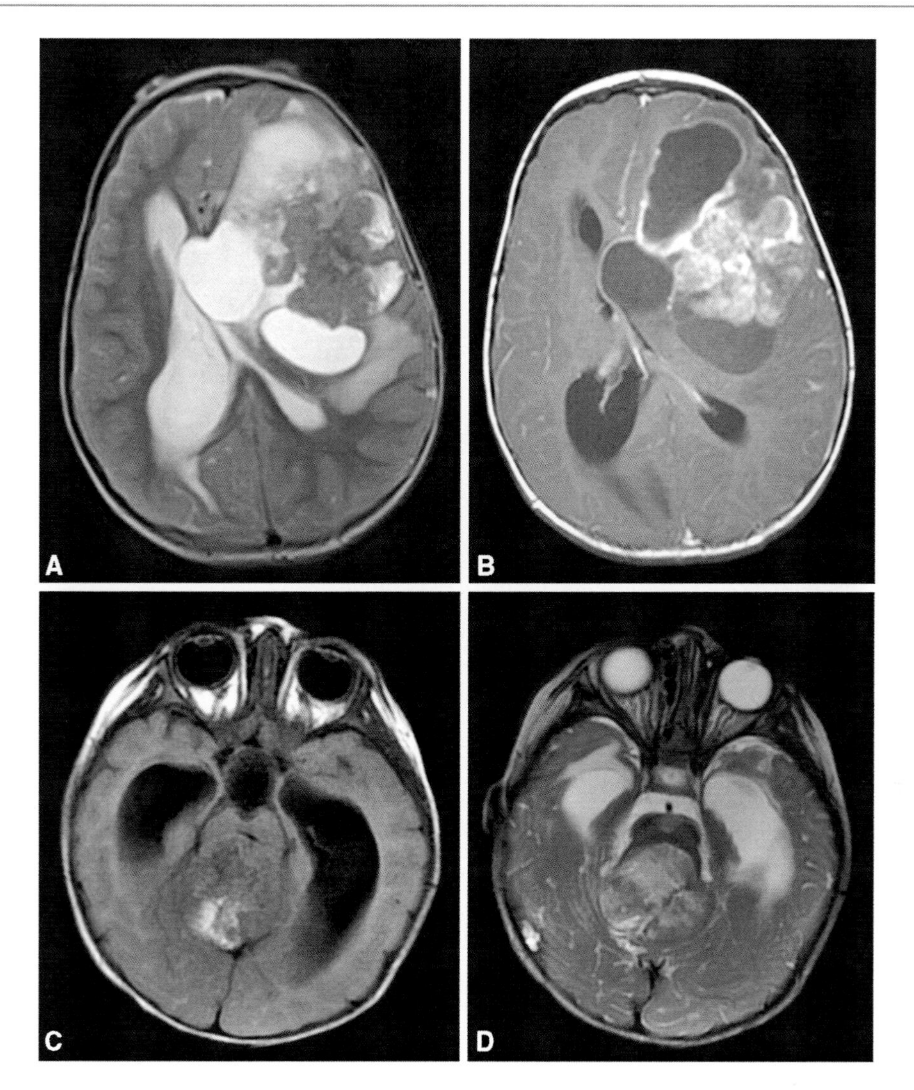

Fig. 2.2 A T2-weighted MRI image of supratentorial *AT/RT* demonstrates a large, mixed cystic and solid mass with significant midline shift and surrounding edema (**a**). A post-contrast T1-weighted image in the same patient reveals variable gadolinium uptake within the solid portion tumor (**b**). In another patient with a posterior fossa *AT/RT*, the mass is isointense on T1-weighted imaging with some bright areas suggestive of intra-tumoral hemorrhage (**c**). The solid portion of the mass has bright areas of T2 signal with some T2-hypointensity reflecting blood products and/or mineralization within the tumor (**d**). Evidence of obstructive hydrocephalus is seen on all images

effects such as weight gain, hypertension, elevated blood glucose and behavior changes.

For the small group of patients who develop seizures (from tumor or associated hemorrhage) at the time of their diagnosis, anticonvulsants should be administered. At the present time, most clinicians consider levitiracetam as the first line anticonvulsant for children with brain tumors as it has a favorable side effect profile and minimal interaction with other medications. The choice of anti-epileptic should be made in conjunction with a pediatric neurologist or neurosurgeon. There has been some controversy surrounding the use of prophylactic anticonvulsants in patients with newly diagnosed brain tumors. For patients who have been prescribed anticonvulsants in the peri-operative period, tapering and discontinuation of the medication within the first post-operative week is recommended in the absence of seizure activity. After immediate stabilization of the patient, surgical resection of the tumor should be performed if possible.

Prior to the development of recent protocols, the prognosis for patients with AT/RT was dismal. Survival rates for patients under 3 years of age were less than 20% at 12 months from diagnosis (MacDonald 2008). Despite aggressive treatments including surgery and chemotherapy, most patients suffered from rapidly progressive disease with a median survival of between 6 and 11 months (Chi et al. 2009). Older patients treated with extensive surgical resections, chemotherapy and radiation therapy had more favorable prognoses (MacDonald 2008). These data are reflective of the fact that patients had been historically treated with chemotherapy according to PNET or medulloblastoma protocols. Further, concerns about long-term neurocognitive effects of radiation therapy on young children precluded its use in most patients with AT/RT (Morgenstern et al. 2010). Contemporary protocols have intensified chemotherapy and investigated the role of high-dose chemotherapy with autologous stem cell transplant, intrathecal chemotherapy and radiation therapy for younger children.

The most significant improvement in outcomes in AT/RT has resulted from a shift to intensive multimodal therapy for patients of all ages. As a result of compelling data from a case series of long term survivors of AT/RT, a recent Phase II multi-center trial was designed by investigators at the Dana Farber Cancer Institute and began enrolling patients in 2004. The chemotherapy utilized in this protocol was based upon a rhabdomyosarcoma regimen and modified to include vincristine, dactinomycin, cyclophosphamide, cisplatin, doxorubicin and temozolomide. Additionally, patients received intrathecal and intraventricular chemotherapy with methotrexate, cytarabine and hydrocortisone. In an attempt to maximally intensify therapy and prevent early relapse, all patients (regardless of age) received radiation therapy early in the course of treatment. Focal radiation was prescribed for patients without metastatic disease to a total dose of 54 Gy. For patients older than 3 years of age with disseminated disease, craniospinal radiation was delivered to dose of 36 Gy with a focal boost up to 54 Gy in the primary tumor location (Chi et al. 2009).

With this intensive regimen, the 1-year progression free survival (PFS) and OS were 70% and 75%, respectively. At 2-years after diagnosis, the PFS was 53% with an OS of 70% (Chi et al. 2009). Though the results of this study are extremely promising, they should be interpreted with caution. The median follow up of the patients was relatively short and the possibility of delayed recurrences exists. Further, no information regarding neurocognitive functioning in this cohort is yet available. There is a potential risk that patients will have significant deficits as a result of radiation therapy to the developing brain.

Simultaneously, another intensive approach to the treatment of AT/RT has been investigated. Many groups in Europe and United States have attempted to replace radiation therapy with high-dose chemotherapy (HDCT) followed by autologous stem cell rescue after case reports in the late 1990s suggested some efficacy of this approach (Garre and Tekautz 2010). Results from these studies have been mixed. A recent report of the Italian experience with 29 cases of AT/RT revealed no difference in OS for patients with treated with transplantation compared to standard chemotherapy (23% versus 18.2%, respectively). HDCT has been prospectively studied by the Children's Oncology Group (COG) in study number 99703 with three cycles of conventional induction chemotherapy followed by three cycles of carboplatin and escalating doses of thiotepa with stem cell rescue. Early results from the study suggest that five of the ten patients are alive at a median of 42 months after diagnosis, however, this data has not yet been reported in its entirety (Garre and Tekautz 2010).

Patients with AT/RT have also been enrolled on the "Head Start II" regimen which included surgical resection, followed by five induction courses of chemotherapy cisplatin, vincristine, cyclophosphamide, etoposide and methotrexate. Consolidation followed with a single autologous stem cell transplant after preparation with carboplatin, thiotepa and etoposide. Of the seven children with AT/RT enrolled on Head Start II regimen, three were long term survivors and never required radiation therapy (Gardner et al. 2008).

Recently, a group from Canada retrospectively reviewed their experience with AT/RT and HDCT followed by autologous transplantation. Of a total of eight identified patients, four patients were alive without evidence of disease at a median follow-up of 52 months. Three of the surviving patients (including two with metastatic disease at diagnosis) were not irradiated. Some of the patients received adjuvant therapy including tamoxifen and intrathecal topotecan; therefore these results are difficult to generalize. Despite the exclusion of radiation therapy, however, the surviving patients in this cohort exhibit some degree of neurocognitive impairment attributed to the effect of surgery and chemotherapy (Finkelstein-Shechter et al. 2010). Another report from Nicolaides et al. (2010) also reported their experience with transplantation for AT/RT. In their cohort of nine children with AT/RT treated with HDCT and autologous transplantation, two patients are long term survivors (Nicolaides et al. 2010). The role of HDCT in the treatment of AT/RT still remains controversial. Taken together, these data suggest that a subset of patients may achieve long term remissions with transplantation and may avoid the need for radiation therapy.

There is limited data on treatment of patients with recurrent AT/RT and outcomes are dismal. For patients who have not had radiation therapy, it is usually considered after a second tumor resection if possible. Several agents have been investigated in early phase clinical trials with disappointing results. One such phase II study was carried out by the Pediatric Brain Tumor Consortium and investigated the use of oxaliplatin for recurrent or refractory AT/RT; though the agent was well tolerated, it had limited activity in this setting (Fouladi et al. 2006).

Prognostic Factors and Outcomes

Given the relative rarity of CNS AT/RT, identification of reliable prognostic factors has been difficult. Generally, it is well accepted that extent of surgical resection is predictive of OS (Morgenstern et al. 2010). This was recently confirmed by the results of the Dana Farber Cancer Institute study, patients with a gross total resection had significantly improved PFS and OS when compared to those with a less than gross total resection (Chi et al. 2009). In contrast, a recent meta-analysis of nearly 80 patients with AT/RT treated with multi-agent chemotherapy did not find similar significant differences with regard to degree of resection (Athale et al. 2009), though they had all been treated with different regimens. Age at the time of diagnosis has also been proposed as a prognostic factor in AT/RT. Historically, patients younger than 3 years of age tend to have less favorable outcomes with a median OS of 17% as compared to OS 89% in older patients (Tekautz et al. 2005) though this does not account for outcomes from recently published studies.

As patients with AT/RT have been treated with various regimens, identification of treatment related prognostic factors has been limited. Athale et al. (2009) reviewed treatment regimen data on approximately 80 cases of AT/RT. With regard to the inclusion of radiation therapy in the treatment algorithm, this meta-analysis revealed no significant difference in mean survival for patients treated with chemotherapy as compared to those who received chemotherapy and radiation. However, for patients under 3 years of age, radiation seemed to have a more beneficial effect with a significantly longer mean survival as compared to chemotherapy alone (Athale et al. 2009). Another treatment approach that appears to be beneficial is the inclusion of intrathecal therapy. In this same review, patients who received intrathecal chemotherapy had significantly longer 2-year OS (64%) as compared to those without intrathecal chemotherapy (17.3%). Additionally, patients who had intrathecal therapy were less likely to have spinal or meningeal relapse (Athale et al. 2009).

Future Directions in Research

Improvement in outcomes in AT/RT will require additional understanding of the complex biology of these tumors. As the number of known biologically active pathways in AT/RT is still low, targeted treatments have not yet reached clinical trials. Cyclin D1 and cyclin dependent kinase inhibitors have been proposed and are currently in development for AT/RT (Garre and Tekautz 2010). Other groups have been attempting to target CD133 positive tumor stem cells. In addition to proliferative and invasive properties, these cells are believed to be resistant to both chemotherapy and radiation therapy as evidenced by their expression of both stem cell and drug resistance genes. One group has considered the use of reservatrol, a naturally derived product that exists in various foods and beverages, in the treatment of AT/RT CD133 positive tumor cells. In cell culture, reservatrol induces apoptosis and increases radiosensitivity in these AT/RT cell lines and may be a promising treatment in the future (Kao et al. 2009). In the search of new developmental mechanisms and therapeutic targets, the role of microRNAs is being investigated in many cancers. MicroRNAs are small non-coding RNAs that operate as modulators of gene expression. In AT/RT, Sredni et al. (2010) found upregulation of microRNAs miR-221/222 which inhibits $p27^{Kip1}$, a known tumor suppressor and inhibitor of cell cycle (Sredni et al. 2010).

Advances in the clinical treatment of patients with AT/RT are focused upon refining the role of HDCT. Several ongoing studies are prospectively considering the use of transplantation for patients with AT/RT. One group in Italy is using ifosfamide, cisplatin and etoposide as induction therapy followed by HDCT with thiotepa, melphalan and autologous stem cell transplantation as consolidation prior to radiation therapy (Garre and Tekautz 2010). Another multi-national study for children older than 3 years of age led by St. Jude Children's Research Hospital stratifies patients based upon a risk group assignment. Low risk patients (those with focal disease) are treated with induction chemotherapy, low dose craniospinal irradiation followed by four autologous transplantation and maintenance vincristine. High risk patients (those with metastatic disease) receive higher doses of craniospinal irradiation in addition to the previously described regimen for low risk patients (www.clinicaltrials.gov, NCT00085202). Finally, the COG is prospectively evaluating the use of autologous transplantation along with radiation therapy in newly diagnosed patients with AT/RT (www.clinicaltrials.gov, NCT00653068).

Discussion

Central nervous system AT/RT is a relatively newly described entity. This rare, malignant tumor often affects young children and historically has been associated with dismal outcomes. Establishing a diagnosis of AT/RT can be challenging as a result of overlapping histological features and expression of multiple epithelial, primitive neuroepithelial and mesenchymal markers with immunohistochemical staining. One feature common to most AT/RTs is a genetic abnormality in the *INI-1* gene on chromosome 22q11. Loss of the INI-1 protein staining is important for distinguishing AT/RT from medulloblastoma or PNET. Treatment of AT/RT was associated with extremely poor outcomes despite surgery, chemotherapy and radiation therapy. However, promising new intensive multimodal therapy approaches have resulted in significantly improved OS. The long term sequelae of these therapies are yet to be determined. Additionally, investigators are considering the role of HDCT followed by autologous stem cell transplantation in AT/RT in an attempt to avoid or delay radiation therapy, especially in very young children. Future strategies in AT/RT are focused on improving our understanding of biologic pathways responsible for tumorigenesis in an attempt to identify therapeutic targets. Clinically, studies are exploring currently available treatments and newer targeted agents with the goal of increasing survival and minimizing treatment related toxicity.

References

Athale UH, Duckworth J, Odame I, Barr R (2009) Childhood atypical teratoid rhabdoid tumor of the central nervous system: a meta-analysis of observational studies. J Pediatr Hematol Oncol 31:651–663

Beckwith JB, Palmer NF (1978) Histopathology and prognosis of Wilms tumors: results from the First National Wilms' Tumor Study. Cancer 41:1937–1948

Biegel JA, Zhou JY, Rorke LB, Stenstrom C, Wainwright LM, Fogelgren B (1999) Germ-line and acquired mutations of INI1 in atypical teratoid and rhabdoid tumors. Cancer Res 59:74–79

Biegel JA, Kalpana G, Knudsen ES, Packer RJ, Roberts CW, Thiele CJ, Weissman B, Smith M (2002a) The role of INI1 and the SWI/SNF complex in the development of rhabdoid tumors: meeting summary from the workshop on childhood atypical teratoid/rhabdoid tumors. Cancer Res 62:323–328

Biegel JA, Tan L, Zhang F, Wainwright L, Russo P, Rorke LB (2002b) Alterations of the hSNF5/INI1 gene in central nervous system atypical teratoid/rhabdoid tumors and renal and extrarenal rhabdoid tumors. Clin Cancer Res 8:3461–3467

Biggs PJ, Garen PD, Powers JM, Garvin AJ (1987) Malignant rhabdoid tumor of the central nervous system. Hum Pathol 18:332–337

Bing F, Nugues F, Grand S, Bessou P, Salon C (2009) Primary intracranial extra-axial and supratentorial atypical rhabdoid tumor. Pediatr Neurol 41:453–456

Biswas A, Goyal S, Puri T, Das P, Sarkar C, Julka PK, Bakhshi S, Rath GK (2009) Atypical teratoid rhabdoid tumor of the brain: case series and review of literature. Childs Nerv Syst 25:1495–1500

Chen ML, McComb JG, Krieger MD (2005) Atypical teratoid/rhabdoid tumors of the central nervous system: management and outcomes. Neurosurg Focus 18:E8

Chi SN, Zimmerman MA, Yao X, Cohen KJ, Burger P, Biegel JA, Rorke-Adams LB, Fisher MJ, Janss A, Mazewski C, Goldman S, Manley PE, Bowers DC, Bendel A, Rubin J, Turner CD, Marcus KJ, Goumnerova L, Ullrich NJ, Kieran MW (2009) Intensive multimodality treatment for children with newly diagnosed CNS atypical teratoid rhabdoid tumor. J Clin Oncol 27:385–389

Finkelstein-Shechter T, Gassas A, Mabbott D, Huang A, Bartels U, Tabori U, Laura J, Hawkins C, Taylor M, Bouffet E (2010) Atypical teratoid or rhabdoid tumors: improved outcome with high-dose chemotherapy. J Pediatr Hematol Oncol 32:e182–e186

Fouladi M, Blaney SM, Poussaint TY, Freeman BB 3rd, McLendon R, Fuller C, Adesina AM, Hancock ML, Danks MK, Stewart C, Boyett JM, Gajjar A (2006) Phase II study of oxaliplatin in children with recurrent or refractory medulloblastoma, supratentorial primitive neuroectodermal tumors, and atypical teratoid rhabdoid tumors: a pediatric brain tumor consortium study. Cancer 107:2291–2297

Gadd S, Sredni ST, Huang CC, Perlman EJ (2010) Rhabdoid tumor: gene expression clues to pathogenesis and potential therapeutic targets. Lab Invest 90:724–738

Gardner SL, Asgharzadeh S, Green A, Horn B, McCowage G, Finlay J (2008) Intensive induction chemotherapy followed by high dose chemotherapy with autologous hematopoietic progenitor cell rescue in young children newly diagnosed with central nervous system atypical teratoid rhabdoid tumors. Pediatr Blood Cancer 51:235–240

Garre ML, Tekautz T (2010) Role of high-dose chemotherapy (HDCT) in treatment of atypical teratoid/rhabdoid tumors (AT/RTs). Pediatr Blood Cancer 54:647–648

Janson K, Nedzi LA, David O, Schorin M, Walsh JW, Bhattacharjee M, Pridjian G, Tan L, Judkins AR, Biegel JA (2006) Predisposition to atypical teratoid/rhabdoid tumor due to an inherited INI1 mutation. Pediatr Blood Cancer 47:279–284

Judkins AR, Mauger J, Ht A, Rorke LB, Biegel JA (2004) Immunohistochemical analysis of hSNF5/INI1 in pediatric CNS neoplasms. Am J Surg Pathol 28:644–650

Kalpana GV, Marmon S, Wang W, Crabtree GR, Goff SP (1994) Binding and stimulation of HIV-1 integrase by a human homolog of yeast transcription factor SNF5. Science 266:2002–2006

Kao CL, Huang PI, Tsai PH, Tsai ML, Lo JF, Lee YY, Chen YJ, Chen YW, Chiou SH (2009) Resveratrol-induced apoptosis and increased radiosensitivity in CD133-positive cells derived from atypical teratoid/rhabdoid tumor. Int J Radiat Oncol Biol Phys 74:219–228

Kleihues P, Louis DN, Scheithauer BW, Rorke LB, Reifenberger G, Burger PC, Cavenee WK (2002) The WHO classification of tumors of the nervous system. J Neuropathol Exp Neurol 61:215–225; discussion 226-219

Ma HI, Kao CL, Lee YY, Chiou GY, Tai LK, Lu KH, Huang CS, Chen YW, Chiou SH, Cheng IC, Wong TT (2010) Differential expression profiling between atypical teratoid/rhabdoid and medulloblastoma tumor in vitro and in vivo using microarray analysis. Childs Nerv Syst 26:293–303

MacDonald TJ (2008) Aggressive infantile embryonal tumors. J Child Neurol 23:1195–1204

Morgenstern DA, Gibson S, Brown T, Sebire NJ, Anderson J (2010) Clinical and pathological features of paediatric malignant rhabdoid tumours. Pediatr Blood Cancer 54:29–34

Nicolaides T, Tihan T, Horn B, Biegel J, Prados M, Banerjee A (2010) High-dose chemotherapy and autologous stem cell rescue for atypical teratoid/rhabdoid tumor of the central nervous system. J Neurooncol 98:117–123

Parmar H, Hawkins C, Bouffet E, Rutka J, Shroff M (2006) Imaging findings in primary intracranial atypical teratoid/rhabdoid tumors. Pediatr Radiol 36:126–132

Parwani AV, Stelow EB, Pambuccian SE, Burger PC, Ali SZ (2005) Atypical teratoid/rhabdoid tumor of the brain: cytopathologic characteristics and differential diagnosis. Cancer 105:65–70

Rorke LB, Packer RJ, Biegel JA (1996) Central nervous system atypical teratoid/rhabdoid tumors of infancy and childhood: definition of an entity. J Neurosurg 85:56–65

Sredni ST, Bonaldo Mde F, Costa FF, Huang CC, Hamm CA, Rajaram V, Tomita T, Goldman S, Bischof JM, Soares MB (2010) Upregulation of mir-221 and mir-222 in atypical teratoid/rhabdoid tumors: potential therapeutic targets. Childs Nerv Syst 26:279–283

Tekautz TM, Fuller CE, Blaney S, Fouladi M, Broniscer A, Merchant TE, Krasin M, Dalton J, Hale G, Kun LE, Wallace D, Gilbertson RJ, Gajjar A (2005) Atypical teratoid/rhabdoid tumors (ATRT): improved survival in children 3 years of age and older with radiation therapy and high-dose alkylator-based chemotherapy. J Clin Oncol 23:1491–1499

Utsuki S, Oka H, Tanaka S, Kondo K, Tanizaki Y, Fujii K (2003) Importance of re-examination for medulloblastoma and atypical teratoid/rhabdoid tumor. Acta Neurochir (Wien) 145:663–666; discussion 666

Versteege I, Sevenet N, Lange J, Rousseau-Merck MF, Ambros P, Handgretinger R, Aurias A, Delattre O (1998) Truncating mutations of hSNF5/INI1 in aggressive paediatric cancer. Nature 394:203–206

Warmuth-Metz M, Bison B, Dannemann-Stern E, Kortmann R, Rutkowski S, Pietsch T (2008) CT and MR imaging in atypical teratoid/rhabdoid tumors of the central nervous system. Neuroradiology 50:447–452

Zhang F, Tan L, Wainwright LM, Bartolomei MS, Biegel JA (2002) No evidence for hypermethylation of the hSNF5/INI1 promoter in pediatric rhabdoid tumors. Genes Chromosomes Cancer 34:398–405

3 Paediatric Teratoid/Rhabdoid Tumours: Germline Deletions of Chromosome 22q11.2

Rachel Beddow

Contents

R. Beddow (✉)
Central and Southern Genetic Services, Wellington Hospital, Private Bag 7902, Wellington, New Zealand
e-mail: Rachel.Beddow@ccdhb.org.nz

Abstract

The highly malignant rhabdoid tumours (MRTs) in particular atypical teratoid/rhabdoid tumours (AT/RT) are generally considered to be a childhood tumour with the majority of patients presenting at younger than 5 years of age. In most cases these tumours arise from inactivation of the *INI1/SMARCB1* gene due to 22q11.2 deletions. Germline alterations of *INI1/SMARCB1* have been found in up to 35% of patients with rhabdoid tumours. Patients with germline alterations generally present at an earlier age and with more aggressive disease, commonly with multiple primary tumours.

The chromosomal region on 22q11 is highly susceptible to microdeletions and microduplications due to the presence of several low copy repeats (LCR) within a 9 Mb region. The proximal deletion at 22q11.2 is the most well known microdeletion syndrome in this region and gives rise to DiGeorge/Velocardiofacial syndrome (DGS/VCFs). However the lesser known distal 22q11.2 deletion syndrome, when it encompasses the *INI1/SMARCB1* gene, confers a high risk of developing AT/RT or MRT. Patients diagnosed with distal 22q11.2 deletion syndrome who also have rhabdoid predisposition syndrome due to loss of *INI1/SMARCB1* should undergo careful monitoring due to their increased risk of developing these type of tumours.

M.A. Hayat (ed.), *Pediatric Cancer, Volume 3: Diagnosis, Therapy, and Prognosis*, Pediatric Cancer 3, DOI 10.1007/978-94-007-4528-5_3, © Springer Science+Business Media Dordrecht 2012

Introduction

Atypical teratoid/rhabdoid tumours (AT/RT) are a highly malignant intracranial, embryonal neoplasm assigned WHO-2007 grade IV. These are composed of cells that exhibit epithelial, neuroepithelial or mesenchymal differentiation and are largely confined to childhood with more than 90% of these tumours being diagnosed in patients younger than 5 years (median onset of 20 months) (Biegel et al. 1999). AT/RT represents 1–2% of all paediatric brain tumours (Rickert and Paulus 2001) and accounts for up to 10% of brain tumours in infants (Biegel 2006).

The development of these tumours was initially associated with monosomy 22 and subsequently deletions and translocations involving 22q11.2 (Biegel et al.1990; Douglass et al. 1990). The *INI1/SMARCB1* gene was later identified by Versteege et al. (1998) as the gene responsible for AT/RT. The majority of AT/RT and malignant rhabdoid tumours (MRT) harbour deletions and/or mutations (somatic or germline) involving the *INI1/SMARCB1* tumour suppressor gene on chromosome 22q11.2. Biallelic inactivation of this gene was shown by Biegel et al. (1999) and Rousseau et al. (1999) to be characteristic of AT/RT.

Inactivation of the *INI1/SMARCB1* gene and resulting protein can be demonstrated using an immunohistochemical (IHC) analysis with an anti-INI1 antibody. INI1 immunohistochemistry has been demonstrated to be sensitive and specific for the diagnosis of malignant rhabdoid tumour, loss of the INI1 protein appears to be rare in other tumours (Hoot et al. 2004). A study by Medijkane et al. (2004) suggested that loss of *INI1/SMARCB1* function affects the actin cytoskeleton, providing a potential explanation for the rhabdoid morphology.

It is widely accepted that 15–20% of AT/RT and MRTs are associated with a germline mutation or deletion involving *INI1/SMARCB1*. However, a recent study conducted Eaton et al. (2011) showed that 35 of the 100 patients studied with rhabdoid tumours had a germline deletion or mutation. This germline mutation or deletion is viewed as the 'first hit' which predisposes these children to malignancies. AT/RT is the first paediatric brain tumour for which a candidate tumour suppressor gene has been identified.

Several constitutional chromosomal conditions are known to confer carriers with an increased susceptibility to various forms of cancer, e.g. Down syndrome with acute myeloid leukaemia (AML) and trisomy 8 with myelodysplasia and acute leukaemia. Constitutional loss of well known tumour suppressor genes *WT1, WT2* and *RB1* are known to be implemented in congenital syndromes which have an increased susceptibility to tumours; loss of *WT1* in 'WAGR' syndrome and loss of *WT2* in Beckwith Wiedemann syndrome leads to susceptibility to Wilms tumours. Constitutional 13q14 deletions which include the *RB1* gene are seen in families with inherited susceptibility to retinoblastoma. These patients tend to present with bilateral tumours unlike the sporadic cases.

Like Retinoblastoma and Wilms tumours, AT/RT and MRT susceptibility is also seen in patients with a congenital syndrome; 22q11.2 distal deletion syndrome. The larger deletion seen in some of the patients with this syndrome encompasses the *INI1/SMRCB1* gene.

The Structure and Function of the *INI1/SMARCB1* Gene

Vesteege et al. (1998) identified the *INI1/SMARCB1* gene, which they called *SNF5/INI1*, within a region frequently deleted in MRT. *SMARCB1* is the HGNC approved gene symbol, its full title is SWI/SNF-related, matrix-associated, actin-dependent regulator of chromatin, subfamily B, member 1. This gene is also commonly called Integrase Interactor 1 or *INI1*. Like many others this gene also has many other synonyms; *Sfh1p, SNF5, hSNF5, Ini1, RDT, BAF47, SNF5L1* and *Snr1*. (OMIM ref 601607, HGNC ref 11103). In keeping with recent publications, for this chapter we will refer to the gene as *INI1/SMARCB1*.

INI1/SMARCB1 is located on chromosome 22 at q11.23 from base pair 22,459,149 to base pair 22,506,704 (NCBI36/hg18) or 24,129,149 to 24,176,704 (NCBI) (GRCh37/hg19). This gene is 47.556kb in total; it comprises of nine exons and has a coding sequence of approximately 1.2kb. *INI1/SMARCB1* encodes a subunit of the SWI/SNF ATP-dependent chromatin remodelling complex. Originally identified in yeast the SWI/SNF complex is present in all eukaryotes and is highly evolutionarily conserved. *INI1/SMARCB1* represents the first member of an ATPase chromatin remodelling complex to be implicated in the genesis of cancer. Studies by Medjkane et al. (2004) and Caramel et al. (2008) aimed to elucidate the mechanism underlying the highly invasive and metastatic nature of rhabdoid tumour identified a role for *INI1/SMARCB1* in controlling the actin cytoskeleton network and found that *INI1/SMARCB1* loss transcriptionally enhances RhoA signalling conferring enhanced migratory potential upon cell lines.

Vries et al. (2005) reported that loss of *INI1/SMARCB1* function in MRT-derived cells leads to polyploidization and chromosomal instability. Chromosomal instability manifests as changes in chromosome structure e.g. rearrangements; translocations, inversions, deletions, duplications and gain and loss of whole chromosomes (aneuploidy). These changes are a hallmark of cancer cells and lead to uncontrolled cell proliferation. Vries et al. (2005) demonstrated that restoration of *INI1/SMARCB1* expression in MRT-derived cells which had lost *INI1/SMARCB1* gene function, leads to purging of the polyploid and aneuploid cells leading to a diploid cell population. However, a study by McKenna et al. (2008) found that *INI1/SMARCB1* cells do not have increased sensitivity to DNA damaging agents, nor altered induction of either γ-H2Ax or repair checkpoints. Further evaluation focused upon primary human MRT found that these aggressive *INI1/SMARCB1*-deficient cancers are diploid and genomically stable. Roberts and Biegel (2009) suggest that disruption of this chromatin remodelling complex can largely substitute for genomic instability in the genesis of this cancer.

In AT/RT and MRT *INI1/SMARCB1* appears to function as a classic tumour suppressor gene; the germline mutation or deletion comprises the 'first-hit' which predispose to the development of these tumours. A 'second-hit' is required for tumour progression, this being caused by somatic loss or mutation of the other allele. Therefore this conforms to Knudson's two hit hypothesis for genetic predisposition caused by inherited mutations in tumour suppressor genes.

Individuals with germline alterations of *INI1/SMARCB1* are predisposed to rhabdoid tumours of the brain, kidney and soft tissues. These patients are often diagnosed at a young age (less than 1 year) and tend to have a worse prognosis. This is in common with two other well known tumour suppressor genes *RB1* in retinoblastoma and *WT1* and *WT2* in Wilms tumours. It is unclear whether the poor prognosis is due to the presence of the mutation/deletion in all the cells or to the fact that these patients often present with multiple primary tumours that are resistant to therapy (Roberts and Biegel 2009).

The most common germline abnormalities detected in the study by Eaton et al. (2011) were point or frameshift mutations resulting in premature truncation of the protein. Other germline abnormalities included heterozygous loss of *INI1/SMARCB1* and duplications or deletions of one or more exons within *INI1/SMARCB1*. The deletions and duplications within *INI1/SMARCB1* encompassed anywhere from one exon to all nine exons, but, exons 4 and 5 appear to be a particular 'hot spots' for both germline and somatic abnormalities. Larger deletions that encompass the whole *INI1/SMARCB1* gene are usually associated with phenotypic abnormalities.

Biegel et al. (1999) reported that patients presenting with multiple primary tumours are usually found to have germline abnormalities of this gene; however, patients who present with an apparently sporadic tumour have also been found to carry germline mutations or deletions of *INI1/SMARCB1*.

Rhabdoid Predisposition Syndrome

Reports of familial associated cases of AT/RT in the literature are limited. Lynch et al. (1983) described the first family, they reported two siblings with para-vertebral tumours. Subsequently, Proust et al. (1999) reported two sisters of consanguineous parents who presented with cerebral AT/RTs within 2 weeks of one another. Sevenet et al. (1999) reported three families with multiple affected siblings who were shown to carry germline mutations of *INI1*. Since these reports there have been other families reported where more than one family member has been affected. This familial inheritance of the mutation/deletion has been termed 'Rhabdoid Predisposition Syndrome'. This syndrome shows variable penetrance, a good example of which is the family reported by Janson et al. (2006) where the two children carrying the identical germline mutation as their mother developed tumours at 17 months and 2 months of age. The mother was unaffected along with the obligate carrier grandmother. The maternal uncle died at 2 years of age from a reported medulloblastoma and renal rhabdoid tumour.

The risk of developing a rhabdoid tumour (or related tumour) for patients carrying a germline mutation/deletion of *INI1/SMARCB1* is unknown. Eaton et al.'s (2011) study demonstrates that some mutations/deletions show variable expressivity and reduced penetrance; having identified several unaffected carriers. The parental origin of mutations/deletions of *INI1/SMARCB1* have not been extensively studied in rhabdoid tumours and hence, whether the risk is affected by the parental origin of the abnormality is unknown. However, children with germline abnormalities involving *INI1/SMARCB1* generally present with rhabdoid tumours at a younger age (median age 5 months) than those with sporadic disease (18 months).

Although *INI1/SMARCB1* abnormalities are responsible for AT/RT and MRT these abnormalities are not specific for rhabdoid tumours and carrier families can present with AT/RT in children but their parents may develop schwannomatosis later in life. Cases of choroid plexus carcinoma, epithelioid sarcoma, peripheral primitive neuroectodermal tumour, undifferentiated sarcoma and epithelioid malignant peripheral nerve sheath tumour have all been reported to demonstrate loss of expression of *INI1/SMARCB1*.

Molecular Structure of 22q11.2

Chromosome 22q11 shows a high frequency of genomic rearrangement. Genomic deletions within the 22q11.2 region are one of the most common microdeletions in humans and occur at a frequency of 1:3000–1:5000. The majority (75–90%) of these deletions occur *de novo* (Perez and Sullivan 2002). This genomic instability is attributed to the presence of several paralogous low copy repeats (LCRs) or segmental duplications (SDs) over a 9Mb region, each containing a complex modular structure and a high degree of sequence identity (96%) over large stretches of the repeat (Shaikh et al. 2007). Guo et al. (2011) found a total of 202 pairs of SD sequences (aka duplicons) to be located in this 9 Mb region.

These SDs or LCRs can mediate meiotic unequal non-allelic homologous recombination (NAHR) events either between homologous chromosomes (interchromosomally), within a single chromatid or between sister chromatids (intrachromosomally). This mechanism can result in genomic rearrangement and sometimes altered gene dosage within the intervening regions. This model accounts for the high number of these deletions which arise *de novo*.

At least eight LCR clusters have been identified at 22q11.2 and have been named by Edelmann et al. (1999) 'LCR22s'.

The four proximal LCRs (LCR22-2, LCR22-3a, LCR22-3b and LCR22-4) have been extensively characterised, given their involvement in recurrent rearrangements of 22q11 that lead to DiGeorge/Velocardiofacial syndrome (DGS/VCFs), the reciprocal duplication syndrome, der(22) syndrome and Cat eye syndrome. Shaikh et al. (2001) reports that these proximal LCRs are larger than the distal ones and have a complex modular structure. The four distal LCRs are smaller with fewer duplicated modules.

The most common microdeletion involves the proximal region and is characterised by a 3 Mb deletion from LCR22-2 to LCR22-4 and this region has been termed the 'Typically Deleted Region' or TDR by Shaikh et al. (2001). Deletions of this region lead to DGS/VCFs and are associated with a broad spectrum of congenital anomalies ranging from cardiac defects, cleft lip and palate, thymic hypoplasia, parathyroid dysfunction, conotruncal anomalies, facial defects, psychotic features and immunodeficiencies (Scambler 2000).

The lesser reported distal 22q11.2 deletion syndrome, however, is caused by deletions typically flanked by LCR22-4 and LCR22-6 or LCR22-7. The phenotype associated with this syndrome is subtle and distinct from that of DGS/VCFs. It includes mild global developmental delay, mild facial dysmorphism with most patients having a smooth philtrum and high arched eyebrows. Only a few patients have so far been reported in the literature and this can most probably be attributed to the non-specific phenotype associated with these deletions. It is anticipated that the detection of patients diagnosed with this syndrome will increase due to the widespread use of microarray technology, which is now used as a 'first-line' test in many centres for investigation of patients with developmental delay, idiopathic mental retardation or/and congenital abnormalities. Array comparative genomic hybridisation (aCGH) allows simultaneous interrogation of numerous DNA probes. Thus, it offers an efficient and high-throughput whole genome test for detecting microdeletions and microduplications.

In addition to congenital anomalies, rearrangements of 22q11 are often detected in malignant conditions; the most common rearrangement on 22q11 is associated with the balanced t(9;22) translocation detected in patients with chronic myeloid leukaemia (CML) and acute lymphocytic leukaemia (ALL). The breakpoint on chromosome 22 is within the LCR22-6 and termed BCR or breakpoint cluster region. The balanced t(8;22) translocation associated with Burkitt's lymphoma (BL) disrupts the immunoglobulin light chain locus (IGL) which again is located at LCR22-6. Other malignancies involving this region include Ewing Sarcoma, meningiomas, schwannomatosis and of course the malignant rhabdoid tumours.

Distal 22q11.2 Deletion Syndrome (Overview)

Distal 22q11.2 deletion syndrome was first identified by Raunch et al.(1999, 2005) and found serendipitously by Ravan et al. (2006) in eight patients with unexplained developmental delay that were being tested by subtelomeric FISH analysis. These patients were noted to have loss of one copy of the BCR (control) probe compatible with an interstitial heterozygous deletion at 22q11.2. The BCR probe is commonly used to identify the t(9;22) translocation detected in CML and ALL. VYSIS (Abbot technologies) also use this probe in the subtelomeric FISH panel 'ToTelVysion' as a 'control probe' in order to identify the chromosome 22s. BCR is located close to *INI1/SMARCB1* and this probe is also used to indicate loss of this gene in AT/RT tumour material.

Since the first report by Raunch et al. (1999) additional cases have been reported by Mikhail et al. (2007), Ben-Shachar et al. (2008), Rødningen et al. (2008) and Beddow et al. (2011). The distal deletion removes the genes located between LCR22-4 and LCR22-6 or LCR22-7 along with the aforementioned *BCR* gene. Ben-Shachar et al. (2008) carried out aCGH analysis on more than 8,000 patients with suspected chromosomal aberrations. Six (10%) of these patients were found to have deletions distal to the TDR (DGS/VCFs common region). The six patients were found to share similar clinical features as well as physical findings. Five were born prematurely with four of these patients having a birth weight below the fifth percentile for gestational age. Five of the patients also showed postnatal growth restrictions. A global developmental delay, more prominent in speech, was found in four of these patients. Minor skeletal abnormalities were found in four of the patients. Two of the patients had a cardiac defect. All six patients showed characteristic facial features; arched eyebrows, deep-set eyes, a smooth philtrum, a thin upper lip, hypoplastic alae nasi, and a small pointed chin.

Distal 22q11.2 Deletion Syndrome and Paediatric Teratoid/Rhabdoid Tumours or Malignant Rhabdoid Tumours

The *INI1/SMARCB1* gene also resides in the segment that has been found to be deleted in some patients with distal 22q11.2 deletion syndrome. Wieser et al. (2005) reported a patient with a micoduplication of the TDR and a microdeletion of the distal region encompassing the *INI1/SMARCB1* gene who developed a fatal MRT. This patient presented with hypacusis (60–80 dB) and at 6 months was referred to hospital with recurrent respiratory tract infections, and later with chronic otitis media. During this time developmental retardation, a ventricular septal defect and dextroposition of the heart were recognised, as well as dysmorphic features suggestive of a syndromic disorder. These features included brachycephaly, almond shaped palpebral fissures, short nose, long philtrum, thin upper lip, retrognathia with low-set, dysplastic, over-folded ears. At 9 months of age the patient had developed a rapidly growing tumour of his right kidney; this was diagnosed as a highly malignant rhabdoid tumour of the kidney. The patient died at the age of 19 months, after extensive cytostatic therapy, from multiple metastases of his tumour. Cytogenetic studies revealed a normal karyotype, 46, XY. However, FISH showed a deletion of the BCR probe on one chromosome 22 along with a duplication of the TDR proximal to the deleted segment.

Since this publication there are now a four further published reports of patients presenting with congenital anomalies consistent with distal 22q11.2 deletion syndrome and aggressive MRT or AT/RT tumours. Jackson et al. (2007) described five patients with germline deletions of 22q11.2 that included the *INI1/SMARCB1* gene, two of whom also had abnormal phenotypic features. The other three infants had highly aggressive disease with multiple tumours at the time of presentation. The patients with the abnormal phenotype were found to have deletions approximately 2.7 Mb in size that correspond with distal 22q11.2 deletion syndrome. The three patients with multiple primary tumours had smaller but overlapping deletions, primarily involving *INI1/SMARCB1*. Both children with phenotypic abnormalities were seen by a clinical geneticist prior to the diagnosis of MRT. The other three patients did not have any obvious phenotypic features consistent with an underlying genomic disorder, although they may have been too young to show developmental delay of other clinical features. Interestingly, the children with the smaller deletions presented early with multiple primary tumours and extremely aggressive disease as opposed to those with the more extensive deletions who developed tumours at a later age. The patient reported by Lafay-Cousin et al. (2009) (with a larger 2.8Mb deletion) also corroborates a possible correlation between size and location of the deletion and the biological course of the tumour, with their patient showing a prolonged continuous remission of 2 years after treatment without radiation. The later onset of an AT/RT tumour is also evident in the patient reported by Beddow et al. (2011) who developed an AT/RT at 18 years of age. This theory however, does not correspond with the patient reported by Toth et al. (2011) whose patient carried the distal 22q11.2 deletion and presented with a rhabdoid tumour at birth. Until further cases are reported with distal 22q11.2 deletion syndrome and AT/RT or MRT the relationship between deletion size and age of onset/severity cannot be fully elucidated. However, it is worth noting that there are published cases of patients with distal 22q11.2 deletion syndrome that do not mention these tumours. It is possible that some of these patients were reported prior to the AT/RT or MRT developing or that these patients' deletions extend only to LCR22-6 and not LCR22-7 and therefore, do not encompass the *INI1/SMARCB1* gene. This situation highlights the need for accurate sizing of this deletion by microarray technology and if the *INI1/SMARCB1*is implicated then careful monitoring of these patients should be initiated.

These six reported cases are summarised in the table below (Table 3.1).

Interestingly, all six reported patients carry near identical deletions of 22q11.2 from LCR22-4 to LCR22-7 (the differences in base pair coordinates is probably due to the wide variety of microarray platforms used). The fact that all six patients' deletions have occurred between LCR22-4 and LCR22-7 (Fig. 3.1) suggest that this deletion arises by NAHR that results from the presence of these LCRs. The phenotypic features associated with distal 22q11.2 deletion syndrome result from heterozygosity of the 22q11.2 region from LCR22-4 to LCR22-6. The larger deletion seen in these six reported patients extends to LCR22-7 and also

Table 3.1 Clinical and molecular features of patients reported with 22q11.2 distal deletion syndrome and MRT or AT/RT

Case	Tumour	Age of onset	Deletion size	Deletion breakpoints NCBI36/hg18	LCRs	ID	Heart defect	Dysmorphism	Small stature	Impaired hearing
Wieser et al.	MRT of the kidney	9 months	2.8Mb	20114134–22944693	LCR22–4 to LCR22–7	+	+ (VSD)	+		+
Jackson et al. (Pt 1)	MRT of the kidney	5 years	2.7Mb		LCR22-4 to LCR22-7	+	+ (VSD)	+		+
Jackson et al. (Pt 2)	MRT of the spine	12 months	2.7Mb		LCR22-4 to LCR22-7		+ (ASD/VSD)	+		
Lafay-Cousin et al.	AT/RT	12 months	2.7Mb	201129573–22880573	LCR22-4 to LCR22-7	+		+	+	Ear tags
Beddow et al.	AT/RT	18 years	2.8Mb	20128705–22961613	LCR22-4 to LCR22-7	+	+ (dilated cardiomyopathy ? inherited)	+		
Toth et al.	MRT of the shoulder	3 weeks	2.8Mb	20138750–22973264	LCR22-4 to LCR22-7		+ (VSD)	+		Ear tags

MRT Malignant rhabdoid tumour, *AT/RT* Atypical teratoid/rhabdoid tumour, *VSD* Ventricular-septal defect, *ASD* Atrial-septal defect

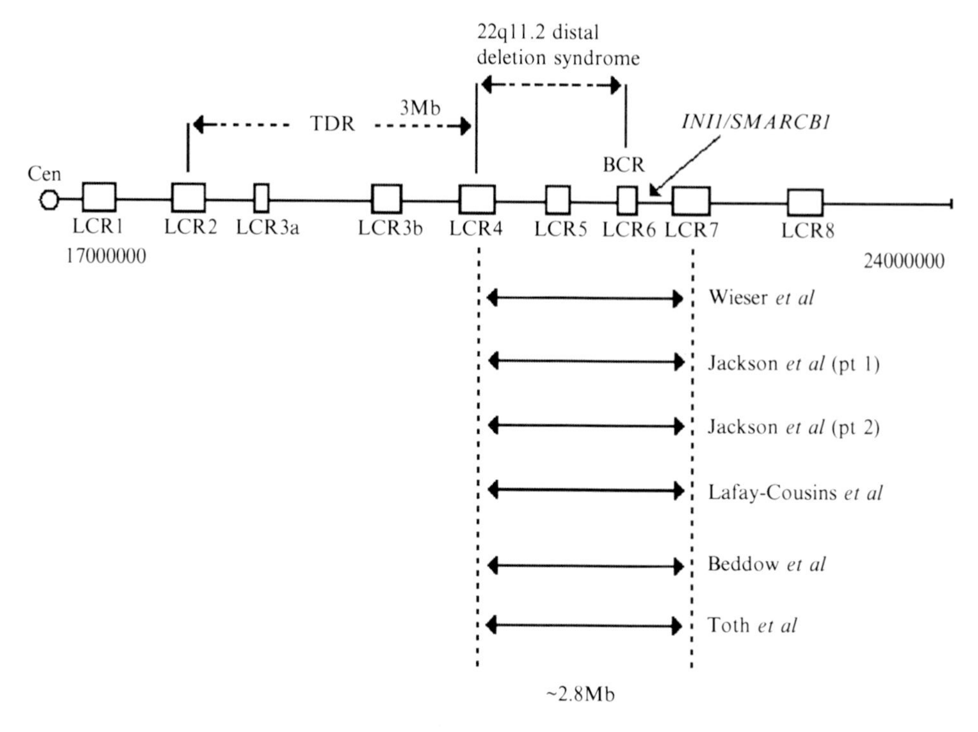

Fig. 3.1 Schematic overview of 22q11.2 region – relative positions according to NCBI36/hg18 showing LCR22s (LCR22-1 to LCR22-8) identifying the 'Typically Deleted Region' or *TDR* which results in DiGeorge/Velocardiofacial syndrome *DGS/VCFs*, the region implicated in distal 22q11.2 deletion syndrome and the relative size and position of the six reported cases

confers rhabdoid predisposition syndrome on these individuals.

Although the facial dysmorphism is mild, the majority of the patients were reported to have a long philtrum with a thin upper lip and downturned corners to the mouth. Small stature/growth retardation was only detected in one of these patients which is in contrast to the other cases of distal 22q11.2 deletion syndrome reported by Ben-Shacher et al. (2008).

The age of onset of MRT or AT/RT in individuals who carry large germline deletions is unclear. The majority of these patients presented with the MRT or AT/RT at 12 months or younger however, one patient was 5 years and one presented at 18 years. These observations suggest that there is variable penetrance for this larger deletion. Indeed, this would account for the fact that only eight patients with a large deletion, encompassing the whole *INI1/SMARCB1*gene, have so far been reported (two of these patients have been excluded in this discussion due to the lack of clinical information).

It is clear from these observations that patients which present with MRT or AT/RT and dysmorphic features should be tested for the distal 22q11.2 deletion. Genetic testing can be carried out by fluorescence in situ hybridisation (FISH) using the BCR probe which is located close to *INI1/SMARCB1* and within the region flanked by LCR22-4 and LCR22-6 or preferably by microarray analysis.

Further family studies should be initiated if a germline deletion is detected. Consultation with a clinical geneticist should be carried out to discuss the implications. Likewise, if a patient displaying dysmorphism and/or developmental delay is diagnosed with distal 22q11.2 deletion syndrome by microarray analysis and the deletion encompasses the *INI1/SMARCB1* gene, careful and prolonged monitoring of these patients should be undertaken. As demonstrated by the examples in the aforementioned papers the second 'hit' in carriers of large 22q11.2 deletion which encompasses *INI1/SMARCB1* could occur at any time.

These patients will require a multidisciplined approach with both the oncology and genetic teams being involved with their management.

While specific guidelines for screening have not yet been established, baseline CNS MRI and renal ultrasounds are standard practice in many centres and if necessary further monitoring can be implemented.

Acknowledgements I would like to thank my friends and colleagues at Central and Southern Regional Genetic Services for their proof reading skills and Kathryn Seally for her help with Fig. 3.1.

References

Beddow RA, Smith M, Kidd A, Corbett R, Hunter AG (2011) Diagnosis of distal 22q11.2 deletion syndrome in a patient with teratoid/rhabdoid tumour. Eur J Med Genet 54:295–298

Ben-Shachar S, Ou Z, Shaw CA, Belmont JW, Patel MS, Hummel M, Amato S, Tartaglia N, Berg J, Reid SV, Lalani SR, Chinault C, Cheung SW, Lupski JR, Patel A (2008) 22q11.2 Distal deletion: a recurrent genomic disorder distinct from DiGeorge syndrome and velocardiofacial syndrome. Am J Hum Genet 82:214–221

Biegel JA (2006) Molecular genetics of atypical teratoid/rhabdoid tumour. Neurosurg Focus 20:E11

Biegel JA, Rourke LB, Packer RJ, Emanuel BS (1990) Monosomy22 in rhabdoid or atypical tumours of the brain. J Neurosurg 73:710–714

Biegel JA, Zhou JY, Rorke LB, Stenstrom C, Wainwright LM, Fogelegren B (1999) Germ-line and acquired mutations of INI1 in atypical teratoid and rhabdoid tumours. Cancer Res 59:74–79

Caramel J, Quignon F, Delattre O (2008) RhoA-dependent regulation of cell migration by the tumour suppressot hSNFs/INI1. Cancer Res 68:6154–6161

Douglass EC, Valentine M, Rowe ST, Parham DM, Williams JA, Sanders JM, Houghton PJ (1990) Malignant rhabdoid tumor: a highly malignant childhood tumor with minimal karyotypic changes. Genes Chromosomes Cancer 2:210–216

Eaton KW, Tooke LS, Wainwright LM, Judkins AR, Biegel JA (2011) Spectrum of *SMARCB1/INI1* mutations in familial and sporadic rhabdoid *tumors*. Pediatr Blood Cancer 56:7–15

Edelmann L, Pandita RK, Spiteri E, Funke B, Goldberg R, Palanisamy N, Chaganti RS, Magenis E, Shprintzen RJ, Morrow BE (1999) A common molecular basis for rearrangement disorders on 22q11. Hum Mol Genet 8:1157–1167

Guo X, Freyer L, Morrow B, Zheng D (2011) Characterization of the past and current duplication activities in the human 22q11.2 region. BMC Genomics 12:71–87

Hoot AC, Russo P, Judkins AR, Perlman EJ, Biegel JA (2004) Immunohistochemical analysis of hSNF5/INI1 distinguishes renal and extra-renal malignant rhabdoid tumours from other pediatric soft tissue tumors. Am J Surg Pathol 28:1485–1791

Jackson EM, Shaikh TH, Gururangan S, Jones MC, Malkin D, Nikkel SM, Zuppan CW, Wainwright LM, Zhang F, Biegel JA (2007) High-density single nucleotide polymorphism array analysis in patients with germline deletions of 22q11.2 and malignant rhabdoid tumour. Hum Genet 122:117–127

Janson K, Nedzi LA, David O, Schorin M, Walsh JW, Bhattacharjee M, Pridjian G, Tan L, Judkins AR, Biegel JA (2006) Predisposition to atypical teratoid/rhabdoid tumor due to an inherited *INI1* mutation. Pediatr Blood Cancer 47:279–284

Lafay-Cousin L, Payne E, Strother D, Chernos J, Chan M, Bernier FP (2009) Goldenhar phenotype in a child with distal 22q11.2 deletion and intracranial atypical teratoid rhabdoid tumour. Am J Med Genet 149A:2855–2859

Lynch HT, Shurin SB, Dahms BB, Izant RJ, Lynch J, Danes BS (1983) Paravertebral malignant rhabdoid tumor in infancy. Cancer 52:290–296

McKenna ES, Sansam CG, Cho YJ, Geulich H, Evans JA, Thom CS, Moreau LA, Biegel JA, Pomeroy SL, Roberts CWM (2008) Loss of the epigenetic tumor suppressor SNF5 leads to cancer without genomic instability. Mol Cell Biol 28:6223–6233

Medjkane S, Novikov E, Verteege I, Delattre O (2004) The tumor suppressor hSNF5/INI1 modulates cell growth and actin cytoskeleton organisation. Cancer Res 64:3406–3413

Mikhail FM, Descartes M, Piotrwski A, Andersson R, Diaz de Ståhl T, Komorowski J, Bruder CE, Dumanski JP, Carroll AJ (2007) A previously unrecognised microdeletion syndrome on chromosome 22 band q11.2 encompassing the BCR gene. Am J Med Genet A 143:2178–2184

Perez E, Sullivan K (2002) Chromosome 22q11.2 Deletion syndrome (DiGeorge and velocardiofacial syndromes). Curr Opin Pediatr 14:678–683

Proust F, Laquerriere A, Costantin B, Ruchoux MM, Vannier JP, Freger P (1999) Simultaneous presentation of atypical teratoid/rhabdoid tumor in siblings. J Neuro Oncol 43:63–70

Raunch A, Pfeiffer RA, Leipold G, Singer H, Tigges M, Hofbeck MA (1999) A novel 22q11.2 Microdeletion in DiGeorge syndrome. Am J Hum Genet 64:659–667

Raunch A, Zink S, Zweier C, Thiel CT, Koch A, Rauch R, Lascorz J, Hüffmeier U, Weyand M, Singer H, Hofbeck M (2005) Systematic assessment of atypical deletions reveals genotype-phenotype correlation in 22q11.2. J Med Genet 42:871–876

Ravan JB, Tepperberg JH, Papenhausen P, Lamb AN, Hedrick J, Eash D, Ledbetter DH, Martin CL (2006) Subtelomere FISH analysis of 11 688 cases: an evaluation of the frequency and pattern of subtelomere rearrangements in individuals with developmental disabilities. J Med Genet 43:478–489

Rickert CH, Paulus W (2001) Epidemiology of central nervous system tumours in childhood and adolescence based on the new WHO classification. Childs Nerv Syst 17:503–511

Roberts CWM, Biegel JA (2009) The role of SMARCB1/INI1 in development of rhabdoid tumor. Cancer Biol Ther 8(5):412–416

Rødningen OK, Prescott T, Eriksson AS, Røsby O (2008) 1.4Mb recurrent 22q11.2 distal deletion syndrome, two new cases expand the phenotype. Eur J Med Genet 51:646–650

Rousseau-Merk MF, Verteege I, Legrand I, Couturier J, Mairal A, Delattre O, Aurias A (1999) hSNF5/INI1 inactivation is mainly associated with homozygous deletions and mitotic recombination in rhabdoid tumour. Cancer Res 59:3152–3156

Scambler PJ (2000) The 22q11 deletion syndromes. Hum Mol Genet 9:2421–2426

Sévenet N, Sheridan E, Amram D, Schneider P, Handgretinge R, Delattre O (1999) Constitutional mutations of the *hSNF/INI1* gene predispose to a variety of cancers. Am J Hum Genet 65:1342–1348

Shaikh TH, Kurahashi H, Emanuel BS (2001) Evolutionarily conserved low copy repeats (LCRs) in 22q11 mediate deletions, duplications, translocations and genomic instability: an update and literature review. Genet Med 3:6–13

Shaikh TH, O'Connor RJ, Pierpont ME, McGrath J, Hacker AM, Nimmakayalu M, Geiger E, Emanuel BS, Saitta SC (2007) Low copy repeats mediate distal chromosome 22q11.2 deletions: sequence analysis predicts breakpoint mechanisms. Genome Res 17:482–491

Toth G, Zraly CB, Thomson TL, Jones C, Lapetino S, Murakas J, Zhang J, Dingwall AK (2011) Congenital anomalies and rhabdoid tumor associated with 22q11 germline deletion and somatic inactivation of the SMARCB1 tumor suppressor. Genes Chromosomes Cancer 50:379–388

Versteege I, Sevenet N, Lange J, Rousseau-Merck M-F, Ambros P, Handgretinger R, Aurias A, Delattre O (1998) Truncating mutations of hSNF5/INI1 in aggressive paediatric cancer. Nature 394:203–206

Vries RGJ, Bezrookove V, Zuijderduijn LMP, Kia SK, Houweling A, Oruetxebarria I, Raap AK, Verrijzer CP (2005) Cancer-associated mutations in chromatin remodeler hSNF5 promote chromosomal instability by compromising the mitotic checkpoint. Genes Dev 19:665–670

Wieser R, Fritz B, Ullmann R, Müller I, Galhuber M, Storlazzi CT, Ramaswamy A, Christiansen H, Shimizu N, Rehder H (2005) Novel rearrangement of chromosome band 22q11.2 causing microdeletion syndrome-like phenotype and rhabdoid tumour of the kidney. Hum Mutat 26:78–83

4 Pediatric Atypical Teratoid/ Rhabdoid Tumor: Role of INI1 Tumor Suppressor Gene

Mariela Carolina Coccé and Marta Susana Gallego

Contents

Abstract

Atypical teratoid/rhabdoid tumor (AT/RT) is a highly aggressive brain tumor of early childhood. Most cases show deletions of chromosome 22 and mutations of the tumor suppressor gene hSNF5/INI1/SMARCB1, located in the chromosome band 22q11.2. The INI1 protein is a core subunit of the SWI/SNF chromatin-remodeling complex and is presumed to function by activating or repressing a variety of target genes involved in cell-cycle control and/or differentiation. We summarize what is currently known regarding the role of INI1 in the development of AT/RT.

Introduction

Rhabdoid tumors (RT) are highly malignant, aggressive, embryonal neoplasms of early infancy and childhood, which may originate from virtually any tissue. In the central nervous system (CNS), these tumors are termed atypical teratoid/rhabdoid tumor (AT/RT) which accounts for 1.3% of paediatric brain tumors (Rickert and Paulus 2001).

Cytogenetic studies of RT provided the first evidence that there was a common genetic event responsible for the pathogenesis of these tumors. Monosomy of chromosome 22 or a deletion or translocation specifically involving chromosome band 22q11.2 were the most frequent chromosomal alterations found in these tumors.

M.C. Coccé (✉) • M.S. Gallego
Cytogenetics Laboratory, Genetics Department, Garrahan Pediatrics Hospital, Combate de los Pozos 1881, 1245 Buenos Aires, Argentina
e-mail: marielacocce@yahoo.com.ar

M.A. Hayat (ed.), *Pediatric Cancer, Volume 3: Diagnosis, Therapy, and Prognosis*, Pediatric Cancer 3,
DOI 10.1007/978-94-007-4528-5_4, © Springer Science+Business Media Dordrecht 2012

These findings were confirmed with molecular approaches by analyzing the loss of heterozygosity (LOH) and by fluorescence in situ hybridization (FISH).

Biegel et al. (1996) applied FISH to a series of RT cell lines and primary tumor samples and based on the results, mapped a rhabdoid tumor locus to the region between the constant region genes of immunoglobulin lambda and BCR in 22q11. Furthermore, the authors proposed that loss or inactivation of a tumor suppressor gene in chromosome 22 was responsible for the initiation or progression of RT.

Using a positional cloning approach, Versteege et al. (1998) identified the INI1 gene as responsible for the initiation of RT. The vast majority of tumors show biallelic somatic inactivation of INI1 as a result of homozygous deletions or truncating non-sense or frameshift mutations. The INI1 protein as a member of the SWI/SNF chromatin remodeling complex regulates transcription of various genes involved in cell signaling, growth, and differentiation. Although the specific function of INI1 in rhabdoid tumor development is unknown, it is hypothesized that INI1 affects its tumor-suppressor function by modulating the transcription of cellular genes.

Biological Functions of INI1

Abrams et al. (1986) identified a Sucrose Non-Fermenting gene number 5 (SNF5) as a gene essential for the expression of glucose-repressible genes in Saccharomyces cerevisiae. Characterization of the SNF5 gene revealed that it encodes a protein which is a glutamine- and proline-rich transcriptional activator that affects the expression of a broad spectrum of genes (Laurent et al. 1990). Several years later, Kalpana et al. (1994) isolated the INI1 protein by the yeast two-hybrid system through its interaction with HIV-1 integrase, and determined that the gene, named INI1 (for integrase interactor 1), encodes a human homolog of yeast SNF5 protein.

Subsequently, Wang et al. (1996) found that hSNF5/INI1 was a component of the SWI/SNF multiprotein complex which remodels nucleosomes in vitro in an ATP-dependent manner. For this reason, this gene is also known as SMARCB1 gene, which stands for SWI/SNF-related, matrix-associated, actin-dependent regulator of chromatin, subfamily B, member 1.

The hSNF5/INI1 gene encodes a 47 KDa protein which contains 27.5% charged residues and is globally acidic. Sequence alignment of the hSNF5/INI1 cDNA with the yeast transcription factor ySNF5 revealed 3 charged regions of high similarity and an absence of the glutamine- and proline-rich domains. These 3 regions collectively define the SNF5 homology domain and share 55% sequence identity and 71% conserved residues with the yeast protein (Kalpana et al. 1994). Two of the charged regions are composed of imperfect repeats 60 amino acids long, named Repeat I (Rpt I) and Repeat II (Rpt II). The third region, located at the carboxyl terminus of the protein, is termed homology region 3 (HR3) and is rich in leucine residues and possesses the secondary structure of a coiled-coil motif (Muchardt et al. 1995). This domain, whose function is unknown, emerges as a critical site for protein–protein interactions.

SWI/SNF Complex

Chromatin remodeling complexes regulate gene expression by modulating access of transcription factors to DNA. The first ATP-dependent chromatin remodeling complex was discovered in yeast cells. This complex was named SWI/SNF because of its requirement for the expression of mating-type switching (SWI) and sucrose non-fermenting (SNF) genes. The SWI/SNF complex is evolutionarily conserved and plays essential roles in a variety of cellular processes including differentiation, proliferation and DNA repair. The mammalian SWI/SNF complex is a ~2 MDa multi-protein complex composed of a collection of core and variable subunits. In human cells, there are 2 classes of SWI/SNF complexes, known as BRG1-associated factor (BAF; also known as SWI/SNF-A) and polybromo BRG1-associate factor (PBAF; also known as SWI/SNF-B), which differ in protein composition.

In addition to ATPase subunits, brahma-related gene I (BRG1) or brahma (BRM), the human complex contains 8–14 proteins, which are referred to as BRM- or BRG1-associated factors or BAFs. The amino-acid sequences of BRM and BRG1 are 75% identical and both are widely expressed. Nonetheless, these subunits are mutually exclusive, as each SWI/SNF complex contains either BRM or BRG1. Mammalian BAF proteins are conventionally identified by their molecular size; hence BAF47 refers to a BRG1-associated protein with an apparent molecular mass of 47 kDa. The BAF47 corresponds to the INI1 protein. This subunit is present in all known variants of the complex.

The BAF complex utilizes either BRM or BRG1 as the ATPase, and is composed of the BRG1/BRM associated factors BAF250, BAF170, BAF155, BAF47/INI1, BAF60a, BAF57, BAF53, and b-Actin. In contrast, the PBAF complex exclusively utilizes BRG1 as the catalytic subunit, and is composed of the factors BAF200, BAF180, BAF170, BAF155, BAF47/INI1, BAF60a, BAF53, and BAF57.

To affect gene regulation, replication, or DNA repair, these enzymes are recruited to DNA through the interaction of distinct members of the SWI/SNF complex and covalently modify histone tails or sequence-specific transcription factors. The current model is that these protein–protein interactions are integral in directing the targeted recruitment of chromatin remodeling complexes to individual genes, rather than broad genomic regions.

The SWI/SNF chromatin remodeling complexes function as a collective unit; however, the individual members play an important role in defining gene-specific targeted recruitment and ensuring appropriate transcriptional regulation. Moreover, BRG1 and BRM have remodeling activity in the absence of other subunits and the addition of other core subunits proteins, such as BAF47, BAF155, and BAF170, increases remodeling activity to a level comparable with that of the whole SWI/SNF complex, indicating that the entire complex is not absolutely necessary for chromatin remodeling.

The complex SWI/SNF plays a critical role in inhibiting S phase entry by repressing the activity of E2F transcription factor by physical interaction and functional Rb and histone deacetylase 1 (HDAC1). The loss of SWI/SNF subunits has been reported in a number of malignant cell lines and tumors, and a large number of experimental observations suggest that this complex functions as a tumor suppressor.

Murine Models

Murine knockout models have provided functional evidence for INI1 as a tumor suppressor gene. In an attempt to identify the mechanisms that cause the formation of these tumors, INI1-knockout mice were generated independently by three groups (Roberts et al. 2000; Klochendler-Yeivin et al. 2000; Guidi et al. 2001). Homozygous inactivation of INI1 results in early embryonic lethality, and heterozygous mice are cancer prone, with 15–30% of animals developing sarcoma-like rhabdoid lesions at a median age of 1 year. As in humans who inherit a mutant INI1 allele, the remaining INI1 allele has been spontaneously lost within the murine tumors. These tumors occur most frequently in the head/neck followed by paraspinal, trunk and extremity locations, all at sites that also occur in humans. Some of the models develop occasional brain tumors although none develop kidney tumors, these two sites being the most frequent location of rhabdoid tumors in humans. The cancers that occur in INI1 heterozygous mice are highly aggressive, always locally invasive and frequently metastatic to regional lymph nodes or lung.

In order to circumvent embryonic lethality and evaluate the effect of bi-allelic loss of INI1, Roberts et al. (2002) constructed a conditional knockout model of INI1 showing that loss of INI1 function resulted in a highly penetrant and extremely short latency development of cancers, in particular lymphomas or rhabdoid tumors, thus demonstrating the extremely powerful oncogenic role of INI1 loss of function. This study, however, also uncovered the requirement of INI1 for survival of most normal, nonmalignant cells. The rapidity with which tumors develop following inducible inactivation of INI1 is unprecedented, 100% of mice develop tumors with a median latency of 11 weeks. In comparison, the time to tumor development with other tumor suppressors is significantly longer, as p53 loss leads to cancer at 20 weeks, p19Arf loss at 38 weeks, p16Ink4a loss at 60 weeks, and loss of p21 does not lead to a detectable increase in tumor formation in mice.

Inactivation of each of the tumor suppressors RB, APC, PTEN, VHL, or NF1 leads to embryonic lethality. Thus, the aggressive cancer-prone phenotype that occurs following reversible inactivation of the INI1 gene is striking when compared to other tumor suppressor knockouts, and indicates a critical role for INI1 in preventing cancer.

Furthermore, the discrepancy observed in the tumor penetrance between the INI1 heterozygous mice and the homozygous conditional knockout mice may be explained by the findings of Guidi et al. (2004) who observed a transcriptional compensation for haploinsufficiency by the remaining INI1 allele. This result in levels of INI1 expression in the heterozygous cells is similar to those in wild-type cells, and supports the hypothesis that bi-allelic loss of INI1 may be required to predispose to cancer.

These mouse models have demonstrated that INI1 prevents tumorigenesis, and paradoxically, it is required for cell survival.

INI1 Mutations in Rhabdoid Tumor

Bi-allelic inactivation of INI1 occurs through different mechanisms including homozygous deletion, cytogenetic deletion, or LOH with a coding-sequence mutation in the remaining allele, or two independent mutations. The bi-allelic inactivating of INI1 observed in RT is consistent with Knudson's 2-hit hypothesis for oncogenesis, which requires the occurrence of 2 random somatic alterations or a germ line alteration and a somatic loss or mutation of the other allele. The germ line alteration can be de novo or inherited from a parent.

In the appropriate clinical setting, germline and somatic mutations and deletions of INI1 may be diagnostic for renal and extra-renal RT as well as AT/RT; however, the role of INI1 inactivation in other CNS tumors, such as choroid plexus carcinoma, remains controversial. Recently, INI1 has also been implicated in the development of familial schwannomatosis, although it is not clear if there is a similar spectrum of mutations and deletions to those seen in classic RT (Eaton et al. 2011).

Patients who present with multiple primary tumors are inevitably found to have a germline alteration; nevertheless, children with apparently sporadic tumors have also been reported to have germline mutations or deletions in INI1. Remarkably, heterozygous germline deletion or mutation of INI1 can be observed in up to 35% of patients with RT, including familial cases described as having RT-predisposition syndrome (Eaton et al. 2011). The mutations and deletions predispose to rhabdoid tumors in all sites, but may show variable expressivity and reduced penetrance. Several unaffected carriers were identified who are thus at risk of developing both benign and malignant tumors, including schwannoma and rhabdoid tumor.

In most patients, the germline mutations or deletions are de novo and parents are reported to be unaffected. Reports of multiple affected siblings with CNS tumors with the same germline mutation, in which neither parent was a carrier, implicated gonadal mosaicism as a mechanism that can result in a familial associated genetic predisposition to cancer.

It has been hypothesized that in patients with a germline INI1 mutation there is an increased period of susceptibility during the first few years of life in which most rhabdoid tumors occur (Janson et al. 2006). Carriers of the INI1 mutation that do not develop such a tumor at young age might be at increased risk of developing other INI1-related but not necessarily malignant tumors later in life. This is also supported by the fact that the manifestation of RT occurs at a very early age, with a median of 5.5 months in children with INI1 germline mutations and a median of 13 months in children without INI1 germline mutations, but it is very rare in older children or adults.

The a priori risk of developing a rhabdoid tumor, or another related tumor, in the setting of a germline mutation is not yet known.

On the other hand, rhabdoid tumors have been seen in the context of a germline chromosome band 22q11.2 deletion that encompasses the INI1 locus. Depending on the size of the deletion, these patients may also be at risk of heart defects, development delay and other congenital abnormalities associated with the loss of additional genes in the 22q11.2 region. As high-density array comparative genomic hybridization or single nucleotide polymorphism (SNP) based oligonucleotide arrays are increasingly being used to screen for genetic disorders in patients with congenital abnormalities and developmental delay, additional individuals will likely be found with germline mutation of INI1 (Jackson et al. 2007).

Identification of constitutional INI1 gene mutations is critical so that parents may be appropriately counseled regarding the chances of recurrence in future children, and given the option for prenatal testing. However, reduced penetrance for INI1, variable risk of developing rhabdoid tumor or schwannoma associated with a germline mutation, gonadal mosaicism and risk of multiple primary tumors all need to be considered in developing recurrence risks for affected families. Study of additional families is warranted in order to better determine the cancer risk for carriers of INI1 germline mutations.

Nowadays, employing a combination of SNP array analysis, MLPA, FISH, and direct sequencing the inactivation of both INI1 alleles on chromosome band 22q11.2 can be identified in most of the pediatric RT (Jackson et al. 2009). The majority of the reported mutations are point or frameshift changes that introduce a novel stop codon, and thus predict premature truncation of the protein. The INI1 gene has nine exons and the mutations reported are distributed throughout the coding sequence of the gene, although they appear to be potential hot spots. Thirty five percent of CNS tumors harbor a somatic mutation in exon 9, which corresponds to a deletion of cytosine or guanine in codon 382. Both delC and delG cause a frameshift change that eliminate the final stop codon and are predicted to result in the addition of 96 amino acids to the C terminal end of the protein. Interestingly, this mutation has not yet been observed in the germline. In primary tumors the altered proteins are not detected by western blot analysis or immunohistochemistry, suggesting that messenger RNA or protein are likely to be unstable. Therefore, another hotspot mutation was identified in exon 5, which involves a transition of a C-to-T in codon 201 and is present in both somatic and germline mutations (Biegel et al. 2002).

Inactivation of both copies of the gene leads to loss of protein expression in the nucleus, which can be detected by immunohistochemistry. This assay for INI1 is currently used as an adjunct to histology in the differential diagnosis of rhabdoid tumors. In contrast, the loss of INI1 expression in the absence of a mutation may identify a subgroup of tumors with epigenetic modification of the INI1 locus or alterations in another gene that could modify INI1 expression.

Alternative mechanism to coding sequence mutations or deletion that have the potential to inactive INI1 include promoter alterations that decrease or inhibit transcription, post-transcriptional modifications, defects in protein translation, and post-translational modification. Hypermethylation of the INI1 promoter does not appear to be the mechanism for decreased expression of INI1 seen in tumors without coding-sequence mutations. On the other hand, it is noteworthy that approximately 2% of AT/RTs express INI1 protein. Recently, it has been demonstrated that genetic alterations of another SWI/SNF chromatin-remodeling complex member, the ATPase subunit BRG1 (also known as SMARCA4) imply the existence of a second locus involved in the pathogenesis of INI1 positive rhabdoid tumors (Hasselblatt et al. 2011).

The INI1 Pathway

Insight into the mechanism of INI1-mediated tumor suppression has been provided by studies performed in cultured RT cells. The identification of downstream target genes regulated in an INI1-dependent manner has been an area of active investigation in recent years. Several in vitro studies have suggested that INI1 suppresses tumor formation by regulation of the p16/CDK4/cyclin D1/Rb/E2F pathway.

Reintroduction of INI1 into INI1-deficient human RT-derived cell lines results in decreased cell proliferation and reduced potential to form colonies as potentiated apoptosis. Furthermore, these cells show dramatic modifications of the cell shape associated with a complete reorganization of the actin cytoskeleton. These cellular phenotypic changes occur concomitantly with the up-regulation of genes involved in the polymerization and organization of the actin cytoskeleton. Even low-level expression of INI1 is enough to cause this effect. Flattened cell morphology is correlated with decrease in the number of cells in S and G2/M phase and respective increase in the number of cells in G0–G1 phase of cell cycle, which suggests that expression of the gene causes G0–G1 arrest. The basis for this arrest is increased expression of the cell-cycle regulator p16Ink4a that occurs following INI1 expression. The INI1 acts as a transcriptional coactivator, which is required for the recruitment of BRG1 containing SWI/SNF chromatin remodeling complex to the p16Ink4a promoter. When the INI1 gene is inactivated, transcription of p16Ink4a is decreased, which causes activation of cyclin D1/CDK4 complex and phosphorylation of Rb. Phosphorylated Rb is inactive and no longer inhibits E2F function, which allows propagation of cell cycle. This may mean that INI1-mediated cell cycle arrest is dependent on p16Ink4a activity.

It is interesting to note that whereas the BRG1 ATPase subunit of SWI/SNF complex is required for Rb-mediated cell-cycle-arrest, INI1 is dispensable for this activity, as Rb can induce cell-cycle arrest in INI1-deficient cells.

Genetic knockout studies have indicated that cyclin D1 is required for genesis of rhabdoid tumors in vivo. It has been reported that INI1-deficient cells over-express cyclin D1. Zhang et al. (2002) found that one of the mechanisms by which INI1 exerts its tumor suppressor function is by mediating the cell cycle arrest due to the direct recruitment of HDAC1 and deacetylation of histones at the cyclin D1 promoter, thereby causing its repression and G0–G1 arrest. On the other hand, it has been found that G1 cell cycle arrest occurred concomitantly with an increase in p21 mRNA and protein levels, and preceded p16Ink4A mRNA and protein up-regulation. Therefore, both p21 and p16Ink4a are targets for INI1. Moreover, the increase in p21 might still require p53 function based on the observation that p53 is recruited to p21 promoter by INI1.

The role of the p53 tumor suppressor in RT is poorly understood. It has been functionally linked to SWI/SNF, whose activity is necessary for p53-mediated transcription activation and p53-mediated cell cycle control (Wang et al. 2007).

Knockdown of INI1 in cell lines and animal models results in activation of p53 without associated TP53 gene mutations. Intriguingly, combined inactivation of INI1 and p53 but not Rb or p16Ink4a leads to accelerated development of RT in mouse models (Isakoff et al. 2005). These data have led to the hypothesis that 2 successive hits involving INI1 and TP53 may contribute to malignant transformation and tumor development. Moreover, it has been found that p53 expression correlates positively with p14Arf expression and negatively with MDM2 in AT/RT cases. This suggests that there is deregulation not only of p16Ink4a but also of the p14Arf pathway (Venneti et al. 2011).

Later studies have revealed that Akt pathway contributes to chromatin remodeling disruption and promoting malignant transformation of AT/RT (Józwiak et al. 2010). Arcaro et al. (2007) found that AT/RT cell lines overexpressed the insulin receptor (IR) and the insulin-like growth factor-I receptor (IGFIR). Insulin potently activates Akt (also called protein kinase B) in AT/RT cells. The Akt activates directly the mTOR (mammalian target of rapamycin) which is a central regulator of cellular state and is often found implicated in tumorigenesis. The mTOR controls the synthesis of essential proteins involved in cell cycle progression, such as cyclin D1, ornithine decarboxylase or survival, like c-Myc. Hence, the Akt/mTOR pathway seems to play an important role in the control of AT/RT proliferation.

Although cell cycle control is the most well-characterized activity of INI1 it may not fully explain its ability to suppress tumor formation. It is possible that INI1 may play independent roles in both development and differentiation pathways. The control of cellular differentiation pathways may be a second mechanism by which INI1 may exert its tumor suppressor activity. Inactivation of INI1 would result in abrogation of cellular differentiation and induction of cell proliferation, consistent with the general observation that tumors tend to be poorly differentiated and display uncontrolled proliferation.

On the other hand, several studies have also suggested that the SWI/SNF complex is involved in DNA damage response (Klochendler-Yeivin et al. 2006). Thus, INI1 loss might contribute to oncogenesis by causing a DNA repair defect and genomic instability. However, the role of INI1 at the level of genetic stability is controversial.

Vries et al. (2005) found that inactivation of INI1 may lead to polyploidy and chromosomal instability due to abnormal chromosomal segregation, suggesting a role for INI1 in mitotic checkpoint control. Morozov et al. (2007) reported that rhabdoid cells over-express Polo like kinase 1 (PLKI), and the INI1 re-expression in RT cells downregulates the expression of this gene. The PLK1 is a highly conserved Ser/Thr kinase in eukaryotes and plays a critical role in various aspects of mitotic events, such as G2/M transition, spindle formation, chromosome congression and segregation, as well as cytokinesis. In later stages of mitosis, PLK1 is involved in the activation of components of the anaphase-promoting complex for mitotic exit and in cytokinesis. One striking consequence of deregulated PLK1 activity is the formation of aberrant centrosomes and mitotic spindle poles, which are tightly correlated with aneuploidy and chromosomal instability in tumor development. The finding that INI1 represses PLK1 expression and in rhabdoid tumors deleted of INI1 exhibits up-regulation of PLK1 supports the idea that INI1 mediates mitotic spindle checkpoint control indirectly via p16/CDK4/cyclin D/Rb/E2F pathway.

Nevertheless, other authors have stated that loss of INI1 can lead to cancer without genomic instability taking into account that the majority of RT display normal diploid karyotypes with alterations occurring almost exclusively at the INI1 locus. They have suggested that the epigenetic role of INI1 in contributing to transcriptional regulation via nucleosome remodeling is the major and perhaps sole mechanism by which INI1 acts as a tumor suppressor gene (Mckenna et al. 2008).

Most recently, a case of AT/RT with a complex karyotype including one cell line showing monosomy 22 and another near-tetraploid one with additional chromosomal abnormalities has been reported. The karyotypic evolution observed in this tumor suggested that INI1 has an epigenetic role in the maintenance of genome integrity by affecting mitotic genes, which could induce chromosomal instability (Cocce et al. 2011). Finally, it is very well recognized that INI1 is the primary gene responsible for the development of rhabdoid tumors; however, additional molecular pathways underlying AT/RT development are poorly understood. Further research is necessary to better understand the pathogenesis of this tumor.

Interactions with Cancer-Related Proteins

Numerous direct interactions have been identified between INI1 and a variety of host proteins such as c-Myc (Cheng et al. 1999), MLL (Rozenblatt-Rosen et al. 1998), GADD34 (Wu et al. 2002) and GLI1 (Jagani et al. 2010), and these associations have been implicated in oncogenesis.

c-Myc

c-MYC is an oncogene that is frequently over-expressed in cancer. The c-Myc binds INI1 to cooperate in transactivation of E box-containing promoters, which suggests that c-Myc-INI1 interactions might specifically recruit the SWI/SNF complex to c-Myc regulated genes. The c-Myc basic helix-loop-helix (bHLH) and leucine zipper (Zip) domains and INI1 Rpt I region are required for this interaction.

Given that c-Myc expression is consistently elevated in INI1-deficient RT (McKenna et al. 2008), the aberrant activation of c-Myc programs either by c-Myc upregulation or by altered nucleosomal positioning at c-Myc target genes may have an important role in SWI/SNF-mutant cancers. The interaction between INI1 and c-Myc could facilitate the transcription of only a discrete subset of c-Myc target genes involved specifically in differentiation or apoptosis, which is consistent with the tumor suppressor activity of INI1.

Mixed Lineage Leukemia

Mixed lineage leukemia (MLL) is translocated and fused in-frame to over 60 partner proteins in aggressive paediatric leukemias, as well as in chemotherapy-induced secondary leukemias, both of which have a poor prognosis. Several lines of evidence indicate that the MLL fusion proteins function through the SWI/SNF complex. MLL binds directly to the INI1 subunit of SWI/SNF. This interaction occurs through the C-terminal SET domain of MLL and the Rpt II region of INI1. Several potential mechanisms exist by which the activity of SWI/SNF might be linked to the action of MLL fusion proteins in oncogenesis. This is noteworthy, since MLL possesses histone methyltransferase activity, directly interacts with INI1, and is recruited by INI1 to cooperatively regulate tumor suppressor loci, raising the possibility of a shared epigenetic mechanism between INI1-mutant and MLL-mutant cancers.

GADD34

Another cellular protein that interacts with INI1 is the growth arrest and DNA damage-inducible protein (GADD34), as its name indicates, the transcript of which is induced by growth arrest or DNA damage (Adler et al. 1999; Wu et al. 2002). GADD34 binds to INI1 through the Rpt II region (residues 305–318). On the other hand, GADD34 binds to protein phosphatase-1 (PP1) and can attenuate the translational elongation of key transcriptional factors through dephosphorylation of eukaryotic initiation factor 2α (eIF2α). The type I serine/threonine phosphatase, PP1, regulates diverse cellular processes such as cell cycle progression, protein synthesis, transcription, and neuronal signaling. The PP1 acquires specificity through its association with targeting regulatory subunits that direct the enzyme to specific cellular compartments and confer substrate specificity. In addition, PP1 is also regulated by inhibitory subunits that control enzyme activity. Wu et al. (2002) found that INI1 can bind independently to the PP1 catalytic subunit and weakly stimulate its phosphatase activity in solution and in complex with GADD34. INI1 and PP1 do not compete for binding to GADD34 but rather form a stable heterotrimeric complex with GADD34. These results implicate INI1 in the function of GADD34 and suggest that INI1 may regulate PP1 activity.

GLI1

In later investigations, Jagani et al. (2010) reported that the INI1 protein interacts specifically with the glioma-associated oncogene family zinc finger-1 (GLI1), a crucial effector of Hedgehog (Hh) signaling, and localized the interaction domain to the C terminus of GLI1 outside of the activation domain. They found that INI1 localizes to GLI1-regulated promoters and that loss of INI1 leads to activation of the Hh pathway, which regulates various aspects of early development and differentiation of central nervous system. In addition, the Hh-GLI1 pathway is critically involved in tumorigenesis, cancer growth and cancer stem cell self-renewal. The authors showed that INI1-deficient RT cells have hyperactivated GLI1 signaling, which has a role in their growth. They suggested a model whereby the SWI/SNF complex physically interacts with GLI1 to directly regulate activity of the Hh pathway via control of chromatin structure at GLI1 target promoters. They also suggested a mechanistic model whereby loss of INI1 drives cancer formation through simultaneous epigenetic perturbation of GLI1 and other key cancer-promoting pathways.

Future Molecular Therapies

Better understanding of the mechanisms by which mutation of INI1 drive oncogenesis has the potential to identify novel therapeutic approaches for rhabdoid tumors and related cancers. Several targets have been identified that may play a role in oncogenic transformation following INI1 loss. Cyclin D1 is expressed at high levels in rhabdoid tumors. Pharmacological inhibitors that reduce the transcription and stability of cyclin D1 have been shown to be effective in reducing the growth of RT cell lines in vitro and in vivo, and further suggest cyclin D1 as a potential therapeutic target for INI1-deficient RT. Loss of INI1 has also been shown to interfere with activation of interferon target genes and treatment with either interferon or inhibition of PLK1 may hold therapeutic promise. More recently, alterations of Hedgehog and Akt/mTOR pathways have been implicated in cancers that are caused by INI1 loss and provide other potential target for designing therapies to treat RT.

References

Abrams E, Neigeborn L, Carlson M (1986) Molecular analysis of SNF2 and SNF5, genes required for expression of glucose-repressible genes in Saccharomyces cerevisiae. Mol Cell Biol 6:3643–3651

Adler HT, Chinery R, Wu DY, Kussick SJ, Payne JM, Fornace AJ Jr, Tkachuk DC (1999) Leukemic HRX fusion proteins inhibit GADD34-induced apoptosis and associate with the GADD34 and hSNF5/INI1 proteins. Mol Cell Biol 19:7050–7060

Arcaro A, Doepfner KT, Boller D, Guerreiro AS, Shalaby T, Jackson SP, Schoenwaelder SM, Delattre O, Grotzer MA, Fischer B (2007) Novel role for insulin as an autocrine growth factor for malignant brain tumour cells. Biochem J 406:57–66

Biegel JA, Allen CS, Kawasaki K, Shimizu N, Budarf ML, Bell CJ (1996) Narrowing the critical region for a rhabdoid tumor locus in 22q11. Genes Chromosomes Cancer 16:94–105

Biegel JA, Tan L, Zhang F, Wainwright L, Russo P, Rorke LB (2002) Alterations of the hSNF5/INI1 gene in central nervous system atypical teratoid/rhabdoid tumors and renal and extrarenal rhabdoid tumors. Clin Cancer Res 8:3461–3467

Cheng SW, Davies KP, Yung E, Beltran RJ, Yu J, Kalpana GV (1999) c-MYC interacts with INI1/hSNF5 and requires the SWI/SNF complex for transactivation function. Nat Genet 22:102–105

Coccé MC, Lubieniecki F, Kordes U, Alderete D, Gallego MS (2011) A complex karyotype in an atypical teratoid/rhabdoid tumor: case report and review of the literature. J Neurooncol 104:375–380

Eaton KW, Tooke LS, Wainwright LM, Judkins AR, Biegel JA (2011) Spectrum of SMARCB1/INI1 mutations in familial and sporadic rhabdoid tumors. Pediatr Blood Cancer 56:7–15

Guidi CJ, Sands AT, Zambrowicz BP, Turner TK, Demers DA, Webster W, Smith TW, Imbalzano AN, Jones SN (2001) Disruption of INI1 leads to peri-implantation lethality and tumorigenesis in mice. Mol Cell Biol 21:3598–3603

Guidi CJ, Veal TM, Jones SN, Imbalzano AN (2004) Transcriptional compensation for loss of an allele of the INI1 tumor suppressor. J Biol Chem 279:4180–4185

Hasselblatt M, Gesk S, Oyen F, Rossi S, Viscardi E, Giangaspero F, Giannini C, Judkins AR, Frühwald MC, Obser T, Schneppenheim R, Siebert R, Paulus W (2011) Nonsense mutation and inactivation of SMARCA4 (BRG1) in an atypical teratoid/rhabdoid tumor showing retained SMARCB1 (INI1) expression. Am J Surg Pathol 35:933–935

Isakoff MS, Sansam CG, Tamayo P, Subramanian A, Evans JA, Fillmore CM, Wang X, Biegel JA, Pomeroy SL, Mesirov JP, Roberts CW (2005) Inactivation of the Snf5 tumor suppressor stimulates cell cycle progression and cooperates with p53 loss in oncogenic transformation. Proc Natl Acad Sci U S A 102:17745–17750

Jackson EM, Shaikh TH, Gururangan S, Jones MC, Malkin D, Nikkel SM, Zuppan CW, Wainwright LM, Zhang F, Biegel JA (2007) High-density single nucleotide polymorphism array analysis in patients with germline deletions of 22q11.2 and malignant rhabdoid tumor. Hum Genet 122:117–127

Jackson EM, Sievert AJ, Gai X, Hakonarson H, Judkins AR, Tooke L, Perin JC, Xie H, Shaikh TH, Biegel JA (2009) Genomic analysis using high-density single nucleotide polymorphism-based oligonucleotide arrays and multiplex ligation-dependent probe amplification provides a comprehensive analysis of INI1/SMARCB1 in malignant rhabdoid tumors. Clin Cancer Res 15:1923–1930

Jagani Z, Mora-Blanco EL, Sansam CG, McKenna ES, Wilson B, Chen D, Klekota J, Tamayo P, Nguyen PT, Tolstorukov M, Park PJ, Cho YJ, Hsiao K, Buonamici S, Pomeroy SL, Mesirov JP, Ruffner H, Bouwmeester T, Luchansky SJ, Murtie J, Kelleher JF, Warmuth M, Sellers WR, Roberts CW, Dorsch M (2010) Loss of the tumor suppressor Snf5 leads to aberrant activation of the Hedgehog-Gli pathway. Nat Med 16:1429–1433

Janson K, Nedzi LA, David O, Schorin M, Walsh JW, Bhattacharjee M, Pridjian G, Tan L, Judkins AR, Biegel JA (2006) Predisposition to atypical teratoid/rhabdoid tumor due to an inherited INI1 mutation. Pediatr Blood Cancer 47:279–284

Józwiak J, Bikowska B, Grajkowska W, Sontowska I, Roszkowski M, Galus R (2010) Activation of Akt/mTOR pathway in a patient with atypical teratoid/rhabdoid tumor. Folia Neuropathol 48:185–189

Kalpana GV, Marmon S, Wang W, Crabtree GR, Goff SP (1994) Binding and stimulation of HIV-1 integrase by a human homolog of yeast transcription factor SNF5. Science 266:2002–2006

Klochendler-Yeivin A, Fiette L, Barra J, Muchardt C, Babinet C, Yaniv M (2000) The murine SNF5/INI1 chromatin remodeling factor is essential for embryonic development and tumor suppression. EMBO Rep 1:500–506

Klochendler-Yeivin A, Picarsky E, Yaniv M (2006) Increased DNA damage sensitivity and apoptosis in cells lacking the Snf5/INI1 subunit of the SWI/SNF chromatin remodeling complex. Mol Cell Biol 26:2661–2674

Laurent BC, Treitel MA, Carlson M (1990) The SNF5 protein of Saccharomyces cerevisiae is a glutamine- and proline-rich transcriptional activator that affects expression of a broad spectrum of genes. Mol Cell Biol 10:5616–5625

McKenna ES, Sansam CG, Cho YJ, Greulich H, Evans JA, Thom CS, Moreau LA, Biegel JA, Pomeroy SL, Roberts CW (2008) Loss of the epigenetic tumor suppressor SNF5 leads to cancer without genomic instability. Mol Cell Biol 28:6223–6233

Morozov A, Lee SJ, Zhang ZK, Cimica V, Zagzag D, Kalpana GV (2007) INI1 induces interferon signaling and spindle checkpoint in rhabdoid tumors. Clin Cancer Res 13:4721–4730

Muchardt C, Sardet C, Bourachot B, Onufryk C, Yaniv M (1995) A human protein with homology to Saccharomyces cerevisiae SNF5 interacts with the potential helicase hbrm. Nucleic Acids Res 23:1127–1132

Rickert CH, Paulus W (2001) Epidemiology of central nervous system tumors in childhood and adolescence based on the new WHO classification. Childs Nerv Syst 17:503–511

Roberts CW, Galusha SA, McMenamin ME, Fletcher CD, Orkin SH (2000) Haploinsufficiency of Snf5 (integrase interactor 1) predisposes to malignant rhabdoid tumors in mice. Proc Natl Acad Sci U S A 97:13796–13800

Roberts CW, Leroux MM, Fleming MD, Orkin SH (2002) Highly penetrant, rapid tumorigenesis through conditional inversion of the tumor suppressor gene Snf5. Cancer Cell 2:415–425

Rozenblatt-Rosen O, Rozovskaia T, Burakov D, Sedkov Y, Tillib S, Blechman J, Nakamura T, Croce CM, Mazo A, Canaani E (1998) The C-terminal SET domains of ALL-1 and TRITHORAX interact with the INI1 and SNR1 proteins, components of the SWI/SNF complex. Proc Natl Acad Sci U S A 95:4152–4157

Venneti S, Le P, Martinez D, Eaton KW, Shyam N, Jordan-Sciutto KL, Pawel B, Biegel JA, Judkins AR (2011) p16INK4A and p14ARF tumor suppressor pathways are deregulated in malignant rhabdoid tumors. J Neuropathol Exp Neurol 70:596–609

Versteege I, Sévenet N, Lange J, Rousseau-Merck MF, Ambros P, Handgretinger R, Aurias A, Delattre O (1998) Truncating mutations of hSNF5/INI1 in aggressive paediatric cancer. Nature 394:203–206

Vries RG, Bezrookove V, Zuijderduijn LM, Kia SK, Houweling A, Oruetxebarria I, Raap AK, Verrijzer CP (2005) Cancer-associated mutations in chromatin remodeler hSNF5 promote chromosomal instability by compromising the mitotic checkpoint. Genes Dev 19:665–670

Wang W, Côté J, Xue Y, Zhou S, Khavari PA, Biggar SR, Muchardt C, Kalpana GV, Goff SP, Yaniv M, Workman JL, Crabtree GR (1996) Purification and biochemical heterogeneity of the mammalian SWI-SNF complex. EMBO J 15:5370–5382

Wang M, Gu C, Qi T, Tang W, Wang L, Wang S, Zeng X (2007) BAF53 interacts with p53 and functions in p53-mediated p21-gene transcription. J Biochem 142:613–620

Wu DY, Tkachuck DC, Roberson RS, Schubach WH (2002) The human SNF5/INI1 protein facilitates the function of the growth arrest and DNA damage-inducible protein (GADD34) and modulates GADD34-bound protein phosphatase-1 activity. J Biol Chem 277:27706–27715

Zhang ZK, Davies KP, Allen J, Zhu L, Pestell RG, Zagzag D, Kalpana GV (2002) Cell cycle arrest and repression of cyclin D1 transcription by INI1/hSNF5. Mol Cell Biol 22:5975–5988

Atypical Teratoid/Rhabdoid Tumors: Diagnosis Using Imaging

5

Atilla Arslanoglu

Contents

A. Arslanoglu, M.D. (✉)
Department of Radiology, Beytepe Military Hospital, Ankara, Turkey
e-mail: atilla02002@yahoo.com

Abstract

Atypical teratoid/rhabdoid tumor (AT/RT) is uncommon malignant intracranial tumor usually during the first 2 years of life with a male predominance. The tumor can arise at any location in the CNS but the posterior fossa is the most common site. The real incidence of the tumor is unknown since these tumors have been misdiagnosed in the past as primitive neuroectodermal tumor/medulloblastoma (PNET/MB) because of overlapping histologic and imaging features. AT/RT can be distinguished from PNET/MB and other childhood tumors by using immunohistochemical markers like EMA, vimentin, actin, hSNF5/INI1 and mutation analysis. Diagnosis of AT/RT is important because these tumors typically have a poor prognosis and need new aggressive therapies.

Detection and diagnosis using imaging is helpful for the extension of the tumor and metastases before immunohistochemistrical and molecular genetics studies. Although the imaging features of the tumor is not specific, awareness of AT/RT is important in making the correct diagnosis of this uncommon but probably underdiagnosed entity. Bulky, heterogeneous masses with calcifications, eccentric cysts, off-midline location in the posterior fossa, presence of disseminated leptomeningeal tumor, restricted diffusion, and eleveted Cholin and decreased N-acetytl aspartat in children younger than 2 years of age should alert the radiologist to the possibility of AT/RT in the differential diagnosis of the mass.

M.A. Hayat (ed.), *Pediatric Cancer, Volume 3: Diagnosis, Therapy, and Prognosis*, Pediatric Cancer 3,
DOI 10.1007/978-94-007-4528-5_5,

Introduction

Atypical teratoid/rhabdoid tumor (AT/RT) is uncommon and aggressive tumor of young children. It occurs mostly during the first 2 years of life with a male predominance. AT/RT is included, in the World Health Organization (WHO) classification of the central nervous system (CNS) in 2000. The tumor has been recognized in early 1980s as a rhabdoid tumor of the CNS (Rorke et al. 1996). Tumors can arise at any location in the CNS but the posterior fossa is the most common site. The real incidence is difficult to determine and it is probably underestimated in children under age 2. In a new study published in August 2010 from Austria, AT/RT is reported being the sixth most common entity (6.1%), and peak incidence was found in the birth to 2 years age group, where they were as common as CNS primitive neuroectodermal tumor/medulloblastoma (PNET/MB). A total of 47.4% of AT/RTs were initially diagnosed, whereas 52.6% were retrospectively detected by the central review (Woehrer et al. 2010). In another study from Taiwan, the ratio of AT/RT to PNET was found to be 1:3.8 among patients younger than 3 years of age and 1:11 for all age groups (Ho et al. 2000). The diagnoses of AT/RT is difficult and is frequently missed due to its similar histologic properties to PNET/MB. The diagnosis of AT/RT is made by light microscopy and immunohistochemistrical findings and can be further analyzed using molecular genetics.

The cell origin of AT/RT is unknown and the tumor composed of rhabdoid cells, undifferentiated cells, malignant mesenchymal, and epithelial tissue. Rhabdoid cells are considered characteristic feature of this tumor and be a unfavor on prognosis (Rorke et al. 1996; Biegel et al. 2002; Burger et al. 1998; Judkins et al. 2004; Parwani et al. 2005; Strother 2005). Rhabdoid cells are plump with eccentric nuclei containing prominent nucleoli within eosinophilic cytoplasm. In rhabdoid cells mitotic activity and necrosis are common and MIB-1 index (proliferating cells) is higher than that of PNET (Ho et al. 2000; Rorke et al. 1996). Besides the rhabdoid tumor cells, AT/RT contains PNET cells, malignant mesenchymal cells, and cells with epithelial differentiation. These diverse elements accounts for naming AT/RT. As much as 70% of the tumor may be made up of PNET-like cells. AT/RTs have no germ cell and tissue differentiation associated with teratomas (Rorke et al. 1996; Biegel et al. 2002; Burger et al. 1998).

Monozomy 22 or deletions of chromosome band 22q11 with alterations of the INI1/hSNF5 gene was demonstrated in AT/RT patients (Biegel et al. 2002; Burger et al. 1998; Dang et al. 2003; Kordes et al. 2010; Packer et al. 2002). INI1/hSNF5, a component of the chromatin remodeling SWI/SNF complex, is a critical tumor suppressor inactivated in rhabdoid tumors. Identification of INI1 as a tumor suppressor has facilitated accurate diagnosis of rhabdoid tumors. This mutation is not present in 100% of AT/RT cases. If the mutation is not present immunohistochemical and morphologic pattern helps for diagnosis of AT/RT. INI1 mutation is important to the diagnosis of ATRT, to the extent that tumors carrying the INI1 mutation and with histological features suggestive of PNET (without a rhabdoid component) are classified as AT/RT (Biegel et al. 2002; Packer et al. 2002).

The immunohistochemical properties of AT/RT are positive epithelial membrane antigen (EMA), vimentin, and smooth-muscle antigen, and negative markers for germ cell tumors (alpha-protein and plesental alkaline protease). Glial fibrillary acidic protein, keratin and neurofilament protein might be positive in AT/RT patients (Biegel et al. 2002; Burger et al. 1998; Judkins et al. 2004; Rorke et al. 1996). Separation of AT/RT from PNET and other pediatric brain tumors is important preoperatively since the former has an unfavorable prognosis and identification of this entity may determine treatment options (Biegel et al. 2002; Dang et al. 2003; Rorke et al. 1996; Strother 2005). The prognosis of patients with AT/RT is poor and mean survival time is in the range of 6–15 months. Diagnosis using imaging is helpful for detection of the tumour and metastases before immunohistochemistrical and molecular genetics studies.

Diagnosis Using Imaging and Discussion

Imaging features of AT/RT have been described in many studies before (Arslanoglu et al. 2004; Bing et al. 2009; Burger et al. 1998; Dang et al. 2003; Evans et al. 2001; Gauvain et al. 2001; Koral et al. 2008; Meyers et al. 2006; Moeller et al. 2007; Niwa et al. 2009; Panigrahy et al. 2010; Parmar et al. 2006; Rorke et al. 1996; Rumboldt et al. 2006; Warmuth-Metz et al. 2008). In larger series, the clinical and histopathological features of AT/RT have been defined with some reference to imaging findings. In 36 out of 53 patients in the study of Burger et al. (1998) and 29 out of 52 patients in the study of Rorke et al. (1996) the tumor was located in the posterior fossa. The rest of the tumors were supratentorial. In a case series of AT/RT by Dang et al. (2003) 52% of the tumors were in cerebellum; 39% were supratentorial, 5% pineal, 2% spinal, and 2%. An unusual case of giant lumbal paraspinal with intraspinal extension and clival-C2 AT/RT are reported recently (Agrawal et al. 2009; Heuer et al. 2010). Multifocal tumors at presentation were described, underscoring the propensity of AT/RT to metastasize via CSF seeding. There has not been an attempt made in the histopathological studies to assign these tumors into specific subsites in the posterior fossa but it appears that AT/RT has a tendency to occur off-midline (Fig. 5.1). This may be helpful in differentiating AT/RT from PNET/MB, which more commonly arises at midline, although the location of both entities is variable and may be difficult to clearly identify due to their large size. Ependymomas and pilocytic astrocytomas (PA) frequently extend to the cerebellopontin angle (CPA) but they are more commonly seen in older children. The location of AT/RT in the supratentorial brain is variable as is PNET's.

All four tumors in our study had readily visible calcifications on CT (Fig. 5.2a) (Arslanoglu et al. 2004). Parmar et al. (2006) found calcification in 36% of their patients. Approximately 15% of PNETs in the posterior fossa contain calcification on histological exam but visible calcification is very rare even on CT studies. Ependymomas, not infrequently, show calcification and are heterogeneous on imaging studies but do not contain large cysts. In the supratentorial compartment, PNETs have visible calcifications on CT in half of the cases.

Eccentrically located cysts between the solid tumor and adjacent brain were presented in our study (Figs. 5.1a and 5.2a) (Arslanoglu et al. 2004). Tumor substance colliquation and CSF entrapment cause the cyst formation speculated and despite the frequent presence of cysts associated with AT/RT has been reported, no specific reference has been made to the location of these cysts relative to the usually bulky mass (Packer et al. 2002; Parmar et al. 2006; Warmuth-Metz et al. 2008). Warmuth-Metz et al. (2008) reported although not as frequent as reported by us, this feature seems to be a regular finding in ATRTs, and they found peripheral cysts twice as frequently as Parmar et al. (2006). This may be an important differentiating point between PNET and AT/RT, since PNETs are usually more uniform tumors, although in about 10% of cases marked heterogeneity and cyst formation can be seen. Pilocytic astrocytomas typically have eccentric cysts but they are not infiltrative in appearance, and more commonly occur in older children. Supratentorial PNET, PA and desmoplastic infantile ganglioglioma (DIG), not infrequently, have cystic components making this finding ineffective in the supratentorial compartment.

Skull invasion was identified on both CT and MRI in one of the hemispheric AT/RTs in our study, which reflects the very aggressive nature of these tumors (Fig. 5.3c, d) (Arslanoglu et al. 2004). A similar occurrence has been reported in association with AT/RT and PNET (Evans et al. 2001). One frontal tumor had destroyed the skull and extended into the galea, this feature reported by Warmuth Metz et al. (2008). Skull invasion is not seen with DIG or PA.

Mild vasogenic edema has been described in association with PNET. No significant edema was observed in any of the our patients when transependymal CSF leak due to hydrocephalus is excluded (Fig. 5.3a) (Arslanoglu et al. 2004). Leptomeningeal spread, although not present in

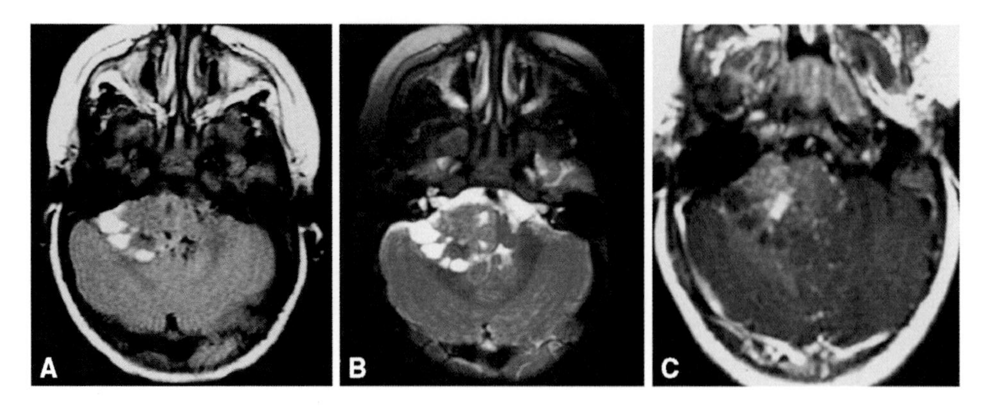

Fig. 5.1 AT/RT in the posterior fossa, off-midline location. (**a**) FLAIR (Fluid attenuation inversion recovery) and (**b**) FSE (fast spin echo) T2 shows a right cerebellopontin angle extra-axial mass with solid and peripheral cystic components. (**c**) Post contrast T1 image demonstrates a mild enhancement with a small relatively more enhancing nodule

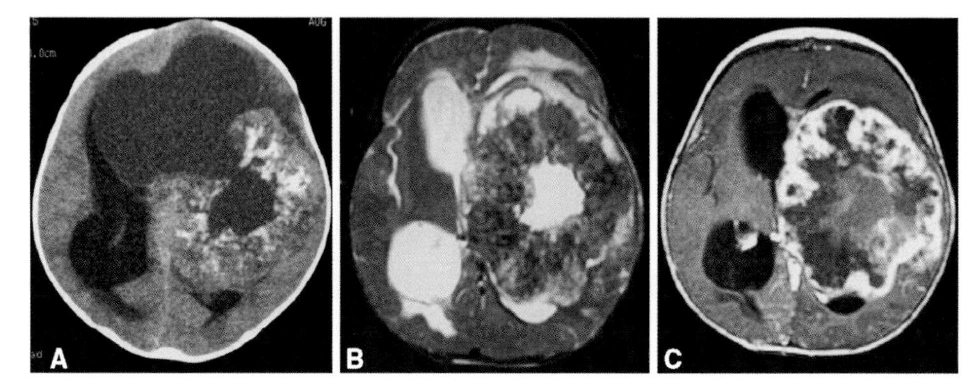

Fig. 5.2 Supratentorial AT/RT with cyst, calcification and a wavy band-like enhancement. (**a**) Non-contrast CT displays a large doughnut shaped mass with central cyst, that opens into an eccentric large cystic component and calcifications. (**b**) FSE T2 demonstrates a large thick walled mass with mild surrounding edema. (**c**) Post contrast T1 axial image reveals typical pattern of a wavy band-like enhancing zone surrounding central necrosis

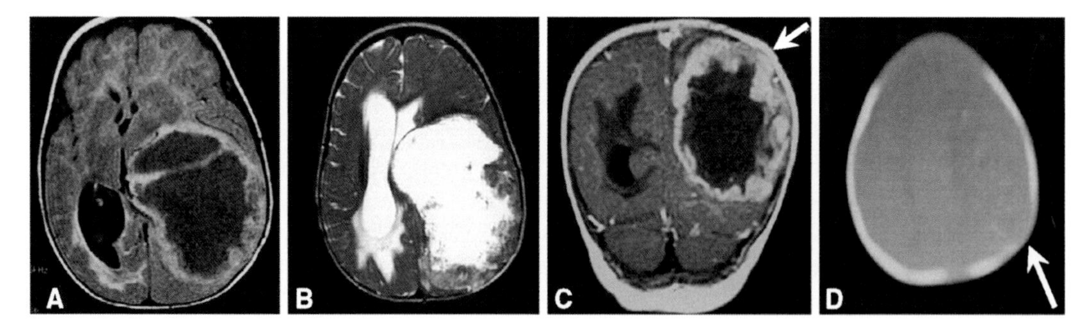

Fig. 5.3 Supratentorial AT/RT with skull invasion. (**a**) FLAIR axial shows a very large cyst mass with thick nodular walls and mass effect but little edema. (**b**) FSE T2 through the same level demonstrates a necrotic mass with thick heterogeneous wall causing midline shift. (**c**) Coronal post contrast image shows a wavy band-like enhancing of tumor. There is remodelling of the calvarium (*arrow*). (**d**) CT bone windows shows erosion of the left parietal bone (*arrow*)

any of our patients, can be seen at presentation. Cerebrospinal fluid involvement via leptomeningeal dissemination is the commonest mode of spread and can be found in greater than 30% patients at initial assessment. Data from Children's Cancer Group and AT/RT registry stated the incidence around 15% (Packer et al. 2002). Disseminated tumor in the leptomeninges and spine is seen with MR imaging (Burger et al. 1998; Packer et al. 2002; Parmar et al. 2006; Rorke et al. 1996).

Since tumor has high cellularity appear hyperdense on CT (Arslanoglu et al. 2004; Koral et al. 2008; Meyers et al. 2006; Moeller et al. 2007; Parmar et al. 2006; Warmuth-Metz et al. 2008). CT attenuation and signal intensity characteristics are similar to PNET/MB. Necrosis, hemorrhage, and calcifications are common. Warmuth-Metz et al. (2008) reported CT density values in the solid parts of the tumors were hyperdense, probably representing a high cellular density. Solid portions of tumor have intermediate-high signal intensity on FLAIR and T2 weighted images. The MR imaging findings are similar to those reported for PNET and are likely related to overlapping histologic features of these hypercellular tumors. Imaging features are often variable secondary to cystic/necrotic changes and hemorrhage. Signal intensity values on T1 and T2-weighted MR images varied widely, and obvious signs of mainly disseminated bleeding were found in a large proportion of tumors (Warmuth-Metz et al. 2008). Spinal imaging findings consistent with the diagnosis include heterogeneity, isointensity/hypointensity to cord on T2-weighted images. AT/RT in the spine is rare but can be considered in the differential diagnosis of spinal canal tumors in children. The tumor can occur anywhere along the spinal axis and may be intramedullary or intradural extramedullary in origin (Moeller et al. 2007).

A variable degree of enhancement was present in all of our cases (Arslanoglu et al. 2004), but this is not a helpful finding in differential diagnosis since most of the other tumors also show enhancement. Warmuth-Metz et al. (2008) reported a considerable number (16%) of tumors did not enhance while most tumors showed enhancement of medium to strong intensity. They found a pattern of enhancement in 38% of their patients that seems to a band-like wavy rim of strong and quite uniform enhancement surrounding a central cystic/necrotic area. Similar enhancement pattern published in several reports on AT/RT including ours (Figs. 5.2c and 5.3c). (Arslanoglu et al. 2004; Bing et al. 2009; Meyers et al. 2006). However, this pattern does not seem to be specific, but at least if it is present it could help in the differential diagnosis.

Published data characterizing diffusion weighted imaging (DWI) in pediatric brain tumors are limited. Meyers et al. (2006) demonstrated that AT/RT present hyperintense signal intensity on DWI, with hypointense signal intensity on apparent diffusion coefficient (ADC) images, indicating restricted diffusion because of the high cellular density of the tumor. Cervical high signal on DWI and low ADC may represent the high cellularity of tumor also reported by Niwa et al. (2009) and Kodama et al. (2007). Gauvain et al. (2001) and Rumboldt et al. (2006) found the same results on DWI. Gauvain et al. (2001) found that PNET/MB and AT/RT have ADC values of $0.72 \pm 0.20 \times 10^{-3}$ mm^2/s (range, $0.538–0.974 \times 10^{-3}$ mm^2/s) and a ratio to normal brain of 1.03 ± 0.26 (range, 0.7–1.26). They suggested ADC values were inversely correlated with tumor cellularity; the apparent diffusion of water was slower in tumors with higher cellularity. In their study, the ADC correlated significantly with both the tumor cellularity and the calculated total nuclear area. In diffusion tensor imaging the anisotropy values were decreased to near zero in all tumors and were not analyzed further (Gauvain et al. 2001). Rumboldt et al. (2006) stated when ADCs between tumor types were compared for creation of cutoffs, a value of greater than 1.40×10^{-3} mm^2/s was 100% specific for JPA, whereas measurements less than 0.90×10^{-3} mm^2/s were 100% specific for medulloblastoma and AT/RT. ADC values of most of ependymomas were between 1.00 and 1.30×10^{-3} mm^2/s. Thus, they suggest that ADC values may play an important role in the presurgical management and proposed that if high ADC values are present, a patient may go directly to surgery without additional imaging, given that pilocytic astrocytomas are unlikely to metastasize. Low ADC values on the other hand suggest that the tumor is either a MB or a AT/RT, and imaging of the spine is necessary to exclude metastases (Rumboldt et al. 2006).

Magnetic Resonance Spectroscopy (MRS) showed elevated levels of choline and decreased N-acetyl aspartate as PNET in the patients with AT/RT (Meyers et al. 2006). Bing et al. (2009) found elevated levels of choline and lipids (indicating aggressive lesion) and decreased N-acetyl aspartate. Taurine has been observed in medulloblastoma (Panigrahy et al. 2010) and reported as an important differentiator of medulloblastoma from other tumors of the posterior fossa including AT/RT. Medulloblastoma also have higher levels of choline than other posterior fossa tumors. A new preliminary data from the research of Panigrahy et al. (2010) indicate that prominent choline and taurine present in medulloblastoma. AT/RTs, on the other hand, appear to have a different metabolic pattern with more moderate choline levels in some cases. Also, there was no evidence for taurine in five cases of AT/RT in their study. The hallmark of pilocytic astrocytomas are very low creatine concentrations, low myo-inositol, and low tCho concentrations consistent with their low cellularity. Ependymomas have higher myo-inositol than medulloblastoma or pilocytic astrocytoma and their choline levels are variable but fall generally between medulloblastoma and pilocytic astrocytoma (Panigrahy et al. 2010).

Bing et al. (2009) reported a metabolic study using DWI, perfusion MRI, and proton MR spectroscopy contributed to a better preoperative diagnosis of a pediatric intracranial tumor. They reported that, in the presence of an aggressive intracranial tumor, a diagnosis of AT/RT must always be evoked in children less than 2 years old, even if the localization is unusual.

The sonographic finding of AT/RT like other brain tumors is a mass that affects adjacent structures and causes hydrocephalus. Although ultrasound findings correlate with CT findings, the sonographic findings of brain tumors are not specific. The distinction between echogenic solid tumors and other intracranial masses may be difficult. Ultrasound is widely used as a screening test in infants with abnormal neurologic examination. When a mass is suspected on ultrasound, further investigation with CT is necessary (Han et al. 1984).

Pozitron Emission Tomography, is a supplementary investigation with radioactive exposure and long scan times, it should be restricted to children with AT/RT and other brain tumors where therapy planning is not possible from CT and MRI (Galldiks et al. 2010).

Differential Diagnosis

Primitive neuroectodermal tumor, commonly medulloblastoma, is the main differential diagnostic entity due to indistinguishable gross, radiologic, and histologic features (Burger et al. 1998; Dang et al. 2003; Koral et al. 2008; Parmar et al. 2006; Rorke et al. 1996). Distinguishing these two tumors is of clinical significance. Patients with AT/RT are younger and present a worse prognosis than those with PNET/MB (Ho et al. 2000; Parmar et al. 2006; Rorke et al. 1996). These tumors can present the same CT and MRI findings. It does not seem possible to differentiate AT/RT from PNET/MB with DWI, perfusion MRI, or MR spectroscopy. The hyperintensity in diffusion-weighted imaging is explained by the hypercellularity of both tumors. Perfusion MRI data in the literature concerning PNET/MB are rare. The MR spectroscopy of PNET may be the same as for AT/RT, revealing aggressive signs with a high peak of choline with decreased creatine and a peak of lipid. The histopathologic differential diagnosis of an AT/RT also focuses on PNET/MB and may be difficult. Since 70% of AT/RT contain histologic fields similar to PNET/MB, which can cause confusion in diagnosis. Moreover, PNET without rhabdoid cells and with a loss of INI1 expression, may mimic AT/RT. The age of the patient, at less than 3 years old, rather than MRI features, favored the diagnosis of AT/RT. Other radiologic differentials include ependymoma, teratoma, choroid plexus tumors, pilocytic astrocytoma, desmoplastic infantile ganglioglioma, and meningioma (Biegel et al. 2002; Burger et al. 1998; Dang et al. 2003; Koral et al. 2008; Meyers et al. 2006; Moeller et al. 2007; Parmar et al. 2006; Rorke et al. 1996).

Treatment and Prognosis

There are different types of treatment options for the patients with AT/RT including surgery, chemotherapy, and radiation. But none of them provide total cure because of highly aggressive nature of the tumor. Although total resection of the tumor is not possible, it is necessary for obtaining tissue to make correct diagnosis. Resection alone is not curative and location of the tumor frequently makes surgical resection difficult. As stated previously disseminated disease at the time of diagnosis is common. There is no standard chemotherapeutic treatment protocols for AT/RT. Patients demonstrated poor survival when treated with standard chemotherapeutic regimens alone. The radiation also has been limited in children younger than three because of the hazards of the radiation to the brain. Thus most patients have been treated with intensive multimodal therapy. A survival of more than 6 years has been reported with a trimodality approach of surgical resection, triple intrathecal chemotherapy, and gamma knife radiosurgery by Hirth et al. (2003). Aggressive therapy can prolong survival in a subset of children with AT/RT reported by Hilden et al. (2004) and Tekautz et al. (2005) respectively. The protocol of the Chi et al. (2009) was the first prospective report with surgery, multiagent systemic and IT chemotherapy, and radiotherapy demonstrating significant progress in survival rates. Morgenstern et al. (2010) conducted a retrospective review of all patients diagnosed with AT/RT at Great Ormond Street Hospital from 1989 to 2009 reporting overall survival was 17.4%, with median survival 10.1 months and outcome in their patients aged <3 years was significantly worse (median survival 6.2 months vs. 19.2 months). They stated there was a clear need for new treatment strategies and the identification of novel molecular targets for AT/RT. Squire et al. (2007) suggested from a computerized bibliographic search conducted using PUBMED that rarity of this disease that no single institution has sufficient experience in treating AT/RT and enrolling a patient on protocol would at least provide the child the combined experiences of multiple institutions to treat well patients with AT/RT in the near future.

The overall outcome for children diagnosed with AT/RT is very poor (Burger et al. 1998; Judkins et al. 2004; Rorke et al. 1996; Biswas et al. 2009). The mean survival in our four patients was only 5 months (Arslanoglu et al. 2004). In their series of 53 patients, Burger et al. (1998) reported a mean survival of 11 months. The presence of disseminated leptomeningeal tumor at diagnosis has been associated with a poor prognosis in patients with AT/RT is reported (Burger et al. 1998; Rorke et al. 1996; Meyers et al. 2006). Meyers et al. (2006) reported disseminated tumor in the leptomeninges was seen with MR imaging in 24% of their patients at diagnosis and occurred in another 35% from 4 months to 2.8 years (mean, 1 year) after surgery and earlier. Spinal AT/RT has also worse prognosis than spinal PNET is reported by Kodama et al. (2007). Treatment data, mostly retrospective studies, for the outcome of AT/RT are limited. According to these data, maximal safe resection should be accomplished. Standard and intensified chemotherapy protocols are curative in a small number of patients. The early radiation therapy was a chance of therapy for the majority of patients who have survived despite of the hazards of the radiation to brain. High-dose chemotherapy protocols (marrow or peripheral blood stem cell rescue) may also be associated with higher chances of cure.

In conclusion, Although the imaging features of the tumor is not specific, awareness of AT/RT is important in making the correct diagnosis of this uncommon but probably underdiagnosed entity. Bulky, heterogeneous masses with calcifications, eccentric cysts, off-midline location in the posterior fossa, presence of disseminated leptomeningeal tumor, restricted diffusion, and moderately eleveted Cholin and decreased N-acetyl aspartate in children younger than 2 years of age should alert the radiologist to the possibility of AT/RT in the differential diagnosis of the mass.

References

Agrawal A, Bhake A, Cincu R (2009) Giant lumbar paraspinal atypical teratoid/rhabdoid tumor in a child. J Cancer Res Ther 5:318–320

Arslanoglu A, Aygun N, Tekhtani D, Aronson L, Cohen K, Burger PC, Yousem DM (2004) Imaging findings of CNS atypical teratoid/rhabdoid tumors. AJNR Am J Neuroradiol 2:476–480

Biegel JA, Tan L, Zhang F, Wainwright L, Russo P, Rorke LB (2002) Alterations of the hSNF5/INI1 gene in central nervous system atypical teratoid/rhabdoid tumors and renal and extrarenal rhabdoid tumors. Clin Cancer Res 8:3461–3467

Bing F, Nugues F, Grand S, Bessou P, Salon C (2009) Primary intracranial extra-axial and supratentorial atypical rhabdoid tumor. Pediatr Neurol 41:453–456

Biswas A, Goyal S, Puri T, Das P, Sarkar C, Julka PK, Bakhshi S, Rath GK (2009) Atypical teratoid rhabdoid tumor of the brain: case series and review of literature. Childs Nerv Syst 25:1495–1500

Burger PC, Yu IT, Tihan T, Friedman HS, Strother DR, Kepner JL, Duffner PK, Kun LE, Perlman EJ (1998) Atypical teratoid/rhabdoid tumor of the central nervous system: a highly malignant tumor of infancy and childhood frequently mistaken for medulloblastoma: a Pediatric Oncology Group study. Am J Surg Pathol 22:1083–1092

Chi SN, Zimmerman MA, Yao X, Cohen KJ, Burger P, Biegel JA, Rorke-Adams LB, Fisher MJ, Janss A, Mazewski C, Goldman S, Manley PE, Bowers DC, Bendel A, Rubin J, Turner CD, Marcus KJ, Goumnerova L, Ullrich NJ, Kieran MW (2009) Intensive multimodality treatment for children with newly diagnosed CNS atypical teratoid rhabdoid tumor. J Clin Oncol 27:385–389

Dang T, Vassilyadi M, Michaud J, Jimenez C, Ventureyra EC (2003) Atypical teratoid/rhabdoid tumors. Childs Nerv Syst 19:244–248

Evans A, Ganatra R, Morris SJ (2001) Imaging features of primary malignant rhabdoid tumour of the brain. Pediatr Radiol 31:631–633

Galldiks N, Kracht LW, Berthold F, Miletic H, Klein JC, Herholz K, Jacobs AH, Heiss WD (2010) [11C]-L-methionine positron emission tomography in the management of children and young adults with brain tumors. J Neurooncol 96:231–239

Gauvain KM, McKinstry RC, Mukherjee P, Perry A, Neil JJ, Kaufman BA, Hayashi RJ (2001) Evaluating pediatric brain tumor cellularity with diffusion-tensor imaging. AJR Am J Roentgenol 177:449–454

Han BK, Babcock DS, Oestreich AE (1984) Sonography of brain tumors in infants. AJR Am J Roentgenol 143:31–36

Heuer GG, Kiefer H, Judkins AR, Belasco J, Biegel JA, Jackson EM, Cohen M, O'Malley BW Jr, Storm PB (2010) Surgical treatment of a clival-C2 atypical teratoid/rhabdoid tumor. J Neurosurg Pediatr 5:75–79

Hilden JM, Meerbaum S, Burger P, Finlay J, Janss A, Scheithauer BW, Walter AW, Rorke LB, Biegel JA (2004) Central nervous system atypical teratoid/rhabdoid tumour: results of therapy in children enrolled in a registry. J Clin Oncol 22:2877–2884

Hirth A, Pedersen PH, Wester K, Mörk S, Helgestad J (2003) Cerebral atypical teratoid/rhabdoid tumor of infancy: long-term survival after multimodal treatment, also including triple intrathecal chemotherapy and gamma knife radiosurgery–case report. Pediatr Hematol Oncol 20:327–332

Ho DM, Hsu CY, Wong TT, Ting LT, Chiang H (2000) Atypical teratoid/rhabdoid tumor of the central nervous system: a comparative study with primitive neuroectodermal tumor/medulloblastoma. Acta Neuropathol 99:482–488

Judkins AR, Mauger J, Ht A, Rorke LB, Biegel JA (2004) Immunohistochemical analysis of hSNF5/INI1 in pediatric CNS neoplasms. Am J Surg Pathol 28: 644–650

Kodama H, Maeda M, Imai H, Matsubara T, Taki W, Takeda K (2007) MRI of primary spinal atypical teratoid/rhabdoid tumor: a case report and literature review. J Neurooncol 84:213–216

Koral K, Gargan L, Bowers DC, Gimi B, Timmons CF, Weprin B, Rollins NK (2008) Imaging characteristics of atypical teratoid-rhabdoid tumor in children compared with medulloblastoma. AJR Am J Roentgenol 190:809–814

Kordes U, Gesk S, Frühwald MC, Graf N, Leuschner I, Hasselblatt M, Jeibmann A, Oyen F, Peters O, Pietsch T, Siebert R, Schneppenheim R (2010) Clinical and molecular features in patients with atypical teratoid rhabdoid tumor or malignant rhabdoid tumor. Genes Chromosomes Cancer 49:176–181

Meyers SP, Khademian ZP, Biegel JA, Chuang SH, Korones DN, Zimmerman RA (2006) Primary intracranial atypical teratoid/rhabdoid tumors of infancy and childhood: MRI features and patient outcomes. AJNR Am J Neuroradiol 27:962–971

Moeller KK, Coventry S, Jernigan S, Moriarty TM (2007) Atypical teratoid/rhabdoid tumor of the spine. AJNR Am J Neuroradiol 28:593–595

Morgenstern DA, Gibson S, Brown T, Sebire NJ, Anderson J (2010) Clinical and pathological features of paediatric malignant rhabdoid tumours. Pediatr Blood Cancer 54:29–34

Niwa T, Aida N, Tanaka M, Okubo J, Sasano M, Shishikura A, Fujita K, Ito S, Tanaka Y, Kigasawa H (2009) Diffusion-weighted imaging of an atypical teratoid/rhabdoid tumor of the cervical spine. Magn Reson Med Sci 8:135–138

Packer RJ, Biegel JA, Blaney S, Finlay J, Geyer JR, Heideman R, Hilden J, Janss AJ, Kun L, Vezina G, Rorke LB, Smith M (2002) Atypical teratoid/rhabdoid tumor of the central nervous system: report on workshop. J Pediatr Hematol Oncol 24:337–342

Panigrahy A, Nelson MD Jr, Blüml S (2010) Magnetic resonance spectroscopy in pediatric neuroradiology: clinical and research applications. Pediatr Radiol 40:3–30

Parmar H, Hawkins C, Bouffet E, Rutka J, Shroff M (2006) Imaging findings in primary intracranial atypical teratoid/rhabdoid tumors. Pediatr Radiol 36:126–132

Parwani AV, Stelow EB, Pambuccian SE, Burger PC, Ali SZ (2005) Atypical teratoid/rhabdoid tumor of the brain: cytopathologic characteristics and differential diagnosis. Cancer 105:65–70

Rorke LB, Packer RJ, Biegel JA (1996) Central nervous system atypical teratoid/rhabdoid tumors of infancy and childhood: definition of an entity. J Neurosurg 85:56–65

Rumboldt Z, Camacho DL, Lake D, Welsh CT, Castillo M (2006) Apparent diffusion coefficients for differentiation of cerebellar tumors in children. AJNR Am J Neuroradiol 27:1362–1369

Squire SE, Chan MD, Marcus KJ (2007) Atypical teratoid/rhabdoid tumor: the controversy behind radiation therapy. J Neurooncol 81:97–111

Strother D (2005) Atypical teratoid rhabdoid tumors of childhood: diagnosis, treatment and challenges. Expert Rev Anticancer Ther 5:907–915

Tekautz TM, Fuller CE, Blaney S, Fouladi M, Broniscer A, Merchant TE, Krasin M, Dalton J, Hale G, Kun LE, Wallace D, Gilbertson RJ, Gajjar A (2005) Atypical teratoid/rhabdoid tumors (ATRT): improved survival in children 3 years of age and older with radiation therapy and high-dose alkylator-based chemotherapy. J Clin Oncol 23:1491–1499

Warmuth-Metz M, Bison B, Dannemann-Stern E, Kortmann R, Rutkowski S, Pietsch T (2008) CT and MR imaging in atypical teratoid/rhabdoid tumors of the central nervous system. Neuroradiology 50:447–452

Woehrer A, Slavc I, Waldhoer T, Heinzl H, Zielonke N, Czech T, Benesch M, Hainfellner JA, Haberler C, Austrian Brain Tumor Registry (2010) Incidence of atypical teratoid/rhabdoid tumors in children: a population-based study by the Austrian Brain Tumor Registry, 1996–2006. Cancer 116(24): 5725–5732

Pediatric Atypical Teratoid/ Rhabdoid Tumor in the Spine: Diagnosis and Treatment

6

Stella Stabouli

Contents

S. Stabouli (✉)
Pediatric Intensive Care Unit, Hippokration General Hospital, 49 Konstantinoupoleos Street, 546 42 Thessaloniki, Greece
e-mail: sstaboul@med.uoa.gr

Abstract

Atypical teratoid/rhabdoid tumor (AT/RT) in the spine is an extremely rare pediatric neoplasm. It usually occurs in very young children and the exact incidence of the disease is not yet known. The differential diagnosis primarily includes primitive neuroectodermal tumor/medulloblastoma. Deletions and mutations of the SMARCB1/INI1/SNF5 locus in chromosome band 22q11.2 characterize the majority of spinal AT/RTs. Cytogenetic and fluorescence in situ hybridization analysis combined with molecular analysis to detect alterations in INI1 gene confirm the diagnosis of disease. Atypical teratoid/rhabdoid tumor in the spine exhibits a very aggressive behavior and long-term survival is reported in very few patients. Despite the lack of optimal treatment guidelines, multimodal therapy including surgery, chemotherapy and radiation therapy are used in the majority of pediatric patients. The efficacy of specific chemotherapy is difficult to evaluate due to the diversity of regimens used and the small number of patients. On the other hand, there is evidence that surgery may improve survival. Finally, the efficacy radiation therapy in pediatric patients needs to be further investigated.

M.A. Hayat (ed.), *Pediatric Cancer, Volume 3: Diagnosis, Therapy, and Prognosis*, Pediatric Cancer 3,
DOI 10.1007/978-94-007-4528-5_6,

Introduction

Atypical teratoid/rhabdoid tumor (AT/RT) is a highly malignant, rare pediatric neoplasm of the central nervous system (CNS). In the past it was often misdiagnosed, because of its resemblance to primitive neuroectodermal tumor (PNET). Atypical teratoid/rhabdoid tumor was first described as a distinct clinicopathologic entity in 1987 (Lefkowitz et al. 1987). The tumor cells present a unique combination of rhabdoid cells, with or without fields, up to 70% primitive neuroepithelial sections, resembling typical PNET, and peripheral/mesenchymal elements that lack divergent tissue differentiation of malignant teratomas (Rorke et al. 1996). The immunohistochemical and cytogenetic profile of AT/RTs allows separation from PNET and other CNS tumors. It is more often located in the posterior fossa, but can arise in any site of CNS. Primary location in the spine is extremely rare. Large size, high tumor stages and dissemination at the time of diagnosis are frequently reported and in spite of intensive treatment outcome is usually unfavorable (Packer et al. 2002). The optimal therapy for spinal AT/RT is not clear from the available data, although occasional cases respond to commonly used malignant CNS therapeutic protocols. As prognosis of AT/RT is extremely poor in children, early and accurate diagnosis is important to ensure appropriate treatment, while prospective trials are needed to design specific protocols for spinal AT/RT.

Epidemiology

Atypical teratoid/rhabdoid tumor accounts for 1.3% of primary CNS neoplasms among the pediatric population (Rickert and Paulus 2001). In the Austrian Brain Tumor Registry, the prevalence is reported higher (6.1%) with an age standardized incidence rate 1.38 per 1,000,000 child-years (Woehrer et al. 2010). Atypical teratoid/rhabdoid tumor usually presents an extremely aggressive nature and primarily affects children younger than 2 years old. Location in the spine is extremely rare and the exact incidence cannot be determined, as there are mainly sporadic cases reported in the literature (Table 6.1). Most patients with spinal AT/RT are under the age of 2 years at the time of diagnosis. Large series of CNS AT/RT included only 1–2 cases of primary spinal AT/RT (Rorke et al. 1996; Cheng et al. 2005; Tekautz et al. 2005). In a meta-analysis of 133 cases of CNS AT/RT in children (median age 2.1 years), 61% of the tumors were located in the posterior fossa, 20% in the cerebral hemispheres, 5% in the ventricular region, 5% in the pineal region and only 1% in the spinal cord (Oka and Scheithauer 1999). A more recent meta-analysis, describing 143 patients, included 10 cases of isolated spinal AT/RT (Athale et al. 2009). Metastases and diffuse disease at diagnosis are found in a significant number of patients with primary spinal AT/RT. Outcome is dismal in the majority of the cases with spinal AT/RT and only few patients are reported as long-term survivors. Patients younger than 3 years old have a poorer prognosis (died of disease within 2–20 months of diagnosis) compared with patients older than 3 years old.

Clinical Presentation and Imaging Findings

The main clinical feature of primary spinal AT/RT is upper or/and lower extremities weakness that progresses to paralysis (hemiplegia/paraplegia), pain, and swelling of the affected region. Ataxia and unstable gait have also been reported at the occurrence of the disease (Rorke et al. 1996; Yano et al. 2008; Niwa et al. 2009; Agrawal et al. 2009; Stabouli et al. 2010).

Atypical teratoid/rhabdoid tumor in the spine can occur all along the spinal canal, intramedullary or extramedullary. Imaging findings are not specific (Niwa et al. 2009; Stabouli et al. 2010). The lesions are usually heterogeneous, reflecting the histopathologic complexity of these tumors. On computed tomography there is usually a hyperdense mass that enhances intensely. Magnetic resonance imaging (MRI) findings may include

Table 6.1 Reported cases of spinal atypical teratoid/rhabdoid tumor in pediatric patients

Case	Authors	Age (mo)	Sex	Location	Therapy	Outcome/time after diagnosis
1	Rosemberg et al. (1994)	24	F	C6-T1	CMT	DOD/2 mo
2	Howlett et al. (1997)	9	M	T5-T10	Surg/CMT/RT	DOD/4 mo
3	Tamiya et al. (2000)	7	F	T7	Surg	DOD/2 mo
4	Bambakidis et al. (2002)	22	M	T11-L3	Surg/CMT/ABMT/RT	DOD/10 mo
5	Bambakidis et al. (2002)	204	M	Diffuse Spinal	RT	DOD/1 mo
6	McManus et al. (2004)	17	F	ND	Surg/CMT	DOD/2 mo
7	Slavac et al. (2005)	ND	ND	ND	Surg/CMT/ABMT/RT	DOD/23 mo
8	Cheng et al. (2005)	24	F	T12	ND	DOD/2 mo
9	Chen et al. (2005)	180	M	ND	Surg/CMT/RT	AWD/34 mo
10	Tanizaki et al. (2006)	10	F	T10	Surg/CMT/RT	DOD/3 mo
11	Bannykh et al. (2006)	48	M	T9-L1	Surg/CMT/RT	NED/18 mo
12	Kodama et al. (2007)	9	M	C4-T6	Surg/CMT/RT	DOD/20 mo
13	Moeller et al. (2007)	108	M	T11-L2	Surg/RT	NED
14	Yang et al. (2007)	84	M	L2-L4	Surg/CMT/RT	DOD/7 mo
15	Seno et al. (2008)	5	F	C4-T3	Surg/CMT	DOD/2 mo
16	Yano et al. (2008)	21	F	Cervical	Surg/CMT/ABMT/RT	NED
17	Tinsa et al. (2008)	48	F	T1	ND	DOD/2 mo
18	Niwa et al. (2009)	72	M	C3-C6	Surg	ND
19	Fridley et al. (2009)	13	F	Cervical	Surg/CMT	DOD/4 mo
20	Agrawal et al. (2009)	18	F	L2	Surg/CMT	DOD
21	Stabouli et al. (2010)	2	M	C1-C5	CMT	DOD/6 mo
22	Mohapatra et al. (2010)	54	F	Cervical	Surg	ND
23	Heuer et al. (2010)	72	M	C2	Surg/CMT/RT	DOD/42 mo
24	Imagama et al. (2011)	24	F	T12-S1	Surg/CMT/RT	DOD/6 mo

F female, *M* male, *Surg* surgery, *CMT* chemotherapy, *RT* radiation therapy, *ABMT* autologous bone marrow transplantation, *ND* not defined, *DOD* died of disease, *mo* months, *NED* no evidence of disease, *AWD* alive with disease

isointensity with hypertintense foci due to intratumoral hemorrhage on T1-weighted images, and heterogeneity (a mix of hypo-, iso-, and hyperintense foci) on T2-weighted images. There is no typical enhancement pattern after intravenous administration of contrast. Cerebrovascular fluid dissemination, edema, cysts, calcification, or necrosis have also been described. Most of these MRI findings are similar to those described in intracranial AT/RTs (Warmuth-Metz et al. 2008). Differential diagnosis includes PNET and ependymoma for intramedulary tumors, while extramedullary tumors may be differentiated from ependymoma, schwannoma, neurofibroma, and meningioma. Imaging findings may not distinguish AT/RT from PNET in many cases, which would require early surgery to establish the AT/RT diagnosis by pathological examination.

Histopathology and Molecular Genetics

Atypical teratoid/rhabdoid tumor in the spine presents similar histological finding as brain AR/RTs and malignant rhabdoid tumors. They are characterized by typical nests or sheets of rhabdoid cells, which have eccentric round nuclei with a prominent nucleolus and a plump cell body with characteristic cytoplasmic filament inclusions (Rorke et al. 1996; Oka and Scheithauer 1999). On immunohistochemical analysis, a wide range of antigens according to the appropriate differential diagnosis are used, in order to establish the diagnosis of CNS AT/RT. Spinal AR/RTs are characteristically positive for vimentin, epithelial membrane antigen (EMA), glial fibrillary acidic protein (GFAP), smooth-muscle antigen (SMA), and in many cases for synaptophysin, cytokeratin, neuron specific enolase (NSE), and cytoplasmic CD99, while they are negative for germ cell markers.

Lack of expression of the SMARCB1 protein, represents a specific means of distinguishing AT/RT from other malignancies with similar histological features. Deletions and mutations of the SMARCB1/INI1/SNF5 locus in chromosome band 22q11.2 characterize the majority of spinal AT/RTs. SMARCB1 (SWI/SNF related, Matrix associated, Actin dependent Regulator of Chromatin, subfamily B, member 1) is a member of the ATP-dependent SW1/SNF chromatin-remodeling complex of proteins and may affect tumor suppressor function by modulating genes transcription.

SMARCB1 loss causes cell cycle progression by downregulation of p16INK4a and upregulation of E2Fs and cyclin D1. In addition, some chromatin remodeling complexes, such as the INO80, SWR1 and RAD54 complexes, may affect DNA repair and maintenance of genome stability (Roberts and Biegel 2009).

Biegel et al. (2002) described homozygous deletions or mutations of INI1 gene in chromosome band 22q11.2 in 75 out of 100 patients with AT/RT. Patients with brain tumors had mutations in exon 5 and a cytosine deletion in exon 9, while the patients with primary spinal tumor (n = 2) had mutations in exon 3 and 5 detected by microsatellite analysis. FISH (fluorescence in situ hybridization) is a sensitive method for detecting SMARCB1/INI1 deletions in AT/RT. As homozygous deletions are not frequent in CNS tumors, cytogenetic and FISH analysis combined with molecular analysis maybe necessary to detect alterations in INI1 gene. Microsatellite analysis for LOH (loss of heterozygosity) can show loss and duplication or mitotic recombination of chromosome 22. Germline mutations of SMARCB1/INI1 predispose to the development of AT/RT, but also rhabdoid tumors of the kidney and soft tissues and affected individuals may present with more than one primary tumor. In most cases, the germline mutations or deletions are de novo as parents are not affected (Roberts and Biegel 2009). However, there are limited reports of inherited SMARCB1/INI1 mutations associated with familial occurrence of AT/RTs and schwannomas (Swensen et al. 2009). A recent study (Eaton et al. 2011) including 100 patients with rhabdoid tumors, among which 65 with AT/RT, estimated that approximately one-third of patients with rhabdoid tumors have an underlying genetic predisposition due to germline mutations.

Treatment

Treatment strategies for CNS AT/RTs are based on small, retrorespective series. Data on therapeutic approaches regarding spinal AT/RT are even scarcer. Most patients had received a variety of combination of multimodal therapy involving surgery, chemotherapy and radiotherapy. Although occasional case reports showed successful treatment, no regimen seems to be consistently efficient with regard to the progression of disease.

The rarity of location in the spine and the poor outcome in most cases result in lack of clear treatment strategies. Most published series include data from therapeutic modalities used to treat pediatric patients with brain AT/RT. Surgery seems to have an important role on outcome. Most cases of spinal AT/RT reported as long-term survivors underwent total or partial resection of the tumor. Moreover, the degree of surgical resection has been associated with longer survival in CNS AT/RT (Zimmerman et al. 2005; Athale et al. 2009).

As diverse chemotherapy regimens have been used in the literature the effect of specific chemotherapy has not been precisely evaluated (Table 6.2). The lack of specific treatment guidelines, mainly because of the rarity of disease, as well as the resemblance to PNET/medulloblastoma, historically favored the use of chemotherapy according to PNET/medulloblastoma protocols. The survival using this approach has been reported less than 12 months (Packer et al. 2002; Rorke et al. 1996). Hilden et al. (2004) evaluated the results of chemotherapy in 42 children with CNS AT/RT enrolled in a registry. The median age at diagnosis in this cohort was 24 months and the median survival reported at 16.75 months, which was significantly

Table 6.2 Published series on chemotherapeutic regimens for pediatric CNS atypical teratoid/rhabdoid tumor

Author	No patients	Location	CMT	No of survivors	Median survival (months)
Olson et al. (1995)	18	Brain	IRS-III	2	ND
Rorke et al. (1996)	52	Brain/1 case spine	baby POG augmented baby POG HDC, ABMT	9	6
Hilden et al. (2004)	42	Brain	CCG 99703 CCG9921 IRS-III SCR	14	16.75
Zimmerman et al. (2005)	4	Brain	DFCI/IRS III	4	37
Tekautz et al. (2005)	37	Brain/1 case spine	ICE SJMB96 CNS14 CCG9921 MOPP1 HDC SCR	12	7 if ≥3 year old 4.8 if <3 year old
Chen et al. (2005)	11	Brain/1 case spine	CCG 99703, ICE	5	ND
Gardner et al. (2008)	13	Brain	HS-I, HS-II	3	10.5
Fidani et al. (2009)	8	Brain	ICE, CECAT, HDC	5	10
Chi et al. (2009)	20	Brain	IRS-III	12	ND
Athale et al. (2009)	143	133 brain/10 cases spine	&	46	17.3
Woehrer et al. (2010)	17	Brain/1 case spine	MUV AT/RT	8	ND
Morgenstern et al. (2010)	15	14 brain/1 case spine	+ ++	1	10.1
Nicolaides et al. (2010)	9	Brain/1 case spine	CCG 99703 HS-II SCR	3	10

Intergroup Rhabdomyosarcoma (IRS)-III regimen 36 cisplatin, vincristine, etoposide, cyclophosphamide, doxorubicin, dacarbazine (or temolomide), actimomycin-D and Intrathecal therapy with methotraxate, hydrocortisone and cytarabine, *DFCI/IRS III* cisplatin, vincristine, etoposide, cyclophosphamide, doxorubicin, temolomide, actimomycin-D, dexrazoxane and Intrathecal therapy with methotraxate, hydrocortisone and cytarabine, *baby POG* cyclophosphamide, vincristine, cisplatinum, and VP-16, *augmented baby POG* higher dose cyclophosphamide and more intensive cisplatinum, *Children's Cancer Group (CCG) 99703* cisplatin, vincristine, cyclophsphamide, etoposide, *CCG9921* carboplatin, Ifosfamide, etoposide, vincristine, *ICE* ifosfamide, carboplatin, etoposide, *SJMB96* topotecan, cisplatin, HD-cyclophaspamide-ABMT, *MOPP1* nitrogen mustard, vincristine, procabazine, prednisone, *Headstart(HS)-II* methotraxate, cisplatin, vincristine, etoposide, cytoxan, *HS-I* cisplatin, vincristine, etoposide, cyclophosphamide, *CECAT* cyclophasphamide, etoposide, carboplatin, thiotepa, *MUV AT/RT* doxorubicin, cyclofosfamide, cisplatin, vincristine, etoposide, ifosfamide, methotraxate+HDC, + cyclospospamide, vincristine, etoposide, carboplatin, ++ vincristine, cisplatin, lomustine, & *v*ariable, *CMT* chemotherapy, *HDC* high dose chemotherapy, *ABMT* autologous bone marrow transplantation, *SCR* stem cell rescue, *ND* not defined

improved compared with previous reports. While most of the patients underwent surgery, approximately one-third of the children received radiotherapy, one-third received intrathecal chemotherapy and one-third high dose chemotherapy with stem cell rescue. The effect of separate modalities could not be determined as patients with prolonged survival received several therapeutic modalities.

In a prospective study (Gardner et al. 2008), 13 children with brain AT/RT were treated with surgery, five cycles of induction chemotherapy (either Head Start I-cisplatin, vinscristine, cyclofosfamide and etoposide or Head Start II-cisplatin, vinscristine, cyclofosfamide, etoposide and methotrexate) followed by a single course of high-dose chemotherapy with autologous hematopoietic progenitor cell rescue. Three children on Head Start II presented long-term remissions providing some evidence that aggressive approaches using multi-drug chemotherapy including myeloablative chemotherapy may result in prolonged survival.

Radiotherapy (RT) could be associated with a better outcome in CNS AT/RT. Tekautz et al. (2005) reported long-term survival in patients older that 3 year treated with high dose alkylator-based chemotherapy (cyclofosfamide/cisplatin/vincristine/etoposide or carboplatin/ifosfamide/etoposide-ICE, high dose cyclophospahmide and topotecan followed by stem cell rescue and oxaliplatin/topotecan) combined with radiotherapy. They reported up to 2.2 years median survival from diagnosis in patients older than 3 years old, compared to 0.4 years in patients younger than 3 years old. Younger patients who usually do not receive radiotherapy, because of its possible effect on neurocognitive development have worse survival rates. Early radiotherapy may have a beneficial effect on disease control with improved survival. Chen et al. (2006) demonstrated on multivariate analysis a significant association between the time of initiation of radiotherapy and outcome. Significant benefit from radiotherapy has also been demonstrated in a cohort of 15 patients with CNS AT/RT (1 with spinal location) in a retrospective analysis of diagnosed cases of AT/RT at Great Ormond Street Hospital over a 20-years period (Morgenstern et al. 2010). All reported cases of primary spinal AT/RT, who presented disease remission received radiation therapy. However, the role of RT is not clear in patients with more aggressive, rapidly progressive disease who usually do not receive radiotherapy for practical reasons and this may have caused a selection bias in the selection of patients for radiotherapy in most published studies.

A meta-analysis of observational studies on childhood CNS AT/RT evaluated 63 reports describing a total of 143 patients (Athale et al. 2009). Among them 10 had isolated spinal disease, age range 0, 6–4, 2 years (50% male). Six patients underwent partial and 1 gross total resection. Most patients received chemotherapy and radiation therapy after surgery. Two patients, who both received radiation therapy after partial and gross total resection, respectively, presented remission of disease. Survival was poorer compared to that of the initial population, including both spinal and brain AT/RT. In the same meta-analysis it was found that radiation therapy positively influenced the overall survival in patients with AT/RT, especially when given with intrathecal chemotherapy in children with CNS AT/RT younger than 3 years of age. On the other hand, the extent of surgical resection did not affect the overall survival. The impact of chemotherapy on survival could not be estimated, as in most published series, because of the variability of therapies performed.

The key role of SMARCB1/INI1 in the development of AT/RT led to new therapeutic insights for CNS AT/RT. Zhang et al. (2002) found that INI1/hSNF5 directly represses the transcription of cyclin D1 gene. Cyclin D1 is a critical protein controlling the G_1 stage of cell cycle and has been implicated in the pathogenesis of human cancer. As cyclin D1 levels are elevated in tumor samples, they suggested that repression of cyclin D1 could be a useful therapeutic target to treat AT/RT. Decreased insulin growth factor I receptor (IGF-IR) expression or impaired function has been reported to induce a reversal of the transformed phenotype, apoptosis and a decrease in cellular radioresistance and chemoresistance. D'cunja et al. (2007) found that IGF-IR was expressed in eight patients with AT/RT. In the same study, treatment with IGF-IR antisense oligonucleotide resulted in significant down-regulation of IGF-IR mRNA and protein expression, induction of apoptosis, and chemosensitisation to doxorubicin and cisplatin. Future research may clarify the potential of these novel therapeutic approaches for pediatric spinal AT/RT.

References

Agrawal A, Bhake A, Cincu R (2009) Giant lumbar paraspinal atypical teratoid/rhabdoid tumor in a child. J Cancer Res Ther 5:318–320

Athale UH, Duckworth J, Odame I, Barr R (2009) Childhood atypical teratoid rhabdoid tumor of the central nervous system: a meta-analysis of observational studies. J Pediatr Hematol Oncol 31:651–663

Bambakidis NC, Robinson S, Cohen M, Cohen AR (2002) Atypical teratoid/rhabdoid tumors of the central nervous system: clinical, radiographic and pathologic features. Pediatr Neurosurg 37:64–70

Bannykh S, Duncan C, Ogle E, Baehring JM (2006) Atypical teratoid/rhabdoid tumor of the spinal canal. J Neurooncol 76:129–130

Biegel JA, Tan L, Zhang F, Wainwright L, Russo P, Rorke LB (2002) Alterations of the hSNF5/INI1 gene in central nervous system atypical teratoid/rhabdoid tumors and renal and extrarenal rhabdoid tumors. Clin Cancer Res 8:3461–3467

Chen ML, McComb JG, Krieger MD (2005) Atypical teratoid/rhabdoid tumors of the central nervous system: management and outcomes. Neurosurg Focus 18:E8

Chen YW, Wong TT, Ho DM, Huang PI, Chang KP, Shiau CY, Yen SH (2006) Impact of radiotherapy for pediatric CNS atypical teratoid/rhabdoid tumor (single institute experience). Int J Radiat Oncol Biol Phys 64:1038–1043

Cheng YC, Lirng JF, Chang FC, Guo WY, Teng MM, Chang CY, Wong TT, Ho DM (2005) Neuroradiological findings in atypical teratoid/rhabdoid tumor of the central nervous system. Acta Radiol 46:89–96

Chi SN, Zimmerman MA, Yao X, Cohen KJ, Burger P, Biegel JA, Rorke-Adams LB, Fisher MJ, Janss A, Mazewski C, Goldman S, Manley PE, Bowers DC, Bendel A, Rubin J, Turner CD, Marcus KJ, Goumnerova L, Ullrich NJ, Kieran MW (2009) Intensive multimodality treatment for children with newly diagnosed CNS atypical teratoid rhabdoid tumor. J Clin Oncol 27:385–389

D'cunja J, Shalaby T, Rivera P, von Büren A, Patti R, Heppner FL, Arcaro A, Rorke-Adams LB, Phillips PC, Grotzer MA (2007) Antisense treatment of IGF-IR induces apoptosis and enhances chemosensitivity in central nervous system atypical teratoid/rhabdoid tumours cells. Eur J Cancer 43:1581–1589

Eaton KW, Tooke LS, Wainwright LM, Judkins AR, Biegel JA (2011) Spectrum of SMARCB1/INI1 mutations in familial and sporadic rhabdoid tumors. Pediatr Blood Cancer 56:7–15

Fidani P, De Ioris MA, Serra A, De Sio L, Ilari I, Cozza R, Boldrini R, Milano GM, Garrè ML, Donfrancesco A (2009) A multimodal strategy based on surgery, radiotherapy, ICE regimen and high dose chemotherapy in atypical teratoid/rhabdoid tumours: a single institution experience. J Neurooncol 92:177–183

Fridley JS, Chamoun RB, Whitehead WE, Curry DJ, Luerssen TG, Adesina A, Jea A (2009) Malignant rhabdoid tumor of the spine in an infant: case report and review of the literature. Pediatr Neurosurg 45:237–243

Gardner SL, Asgharzadeh S, Green A, Horn B, McCowage G, Finlay J (2008) Intensive induction chemotherapy followed by high dose chemotherapy with autologous hematopoietic progenitor cell rescue in young children newly diagnosed with central nervous system atypical teratoid rhabdoid tumors. Pediatr Blood Cancer 51:235–240

Heuer GG, Kiefer H, Judkins AR, Belasco J, Biegel JA, Jackson EM, Cohen M, O'Malley BW Jr, Storm PB (2010) Surgical treatment of a clival-C2 atypical teratoid/rhabdoid tumor. J Neurosurg Pediatr 5:75–79

Hilden JM, Meerbaum S, Burger P, Finlay J, Janss A, Scheithauer BW, Walter AW, Rorke LB, Biegel JA (2004) Central nervous system atypical teratoid/rhabdoid tumor: results of therapy in children enrolled in a registry. J Clin Oncol 22:2877–2884

Howlett DC, King AP, Jarosz JM, Stewart RA, al-Sarraj ST, Bingham JB, Cox TC (1997) Imaging and pathological features of primary malignant rhabdoid tumours of the brain and spine. Neuroradiology 39:719–723

Imagama S, Wakao N, Ando K, Hirano K, Tauchi R, Muramoto A, Matsui H, Matsumoto T, Ukai J, Kobayashi K, Shinjo R, Nakashima H, Maruyama K, Matsuyama Y, Ishiguro N (2011) Treatment for primary spinal atypical teratoid/rhabdoid tumor. J Orthop Sci. doi:10.1007/s00776-011-0122-7 [Epub ahead of print]

Kodama H, Maeda M, Imai H, Matsubara T, Taki W, Takeda K (2007) MRI of primary spinal atypical teratoid/rhabdoid tumor: a case report and literature review. J Neurooncol 84:213–216

Lefkowitz IB, Rorke LB, Packer RJ, Sutton LN, Siegel KR, Katnick RJ (1987) Atypical teratoid/rhabdoid tumor of infancy: definition of an entity. Ann Neurol 22:448–449

McManus MJ, Puccetti DM, Koehn MA (2004) Atypical teratoid/rhabdoid tumors: resistance to multiple chemotherapeutic agents. In: Proceedings of 11th international symposium on pediatric neuro-oncology, Boston, p 166

Moeller KK, Coventry S, Jernigan S, Moriarty TM (2007) Atypical teratoid/rhabdoid tumor of the spine. AJNR Am J Neuroradiol 28:593–595

Mohapatra I, Santosh V, Chickabasaviah YT, Mahadevan A, Tandon A, Ghosh A, Chidambaram B, Sampath S, Bhagavatula ID, Chandramouli BA, Kolluri SV, Shankar SK (2010) Histological and immunohistochemical characterization of AT/RT: a report of 15 cases from India. Neuropathology 30:251–259

Morgenstern DA, Gibson S, Brown T, Sebire NJ, Anderson J (2010) Clinical and pathological features of paediatric malignant rhabdoid tumours. Pediatr Blood Cancer 54:29–34

Nicolaides T, Tihan T, Horn B, Biegel J, Prados M, Banerjee A (2010) High-dose chemotherapy and autologous stem cell rescue for atypical teratoid/rhabdoid tumor of the central nervous system. J Neurooncol 98:117–123

Niwa T, Aida N, Tanaka M, Okubo J, Sasano M, Shishikura A, Fujita K, Ito S, Tanaka Y, Kigasawa H (2009) Diffusion-weighted imaging of an atypical teratoid/rhabdoid tumor of the cervical spine. Magn Reson Med Sci 8:135–138

Oka H, Scheithauer BW (1999) Clinicopathological characteristics of atypical teratoid/rhabdoid tumor. Neurol Med Chir (Tokyo) 39:510–517

Olson TA, Bayar E, Kosnik E, Hamoudi AB, Klopfenstein KJ, Pieters RS, Ruymann FB (1995) Successful treatment of disseminated central nervous system malignant rhabdoid tumor. J Pediatr Hematol Oncol 17:71–75

Packer RJ, Biegel JA, Blaney S, Finlay J, Geyer JR, Heideman R, Hilden J, Janss AJ, Kun L, Vezina G, Rorke LB, Smith M (2002) Atypical teratoid/rhabdoid tumor of the central nervous system: report on workshop. J Pediatr Hematol Oncol 24:337–342

Rickert CH, Paulus W (2001) Epidemiology of central nervous system tumors in childhood and adolescence based on the new WHO classification. Childs Nerv Syst 17:503–511

Roberts CW, Biegel JA (2009) The role of SMARCB1/INI1 in development of rhabdoid tumor. Cancer Biol Ther 8:412–416

Rorke LB, Packer RJ, Biegel JA (1996) Central nervous system atypical teratoid/rhabdoid tumors of infancy and childhood: definition of an entity. J Neurosurg 85:56–65

Rosemberg S, Menezes Y, Sousa MR, Plese P, Ciquini O (1994) Primary malignant rhabdoid tumor of the spinal dura. Clin Neuropathol 13:221–224

Seno T, Kawaguchi T, Yamahara T, Sakurai Y, Oishi T, Inagaki T, Yamanouchi Y, Asai A, Kawamoto K (2008) An immunohistochemical and electron microscopic study of atypical teratoid/rhabdoid tumor. Brain Tumor Pathol 25:79–83

Slavac L, Czech T, Widhalm G et al (2005) Atypical teratoid/rhabdoid tumor of the CNS – therapeutic management and outcome in four patients. In: Proceedings of SIOP XXXVII annual conference, PD 05

Stabouli S, Sdougka M, Tsitspoulos P, Violaki A, Anagnostopoulos I, Tsonidis Ch, Koliouskas D (2010) Primary atypical teratoid/rhabdoid tumor of the spine in an infant. Hippokratia 14:286–288

Swensen JJ, Keyser J, Coffin CM, Biegel JA, Viskochil DH, Williams MS (2009) Familial occurrence of schwannomas and malignant rhabdoid tumour associated with a duplication in SMARCB1. J Med Genet 46:68–72

Tamiya T, Nakashima H, Ono Y, Kawada S, Hamazaki S, Furuta T, Matsumoto K, Ohmoto T (2000) Spinal atypical teratoid/rhabdoid tumor in an infant. Pediatr Neurosurg 32:145–149

Tanizaki Y, Oka H, Utsuki S, Shimizu S, Suzuki S, Fujii K (2006) Atypical teratoid/rhabdoid tumor arising from the spinal cord–case report and review of the literature. Clin Neuropathol 25:81–85

Tekautz TM, Fuller CE, Blaney S, Fouladi M, Broniscer A, Merchant TE, Krasin M, Dalton J, Hale G, Kun LE, Wallace D, Gilbertson RJ, Gajjar A (2005) Atypical teratoid/rhabdoid tumors (ATRT): improved survival in children 3 years of age and older with radiation therapy and high-dose alkylator-based chemotherapy. J Clin Oncol 23:1491–1499

Tinsa F, Jallouli M, Douira W, Boubaker A, Kchir N, Hassine DB, Boussetta K, Bousnina S (2008) Atypical teratoid/rhabdoid tumor of the spine in a 4-year-old girl. J Child Neurol 23:1439–1442

Warmuth-Metz M, Bison B, Dannemann-Stern E, Kortmann R, Rutkowski S, Pietsch T (2008) CT and MR imaging in atypical teratoid/rhabdoid tumors of the central nervous system. Neuroradiology 50:447–452

Woehrer A, Slavc I, Waldhoer T, Heinzl H, Zielonke N, Czech T, Benesch M, Hainfellner JA, Haberler C, Registry Austrian Brain Tumor (2010) Incidence of atypical teratoid/rhabdoid tumors in children: a population-based study by the Austrian Brain Tumor Registry, 1996–2006. Cancer 116:5725–5732

Yang CS, Jan YJ, Wang J, Shen CC, Chen CC, Chen M (2007) Spinal atypical teratoid/rhabdoid tumor in a 7-year-old boy. Neuropathology 27:139–144

Yano S, Hida K, Kobayashi H, Iwasaki Y (2008) Successful multimodal therapies for a primary atypical teratoid/rhabdoid tumor in the cervical spine. Pediatr Neurosurg 44:406–413

Zhang ZK, Davies KP, Allen J, Zhu L, Pestell RG, Zagzag D, Kalpana GV (2002) Cell cycle arrest and repression of cyclin D1 transcription by INI1/hSNF5. Mol Cell Biol 22:5975–5988

Zimmerman MA, Goumnerova LC, Proctor M, Scott RM, Marcus K, Pomeroy SL, Turner CD, Chi SN, Chordas C, Kieran MW (2005) Continuous remission of newly diagnosed and relapsed central nervous system atypical teratoid/rhabdoid tumor. J Neurooncol 72:77–84

Early Childhood Clival-C2 Atypical Teratoid/Rhabdoid Tumor: Gross Total Resection Followed by Aggressive Chemotherapy and Radiation

7

Michael J. Kramarz, Eric M. Jackson, Adam C. Resnick, and Phillip B. Storm

Contents

M.J. Kramarz (✉) • A.C. Resnick • P.B. Storm
Department of Neurosurgery, Children's Hospital of Philadelphia, University of Pennsylvania Medical Center, Philadelphia, PA, USA
e-mail: mkramarz@mail.med.upenn.edu

E.M. Jackson
Department of Neurosurgery, Nationwide Children's Hospital, Columbus, OH, USA
e-mail: STORM@email.chop.edu

Abstract

Atypical teratoid/rhabdoid tumors (AT/RTs) are rare and aggressive tumors that most often occur in early childhood. These tumors usually are located in the cerebellum or cerebral hemispheres, but can occur in unusual locations. Prior to genetic analysis demonstrating a deletion of the tumor suppressor gene *INI-1*, these tumors were often misdiagnosed as primitive neuroectodermal tumors (PNETs). The patient presented here is a 7 year-old boy with an extradural clival-C2 AT/RT who was treated with a gross total resection (GTR) using an aggressive transoral resection. He was then stabilized with a halo and an instrumented fusion from occiput to C5, and received adjuvant therapy consisting of chemotherapy, radiation therapy, and a bone marrow transplant with a stem cell rescue. The patient survived an additional 42 months after surgery before dying of disseminated disease. Given the very small number of extradural spinal AT/RTs, the best treatment and prognosis is unknown. However, an aggressive approach of GTR followed by intensive chemotherapy and radiation therapy regimens appears to provide the best option at this point in time.

Introduction

Atypical teratoid/rhabdoid tumors (AT/RTs) are extremely rare, aggressive tumors of early childhood that can occur in a number of locations

M.A. Hayat (ed.), *Pediatric Cancer, Volume 3: Diagnosis, Therapy, and Prognosis*, Pediatric Cancer 3, DOI 10.1007/978-94-007-4528-5_7, © Springer Science+Business Media Dordrecht 2012

throughout the central nervous system (CNS) (Burger et al. 1998; Heuer et al. 2007; Packer et al. 2002; Rorke et al. 1996). The majority of AT/RTs present in the posterior fossa, followed by other intracranial locations; even fewer occur in extracranial locations (Packer et al. 2002). These lesions were considered neuroectodermal in origin, but more recently they have been given their own classification based on their unique histology and genetics (Biegel 2006; Rorke et al. 1996). The genetic alteration of AT/RTs is a loss of the putative tumor suppressor gene *INI-1* using fluorescent *in situ* hybridization (FISH) (Rorke et al. 1996). Patients diagnosed with an AT/RT carry a dismal prognosis. Historically, median survival was estimated between 6 and 11 months (Burger et al. 1998; Packer et al. 2002). More recently, median survival estimates seem to have been extended to around 17 months (Hilden et al. 2004; Athale et al. 2009). Because these tumors typically occur in children less than 3 years of age, these patients cannot be treated with craniospinal radiation therapy and their 5 year survival rates approach zero (Squire et al. 2007; Tekautz et al. 2005).

Treatment recommendations and outcomes for older patients with extra-CNS disease are not well described because of the paucity of patients. To our knowledge there is only one other published report of a patient presenting with a clival region AT/RT (Kazan et al. 2007). That patient was 4 years-old and treated with a limited resection and no adjuvant therapy at the family's request; the patient died 6 months after presentation. Recently, a 4 year-old male presented to an outside hospital with neck pain. Five months after removal of purulent adenoids, imaging and history were suggestive of acute osteomyletitis involving C1-C2; however, needle biopsy was consistent with a diagnosis of AT/RT based on histology, immunochemistry, and loss of *INI-1*.

There are a growing number of studies of CNS and extra-CNS AT/RTs reporting significantly improved survival of older patients undergoing a gross total resection (GTR) and aggressive adjuvant chemotherapy and radiation therapy (Tekautz et al. 2005; Hirth et al. 2003; Howes et al. 2005; Chi et al. 2009; Zimmerman et al. 2005). One patient, who was 2 years-old at the time of diagnosis with an intradural AT/RT in the cervical spine, was reported to be in complete remission over 2 years after surgery and multimodal treatment (Yano et al. 2008). Furthermore, there are data showing that patients with atypical presentations of AT/RTs can have a prolonged survival compared with patients with typical presentations (Chi et al. 2009; Hilden et al. 2004; Tekautz et al. 2005; Zimmerman et al. 2005). The case presented here is the first instance of managing a clival region AT/RT with en bloc resection followed by aggressive chemotherapy and radiation therapy.

Case Report

History and Examination

A 7 year-old boy presented with an 11 month history of neck pain on turning his head and a 4 month history of photophobia (Heuer et al. 2010). He presented after plain radiographs had shown a widened atlantodens interval, and subsequent magnetic resonance (MR) imaging revealed an enhancing mass compressing the brainstem and upper spinal cord from the clivus to C2 (Fig. 7.1a, b). The patient was determined to be M0 following a metastatic workup. He was admitted to the Children's Hospital of Philadelphia (CHOP) for a transoral needle biopsy procedure with the pathology results indicating numerous rhabdoid cells with a mixture of neuroepithelial and mesenchymal components and the loss of *INI-1* expression. These histological and genetic findings are consistent with AT/RT (Judkins et al. 2004; Biegel 2006). Molecular genetic studies later demonstrated a homozygous loss of the 22q11.2 region containing the *INI-1* gene.

The family was given the options of nonsurgical management, a low-morbidity debulking procedure, or an aggressive two-stage anterior/posterior procedure to remove the tumor en bloc. The family opted for complete resection, and given the patient's older age and atypical tumor location, there was consensus between all treating physicians that this procedure was the best option.

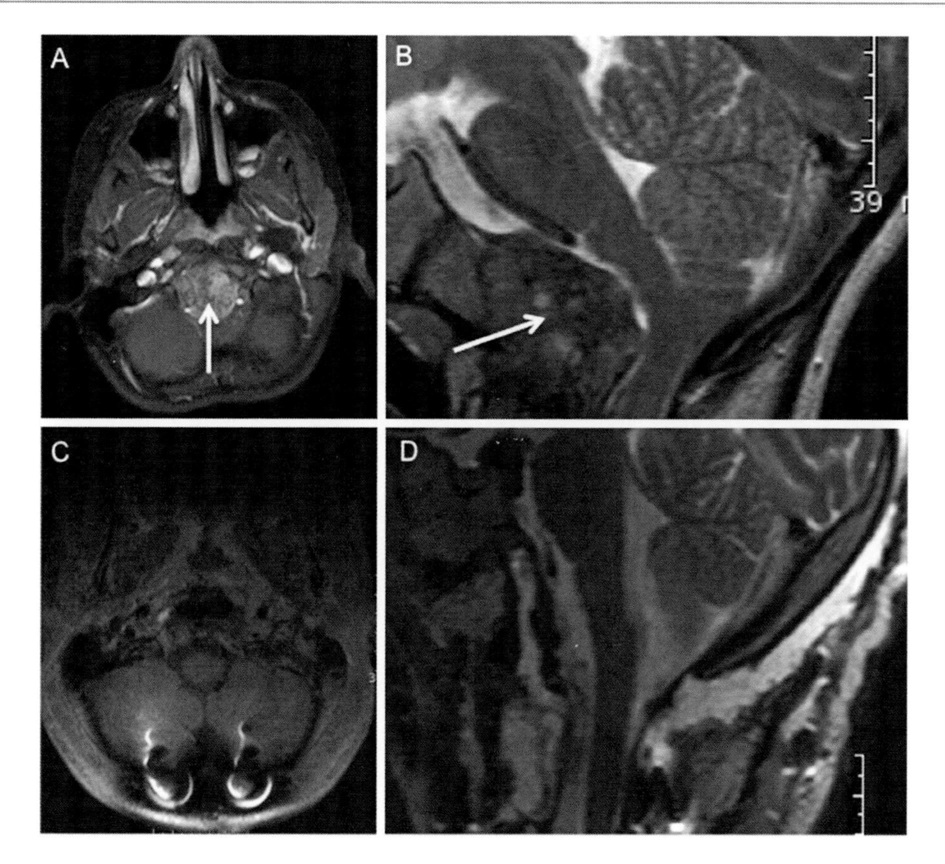

Fig. 7.1 (**a**) Axial T1WI post gadolinium-enhancement showing clival-C2 enhancing AT/RT (*arrow*) (**b**) Sagittal T2WI showing heterogeneous mass in the clival-C2 region displacing the cervicomedullary junction posteriorly (*arrow*) (**c**) Postoperative axial T1W1, post gadolinium -enhancement showing GTR after transoral approach. (**d**) Postoperative sagittal T2WI after transoral approach

The goal of the posterior approach was stabilization, whereas the goal of the anterior approach was en bloc resection.

Treatment

The procedure was performed in two stages. Prior to the en bloc resection of the clival neoplasm, the patient underwent a posterior instrumented fusion from the occipital bone down to C5. Synthes Axon occipital screws, lateral mass screws, and rods were used in this procedure. C1 and C2 were not instrumented due to the amount of bone and tumor at these levels that would need to be removed during the anterior approach in order to achieve complete resection of the clival-C2 mass. Two days later, an anterior resection was performed with the goal of gross total resection. In order to achieve maximum exposure for a safe GTR, a tracheostomy tube was placed, the patient's mandible was split, and his tongue was pushed inferiorly (Balasingam et al. 2006; Di Lorenzo 1989; Menezes 2008; Pollack et al. 1995). Subsequent to removing the anterior arch of C1, a high-speed bur was employed to remove bone from the clivus and the body of C2 until pristine dura was visualized. The tumor was completely extradural and resected en bloc with complete preservation of neurological function and without any evidence of CSF leakage. We typically do not place our patients in a halo after an occipital cervical fusion (Bauman et al. 2011), but given the aggressive nature of the adjuvant radiation therapy, the patient was placed in a halo after the

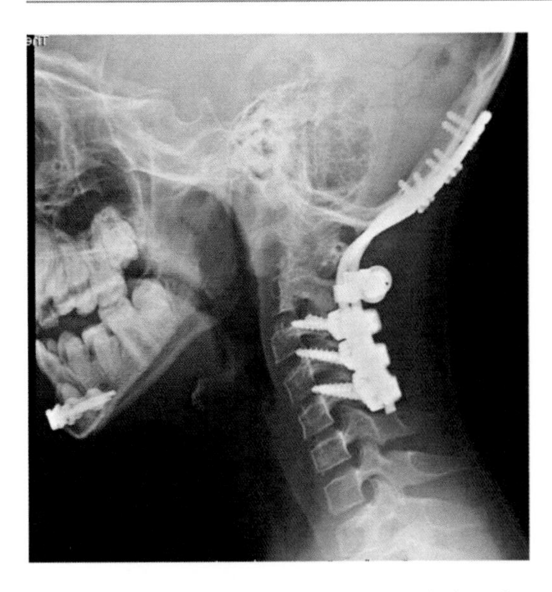

Fig. 7.2 Lateral radiograph showing bony fusion after O-C5 posterior instrumentation. Note the mandibular plate used after mandibular splitting

anterior procedure. The halo was removed after bony fusion (Fig. 7.2).

Posttreatment Course

Postoperative imaging confirmed GTR (Fig. 7.1c, d) and 10 days after surgery the patient's tracheostomy tube was decannulated. Today, the standard treatment for AT/RT includes radiation and chemotherapy following surgical biopsy or resection (complete or partial). However, these treatment modalities are not particularly effective at preventing local recurrence, metastasis, or both, and most patients eventually develop one or more of these. Our patient underwent treatment according to the Boston AT/RT CNS clinical trial guidelines, receiving vincristine, doxorubicin, cyclophosphamide, cisplatinum, etoposide, and intrathecal methotrexate, hydrocortisone, and ARA-C prior to the initiation of radiation. Two months following resection, he received 5,400 cGy of involved-field radiation for 6 weeks. While receiving radiation, he also received vincristine, cisplatin, etoposide, and cyclophosphamide. No further doxorubicin was administered until after the radiation therapy was concluded. Treatment was finished with intrathecal chemotherapy, as well as systemic courses of vincristine/doxorubicin and ultimately actinomycin/cyclophosphamide, and additional courses of temozolomide and actinomycin. The patient experienced mucositis, radiodermatitis, and myelosuppression, which are characteristic side effects of the regimen, but overall tolerated this therapy quite well. A gastrostomy tube was placed for nutrition because of the morbidity related to the chemotherapy and radiation therapy. Chemotherapy was continued for 16 months after surgery.

The patient re-presented 27 months after the original resection with left posterolateral thigh pain accompanied by somewhat decreased strength in his left lower extremity. An MR image demonstrated no tumor at the clival-C2 site of the original tumor; however, another MR image revealed a 2-cm intradural, extramedullary mass filling the thecal sac at the L1 level. The patient underwent a laminectomy from T12 to L1, and the tumor was removed. The diagnosis of this lesion was metastatic AT/RT. The patient underwent high-dose chemotherapy and a stem cell rescue clinical trial following surgery. Unfortunately, the boy relapsed yet again, this time with disseminated disease, and ended up dying 42 months after the initial resection.

Discussion

The patient presented several management issues. First, a diagnosis needed to be established before an intervention could be recommended. In patients of this age group, tumors in this location (clival-C2) are quite rare. Based on the patient's preoperative plain radiography, computed tomography (CT), and MR imaging, the differential diagnosis included chordoma, neuroblastoma, Ewing sarcoma, Langerhans cell histiocytosis, lymphoma, and rhabdoid tumor. The treatment regimen for these diagnoses is considerably different. Some are treated with upfront chemotherapy, radiation or both, while others are treated with aggressive resection followed by adjuvant therapy. We performed a transoral needle biopsy to rule out lesions that should be treated either by the oncology service alone or prior to attempting a complete resection. The diagnosis of AT/RT was confirmed based on the deletion of *INI-1* in the biopsy specimen. The second management issue was the timing of surgical intervention within the treatment regimen. The standard of care for AT/RTs is upfront GTR followed by intensive chemotherapy and radiation therapy (Zimmerman et al. 2005). After detailed discussions between the team (neurosurgery, neurooncology, and general oncology services) and the family, a consensus of upfront surgery with the goal of complete resection was reached.

The next decision to be made was the surgical approach to the lesion. While our institution has extensive experience with both open and endoscopic skull base surgeries, it was decided that in this case a large open anterior approach to the tumor would be best. This decision was made based on the degree of bony erosion of the clivus and the odontoid process, as well as the existence of tumor both anterior and posterior to C2, which would necessitate fusion for stabilization after the resection. It should be noted that although not done in this case, lesions of the clivus have been effectively approached via an endoscopic, endonasal approach, even in children (Al-Mefty et al. 2008; Fraser et al. 2010; Jho et al. 1997; Solares et al. 2005; Kelley et al. 1999). Endoscopic assistance in open, transoral approaches to the clivus have also been employed with success to date (Frempong-Boadu et al. 2002).

We felt that the best chance of a safe, complete resection was through maximum exposure via a mandible-splitting, tongue-sparing approach. This approach has been extensively used by other authors for similarly aggressive tumors in this location (Youssef and Sloan 2010; Menezes 2008), and provided outstanding exposure, allowing for safe GTR of the lesion. Overall, the patient tolerated the procedure extremely well, and no long-term surgical morbidity from the anterior approach was appreciated. He did require a gastrostomy tube for nutrition, but the cause of this intervention was the adjuvant chemotherapy and radiation therapy, not the surgery. After completing the chemotherapy regimen without interruption, the patient resumed his normal activities and was well enough to return to school fulltime.

Unfortunately, 27 months after the resection, the patient returned with a metastatic lesion to his lumbar spine without local recurrence. The metastasis occurred despite the aggressive, multimodal treatment regimen he obtained upon initial presentation: gross total resection, aggressive chemotherapy, and radiation therapy. Because only one metastatic lesion was present, the patient underwent resection and again fared well. However, 13 months later he represented with disseminated disease and died shortly thereafter. The patient survived 42 months after the initial resection of his lesion.

This case is now only the second of three reported instances of an AT/RT appearing as a clival-C2 mass, and is the first report of treatment involving an en bloc resection. In a previous case-report, a posterior open biopsy procedure was performed solely to confirm the diagnosis. The patient neither underwent a radical resection nor received additional treatment and was dead 6 months after the original diagnosis (Kazan et al. 2007). Our patient, on the other hand, underwent both GTR, aggressive chemotherapy and radiation therapy, and had a substantial improvement in survival. While his survival was increased substantially relative to the first patient with a clival AT/RT described in Kazan et al., the tumor recurred and was fatal, as is common with the aggressive nature of AT/RTs. We do not have long-term follow-up for the third patient, who presented with a circumferential AT/RT at the level of C2 (Fig. 7.3). Given the difficult nature of a GTR, this patient is being treated with upfront chemotherapy and will be reevaluated radiographically thereafter. If at that time there is dramatic reduction in the tumor burden, GTR will be attempted prior to initiation of radiation therapy.

Given the rarity of AT/RTs in general and their occurrence at the clivus and upper cervical spine in particular, it is difficult to make firm recommendations for their management. However, despite the dismal prognosis of AT/RT and many other pediatric brain tumors, there is reason to be optimistic. Several reports show that pediatric CNS tumors have different and far fewer mutations

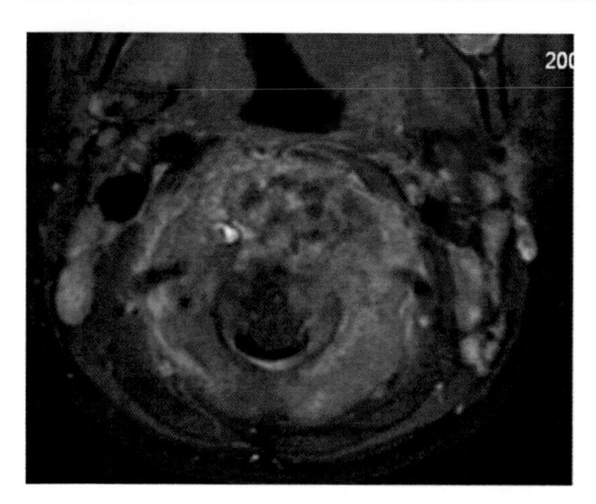

Fig. 7.3 Axial T1WI with gadolinium-enhancement showing a circumferential invasive and destructive C2 lesion

than their adult counterparts (Dougherty et al. 2010; Parsons et al. 2011; Sievert et al. 2009). Hopefully, this will allow for more effective therapies to be developed and introduced into practice in the coming years.

In conclusion, the AT/RT is a rare and aggressive tumor of early childhood and can occur in unusual locations. Although these lesions are associated with a poor outcome, the overall prognosis for AT/RTs located outside the posterior fossa in older patients is unclear given their rarity. Based on reports showing prolonged survival with this subset of AT/RTs that are treated with complete resection, and based on our own experience, we advocate GTR followed by aggressive chemotherapy and radiation.

References

Al-Mefty O, Kadri PAS, Hasan DM, Isolan GR, Pravdenkova S (2008) Anterior clivectomy: surgical technique and clinical applications. J Neurosurg 109(5):783–793

Athale UH, Duckworth J, Odame I, Barr R (2009) Childhood atypical teratoid rhabdoid tumor of the central nervous system: a meta-analysis of observational studies. J Pediatr Hematol Oncol 31(9):651–663

Balasingam V, Anderson GJ, Gross ND, Cheng CM, Noguchi A, Dogan A, McMenomey SO, Delashaw JB Jr, Andersen PE (2006) Anatomical analysis of transoral surgical approaches to the clivus. J Neurosurg 105(2):301–308

Bauman JA, Hardesty DA, Heuer GG, Storm PB (2011) Use of occipital bone graft in pediatric posterior cervical fusion: an alternative paramedian technique and review of the literature. J Neurosurg Pediatr 7(5):475–481. doi:10.3171/2011.2.PEDS10331

Biegel JA (2006) Molecular genetics of atypical teratoid/rhabdoid tumor. Neurosurg Focus 20(1):E11

Burger PC, Yu IT, Tihan T, Friedman HS, Strother DR, Kepner JL, Duffner PK, Kun LE, Perlman EJ (1998) Atypical teratoid/rhabdoid tumor of the central nervous system: a highly malignant tumor of infancy and childhood frequently mistaken for medulloblastoma: a pediatric oncology group study. Am J Surg Pathol 22(9):1083–1092

Chi SN, Zimmerman MA, Yao X, Cohen KJ, Burger P, Biegel JA, Rorke-Adams LB, Fisher MJ, Janss A, Mazewski C, Goldman S, Manley PE, Bowers DC, Bendel A, Rubin J, Turner CD, Marcus KJ, Goumnerova L, Ullrich NJ, Kieran MW (2009) Intensive multimodality treatment for children with newly diagnosed CNS atypical teratoid rhabdoid tumor. J Clin Oncol 27(3):385–389

Di Lorenzo N (1989) Transoral approach to extradural lesions of the lower clivus and upper cervical spine: an experience of 19 cases. Neurosurgery 24(1):37–42

Dougherty MJ, Santi M, Brose MS, Ma C, Resnick AC, Sievert AJ, Storm PB, Biegel JA (2010) Activating mutations in BRAF characterize a spectrum of pediatric low-grade gliomas. Neuro Oncol 12(7):621–630

Fraser JF, Nyquist GG, Moore N, Anand VK, Schwartz TH (2010) Endoscopic endonasal transclival resection of chordomas: operative technique, clinical outcome, and review of the literature. J Neurosurg 112(5):1061–1069

Frempong-Boadu AK, Faunce WA, Fessler RG (2002) Endoscopically assisted transoral-transpharyngeal approach to the craniovertebral junction. Neurosurgery 51(5 Suppl):S60–S66

Heuer GG, Jackson EM, Magge SN, Storm PB (2007) Surgical management of pediatric brain tumors. Expert Rev Anticancer Ther 7(12 Suppl):S61–S68

Heuer GG, Kiefer H, Judkins AR, Belasco J, Biegel JA, Jackson EM, Cohen M, O'Malley BW Jr, Storm PB (2010) Surgical treatment of a clival-C2 atypical teratoid/rhabdoid tumor. J Neurosurg Pediatr 5(1):75–79

Hilden JM, Meerbaum S, Burger P, Finlay J, Janss A, Scheithauer BW, Walter AW, Rorke LB, Biegel JA (2004) Central nervous system atypical teratoid/rhabdoid tumor: results of therapy in children enrolled in a registry. J Clin Oncol 22(14):2877–2884

Hirth A, Pedersen P-H, Wester K, Mork S, Helgestad J (2003) Cerebral atypical teratoid/rhabdoid tumor of infancy: long-term survival after multimodal treatment, also including triple intrathecal chemotherapy and gamma knife radiosurgery–case report. Pediatr Hematol Oncol 20(4):327–332

Howes TL, Buatti JM, O'Dorisio MS, Kirby PA, Ryken TC (2005) Atypical teratoid/rhabdoid tumor case report: treatment with surgical excision, radiation therapy, and alternative medicines. J Neurooncol 72(1):85–88

Jho HD, Carrau RL, McLaughlin MR, Somaza SC (1997) Endoscopic transsphenoidal resection of a large chordoma in the posterior fossa. Acta Neurochir (Wien) 139(4):343–347; discussion 347–348

Judkins AR, Mauger J, Ht A, Rorke LB, Biegel JA (2004) Immunohistochemical analysis of hSNF5/INI1 in pediatric CNS neoplasms. Am J Surg Pathol 28(5):644–650

Kazan S, Goksu E, Mihci E, Gokhan G, Keser I, Gurer I (2007) Primary atypical teratoid/rhabdoid tumor of the clival region. Case report. J Neurosurg 106(4 Suppl):308–311

Kelley TF, Stankiewicz JA, Chow JM, Origitano TC (1999) Endoscopic transsphenoidal biopsy of the sphenoid and clival mass. Am J Rhinol 13(1):17–21

Menezes AH (2008) Craniovertebral junction neoplasms in the pediatric population. Childs Nerv Syst 24(10):1173–1186

Packer RJ, Biegel JA, Blaney S, Finlay J, Geyer JR, Heideman R, Hilden J, Janss AJ, Kun L, Vezina G, Rorke LB, Smith M (2002) Atypical teratoid/rhabdoid tumor of the central nervous system: report on workshop. J Pediatr Hematol Oncol 24(5):337–342

Parsons DW, Li M, Zhang X, Jones S, Leary RJ, Lin JC, Boca SM, Carter H, Samayoa J, Bettegowda C, Gallia GL, Jallo GI, Binder ZA, Nikolsky Y, Hartigan J, Smith DR, Gerhard DS, Fults DW, VandenBerg S, Berger MS, Marie SK, Shinjo SM, Clara C, Phillips PC, Minturn JE, Biegel JA, Judkins AR, Resnick AC, Storm PB, Curran T, He Y, Rasheed BA, Friedman HS, Keir ST, McLendon R, Northcott PA, Taylor MD, Burger PC, Riggins GJ, Karchin R, Parmigiani G, Bigner DD, Yan H, Papadopoulos N, Vogelstein B, Kinzler KW, Velculescu VE (2011) The genetic landscape of the childhood cancer medulloblastoma. Science 331(6016):435–439

Pollack IF, Welch W, Jacobs GB, Janecka IP (1995) Frameless stereotactic guidance. An intraoperative adjunct in the transoral approach for ventral cervicomedullary junction decompression. Spine (Phila Pa 1976) 20(2): 216–220

Rorke LB, Packer RJ, Biegel JA (1996) Central nervous system atypical teratoid/rhabdoid tumors of infancy and childhood: definition of an entity. J Neurosurg 85(1):56–65

Sievert AJ, Jackson EM, Gai X, Hakonarson H, Judkins AR, Resnick AC, Sutton LN, Storm PB, Shaikh TH, Biegel JA (2009) Duplication of 7q34 in pediatric low-grade astrocytomas detected by high-density single-nucleotide polymorphism-based genotype arrays results in a novel BRAF fusion gene. Brain Pathol 19(3):449–458

Solares CA, Fakhri S, Batra PS, Lee J, Lanza DC (2005) Transnasal endoscopic resection of lesions of the clivus: a preliminary report. Laryngoscope 115(11):1917–1922

Squire SE, Chan MD, Marcus KJ (2007) Atypical teratoid/rhabdoid tumor: the controversy behind radiation therapy. J Neurooncol 81(1):97–111

Tekautz TM, Fuller CE, Blaney S, Fouladi M, Broniscer A, Merchant TE, Krasin M, Dalton J, Hale G, Kun LE, Wallace D, Gilbertson RJ, Gajjar A (2005) Atypical teratoid/rhabdoid tumors (ATRT): improved survival in children 3 years of age and older with radiation therapy and high-dose alkylator-based chemotherapy. J Clin Oncol 23(7):1491–1499

Yano S, Hida K, Kobayashi H, Iwasaki Y (2008) Successful multimodal therapies for a primary atypical teratoid/rhabdoid tumor in the cervical spine. Pediatr Neurosurg 44(5):406–413

Youssef AS, Sloan AE (2010) Extended transoral approaches: surgical technique and analysis. Neurosurgery 66(3 Suppl):126–134

Zimmerman MA, Goumnerova LC, Proctor M, Scott RM, Marcus K, Pomeroy SL, Turner CD, Chi SN, Chordas C, Kieran MW (2005) Continuous remission of newly diagnosed and relapsed central nervous system atypical teratoid/rhabdoid tumor. J Neurooncol 72(1):77–84

8 Pediatric Atypical Teratoid/ Rhabdoid Tumors: Dissemination to the Cerebrospinal Fluid

Junjeong Choi, Hyosun Kim, and Se Hoon Kim

Contents

J. Choi
Department of Pathology, Yonsei University Wonju College of Medicine, 162 Ilsadong Wonju, 220-701, Wonju, Republic of Korea
e-mail: junjeong@yonsei.ac.kr

H. Kim
Department of Pediatrics, Yonsei University College of Medicine, 50 Yonsei-ro Seodaemun-gu, Seoul, 120-752, Republic of Korea
e-mail: pseudosanta@yuhs.ac

S.H. Kim (✉)
Department of Pathology, Yonsei University College of Medicine, 50 Yonsei-ro Seodaemun-gu, Seoul, 120-752, Republic of Korea
e-mail: paxco@yuhs.ac

Abstract

About a third of the patients of atypical teratoid rhabdoid tumor (AT/RT) present with positive CSF cytology at the time of first diagnosis and spinal and leptomeningeal spread ultimately develops in more than a half of the patients regardless of the local recurrence of the disease. Thus, CSF cytology is clinically important in terms of the assessment of the disease and the determination of treatment modalities as well as monitoring the course of the disease and the response to the therapy. Most of the reported AT/RT cases described large atypical cells, abundant cytoplasm, eccentrically placed nuclei, and prominent nucleoli with cellular clustering in the CSF cytology. A potential association of E-cadherin in the cellular clustering in AT/RT was suggested with comparison of medulloblastoma cases. Chang's M staging has been used for AT/RT staging, but it is likely that the application of this system to all AT/RTs in diverse anatomical location has limitations. Accordingly, a new staging system should be developed. Liquid based cytology preparation is satisfactory for the morphologic diagnosis of AT/RT in CSF.

Introduction

Because of a dismal clinical course (Burger et al. 1998; Packer et al. 2002), intensive treatment with multimodalities was suggested for children

M.A. Hayat (ed.), *Pediatric Cancer, Volume 3: Diagnosis, Therapy, and Prognosis*, Pediatric Cancer 3,
DOI 10.1007/978-94-007-4528-5_8,

with newly diagnosed CNS atypical teratoid rhabdoid tumor (AT/RT) (Chi et al. 2009). This treatment consists of five phases; preirradiation, chemoradiation, consolidation, maintenance, and continuation therapy. Usually the dosage of chemo-agents or irradiation is adjusted based on the M staging and tumor extension of the patients. The patients with M0 disease receive intrathecal (IT) chemotherapy with a cycle of systemic chemotherapy, whereas the patients with positive CSF cytology at the time of diagnosis receive (IT) chemotherapy until two consecutive CSF samples are negative for malignant cells. Thus, CSF cytology of AT/RT is crucial in terms of diagnosis and monitoring the disease. In this chapter, we will discuss the general features of AT/RT dissemination to CSF.

Clinical Aspects of CSF Dissemination

The incidence of leptomeningeal dissemination of AT/RT at the time of diagnosis was reported to be up to 31% when assessed by CSF cytology (Burger et al. 1998; Athale et al. 2009). In spite of this, it is reported that only five of eight patients who were diagnosed as positive on imaging study diagnosed in the CSF cytology (Burger et al. 1998). Regardless of local recurrence of the disease, more than a half of the patients ultimately develop leptomeningeal and spinal spread (Rorke et al. 1996; Burger et al. 1998; Athale et al. 2009). Although the sensitivity of the CSF cytology is limited, it is clinically important in terms of the assessment of the disease and the determination of treatment modalities as well as monitoring the course of the disease and the response to the therapy. Thus Athale et al. (2009) proposed evaluating of CSF at diagnosis and intensifying treatment with IT medication.

Cytopathologic Features of AT/RT

The cytopathological features of AT/RT in CSF had been sporadically reported (Lu et al. 2000; Parwani et al. 2005; El-Nabbout et al. 2010; Huddleston et al. 2010). All reported cases commonly described cytological features, such as large atypical cells, abundant cytoplasm, eccentrically placed nuclei, and prominent nucleoli (Fig. 8.1). As AT/RT shows very diverse morphological features in histology, it may show various morphologies with wide spectrum in CSF. Huddleston et al. (2010) described a second population of smaller mononuclear cells with minimal cytoplasm as well as cells with typical morphologies.

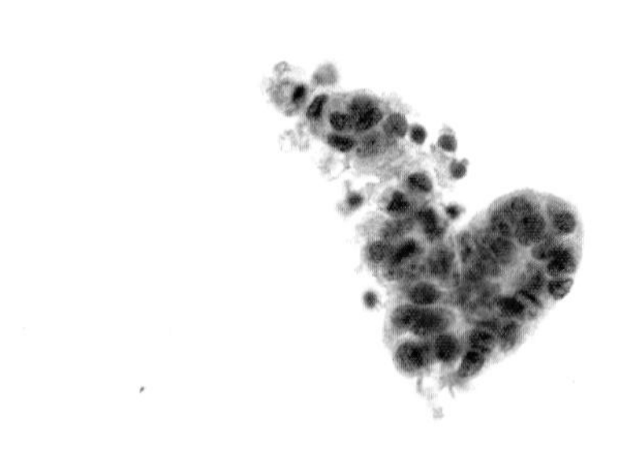
A

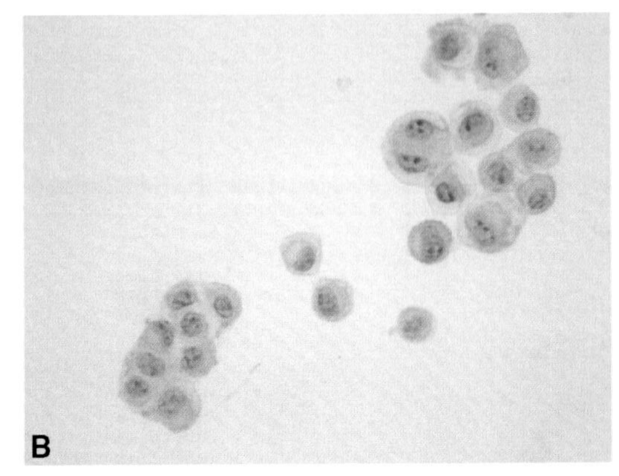
B

Fig. 8.1 Typical cellular cluster of AT/RT. (**a**, **b**) Tumor cell clusters with eccentric nuclei with prominent nucleoli and abundant cytoplasms (×600)

A recent collective review (Choi et al. 2010) compared many diverse features of cytomorphologies of AT/RT in CSF to their mimickers such as medulloblastoma, PNET, and metastatic carcinoma, malignant lymphoma, malignant melanoma, and germinoma. Especially, they proposed "clustering of tumor cells" as a specific cytological feature of AT/RT in CSF. They did

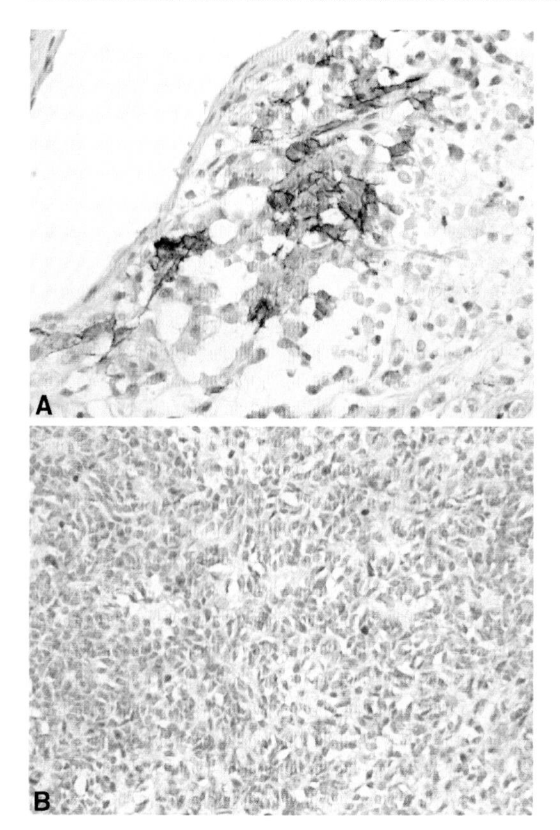

Fig. 8.2 E-cadherin immunohistochemical staining of AT/RT (**a**) and Medulloblastoma (**b**). (**a**) E-cadherin immunohistochemistry shows focal areas of positive reactions with membranous pattern in AT/RT (×400). (**b**) However there is no positive reaction in medulloblastoma (×400)

not elaborate the mechanism in the article, but the potential role of E-cadherin expression in the clustering of tumor cells was suggested in AT/RT since the expression is specific in AT/RT while medulloblastoma did not express E-cadherin (Utsuki et al. 2004) (Fig. 8.2).

Certainly, it is nearly impossible to diagnose AT/RT solely based on CSF cytology without clinical information, and the assessment of malignancy might be sufficient information. However, the cytological characteristics may help the diagnosis in certain specific cases such as the reported case of primary diffuse cererebral leptomeningeal AT/RT where tumor did not form discrete detectable mass like lesion (El-Nabbout et al. 2010). In this case, atypical cells in CSF were the major diagnostic clue clinically available. Thus, cytopathology may provide diagnostic information in a certain clinical situation.

Prospectives

The staging system for AT/RT was adopted from the previously known M staging for medulloblastoma (Chang et al. 1969; Chi et al. 2009). Staging of tumor is performed by assessing the extent of tumor in the neuroaxis. Although patients with a high risk of disseminated disease at presentation showed a high rate of relapse, the M stage of AT/RT did not seem to affect the patients' overall survival statistically (Chi et al. 2009). The result from metaanalysis suggested no relation of CSF positivity with the overall survival of the patients (Athale et al. 2009). Since most of the reported studies were performed in a limited number of patients and a standard treatment protocol has not been defined in the disease, the conclusion should be accepted with caution. It seems that the application of Chang's M staging to AT/RT without modification has limitations considering that the biological behaviors of AT/RTs seem quite different from those of medulloblastoma; for example, AT/RT occurs in various anatomical locations and some cases even showed multifocal nature of the tumors (Rorke et al. 1996). AT/RT accompanied with extra-CNS tumor adds additional complexities (Rorke et al. 1996). Thus, a new clinical staging system reflecting biological behavior of the disease should be developed.

Transitionally, CSF cytological evaluation was routinely performed with cytospin preparation. Liquid-based preparations (e.g., Thinprep and SurePath) were applied to many areas of non-gynecological specimens such as the thyroid and the lungs. Although this method had some limitations and disadvantages (Hoda 2007), it is endorsed as a satisfactory method for the assessment of cytomorphology. This preparation method can be applied to detect AT/RT in CSF.

References

Athale UH, Duckworth J, Odame I, Barr R (2009) Childhood atypical teratoid rhabdoid tumor of the central nervous system: a meta-analysis of observational studies. J Pediatr Hematol Oncol 31:651–663

Burger PC, Yu IT, Tihan T, Friedman HS, Strother DR, Kepner JL, Duffner PK, Kun LE, Perlman EJ (1998) Atypical teratoid/rhabdoid tumor of the central nervous system: a highly malignant tumor of infancy and childhood frequently mistaken for medulloblastoma: a pediatric oncology group study. Am J Surg Pathol 22:1083–1092

Chang CH, Housepian EM, Herbert C Jr (1969) An operative staging system and a megavoltage radiotherapeutic technic for cerebellar medulloblastomas. Radiology 93:1351–1359

Chi SN, Zimmerman MA, Yao X, Cohen KJ, Burger P, Biegel JA, Rorke-Adams LB, Fisher MJ, Janss A, Mazewski C, Goldman S, Manley PE, Bowers DC, Bendel A, Rubin J, Turner CD, Marcus KJ, Goumnerova L, Ullrich NJ, Kieran MW (2009) Intensive multimodality treatment for children with newly diagnosed CNS atypical teratoid rhabdoid tumor. J Clin Oncol 27:385–389

Choi J, Kim H, Kim SH (2010) Atypical teratoid/rhabdoid tumor: analysis of cytomorphologic features in CSF, focused on the differential diagnosis from mimickers. Diagn Cytopathol. doi:10.1002/dc.21594

El-Nabbout B, Shbarou R, Glasier CM, Saad AG (2010) Primary diffuse cerebral leptomeningeal atypical teratoid rhabdoid tumor: report of the first case. J Neurooncol 98:431–434

Hoda RS (2007) Non-gynecologic cytology on liquid-based preparations: a morphologic review of facts and artifacts. Diagn Cytopathol 35:621–634

Huddleston BJ, Sjostrom CM, Collins BT (2010) Atypical teratoid/rhabdoid tumor involving cerebrospinal fluid: a case report. Acta Cytol 54:958–962

Lu L, Wilkinson EJ, Yachnis AT (2000) CSF cytology of atypical teratoid/rhabdoid tumor of the brain in a two-year-old girl: a case report. Diagn Cytopathol 23:329–332

Packer RJ, Biegel JA, Blaney S, Finlay J, Geyer JR, Heideman R, Hilden J, Janss AJ, Kun L, Vezina G, Rorke LB, Smith M (2002) Atypical teratoid/rhabdoid tumor of the central nervous system: report on workshop. J Pediatr Hematol Oncol 24:337–342

Parwani AV, Stelow EB, Pambuccian SE, Burger PC, Ali SZ (2005) Atypical teratoid/rhabdoid tumor of the brain: cytopathologic characteristics and differential diagnosis. Cancer 105:65–70

Rorke LB, Packer RJ, Biegel JA (1996) Central nervous system atypical teratoid/rhabdoid tumors of infancy and childhood: definition of an entity. J Neurosurg 85:56–65

Utsuki S, Oka H, Sato Y, Tsutiya B, Kondo K, Tanizaki Y, Tanaka S, Fujii K (2004) E, N-cadherins and beta-catenin expression in medulloblastoma and atypical teratoid/rhabdoid tumor. Neurol Med Chir (Tokyo) 44:402–406; discussion 407

Part II

Medulloblastoma

9 Teratoid Pediatric Medullomyoblastoma

Uygur Er

Contents

Abstract

Cerebellar midline primitive neuroectodermal tumours containing muscle fibers generally referred to as medullomyoblastoma. Medullomyoblastoma is almost exclusively seen in children. The clinical findings are similar to the every midline posterior fossa tumour. Clinical history is typically brief, the prognosis is very poor. Medullomyoblastomas are seen as solid lesion on computerized tomography and magnetic resonance imaging. They enhance with intravenous contrast media on all imaging sequences. There are four main theories considering histogenesis of the muscle fibers within the tumour. It is accepted as a teratoma or a teratoid tumour widely. Surgical debulking is essential part of the treatment. Postoperative radiotherapy and chemotherapy may be beneficial for lengthening of the survival time. Pathologic examination generally shows two distinct patterns in different areas. Both malignant apparent striated and smooth muscle fibers can be found within the tumour. The documented myogenic differentiation is necessary for the definitive diagnosis.

Introduction

Primary tumours of the central nervous system (CNS) containing muscle elements are exceptional. These tumours generally tend to occur in the cerebellum but may also found in other sites in the CNS. Medullomyoblastoma (MMB) was

U. Er (✉)
Neurosurgery Clinic, TOBB ETU Hospital, The Union of Chambers and Commodity Exchanges of Turkey, Economics and Technology University, Sogutozu C., Fourth Sk., No. 22/7, 06510 Cankaya, Ankara, Turkey
e-mail: uygurer@gmail.com

M.A. Hayat (ed.), *Pediatric Cancer, Volume 3: Diagnosis, Therapy, and Prognosis*, Pediatric Cancer 3,
DOI 10.1007/978-94-007-4528-5_9,

described firstly by Marinesco and Goldstein (1933) that a tumour consisting medulloblastic and myogenic elements. It was firstly suggested by these authors that skeletal muscle differentiation in medulloblastoma (MB) resulted from metaplasia of smooth muscle within blood vessels of the brain. Subsequently some authors classified these tumours as teratoma because of its skeletal muscle including (Ingraham and Bailey 1946). Primitive neuroectodermal tumours (PNET) containing muscle fibers and localized to the cerebellar vermis generally referred to as MMB (Smith and Davidson 1984). Some authors have preferred to classify them as variants of malignant teratoma or teratoid tumour (Er et al. 2008). Controversies on exact origin of cells and categorization of MMB are still continuing.

Epidemyology and Clinic

The most frequent embryonal neoplasm of the neuroepithelial tissue in children is MB (Er et al. 2008). In children, MB comprises about 15–20% of intracranial tumours (Laurent and Cheek 1985), 30–55% of posterior fossa tumours (Allen 1985). It was estimated by Cheema et al. (2001) that its annual incidence is 0.5 per 100,000 children younger than 15 years. The median age at diagnosis is 4.5 years and male to female ratio is changing from 2 to 4.5. MMB is a quite-rarely reported biphasic histological variant of this frequent pathology (Er et al. 2008). Since Marinesco and Goldstein's first report, too little cases have been reported in the literature. MMB is almost exclusively seen in children, only a few adult MMB cases can be found in the literature (Rao et al. 1990).

The clinical findings of a MMB are similar to the every midline posterior fossa tumour. Clinical history is typically brief (6–12 weeks). Patients with MMB tend to develop early obstructive hydrocephalus. Headache, nausea and vomiting, truncal and appendicular ataxia are typical presenting symptoms. Drop metastases may produce back pain, urinary retention and paraparesias. Papilledema, extraocular muscle palsies, ataxia and nystagmus are common signs. The prognosis of MMB is very poor with less than 2 years average survival time (Er et al. 2008).

Diagnosis

MMBs are usually seen as solid lesion on computerized tomography (CT) and magnetic resonance imaging (MRI). Tumour is hyperdense on noncontrast CT, hypo- to isointense on T1-Weighted images (T1-WI) and heterogeneous on T2-WI of MRI. Some MMBs can be seen heterogeneously hyperintense on T1-WI (Fig. 9.1), (Er et al. 2008). Majority of tumours enhance with intravenous contrast media on all sequences. Postcontrast sequences may also reveal slight peripheral oedema (Er et al. 2008). All midline posterior fossa tumours should consider for differential diagnosis. The documented myogenic differentiation is necessary for the definitive diagnosis.

Histogenesis of Muscle Fibers in MMB

Muscle fibers in MMB were considered by Marinesco and Goldstein (1933) that they have originated through a dysembryogenetic process or from the metaplastic transformation of

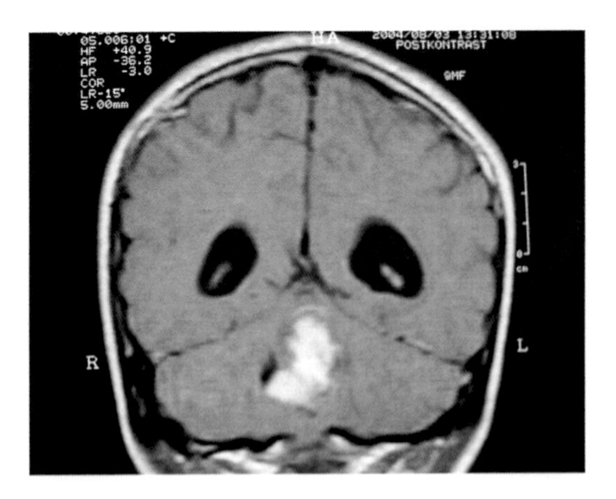

Fig. 9.1 A coronal T1-WI, postcontrast MRI reveals a heterogeneously enhanced hyperintense vermian mass and slight brain stem compression

vascular smooth muscle cells. Ingraham and Bailey (1946) proposed that this tumour was a variant of malignant teratoma or a teratoid tumour. The concept that the muscle fibers in MMB may be derived from unstable pluripotential mesenchymal cell within or vicinity of the tumour was suggested by Lewis (1973) and Stahlberger and Friede (1977). It has been implied that the neoplastic MB cells induce perivascular ecto-mesenchymal cells to differentiate into muscle fibers (Smith and Davidson 1984). Walter and Brucher (1979) proposed the third hypothesis. According to this hypothesis, the myoblastic component is derived from the multipotential endothelial cells. Another hypothesis about the histogenesis of the muscle fibers in MMB takes into account that they derive directly from the primitive neuroepithelial cells (Smith and Davidson 1984). This hypothesis is based on the concept that the primitive neuroectodermal cells are pluripotential and possess myogenic capabilities.

Treatment

Surgical debulking is essential part of the treatment. Resection as much tumour as possible without neurological deficits may augment the benefit of postsurgery treatments. There are some evidences that radiotherapy (RT) after a total removal of MMB may lengthen survival time to 4 years at least (Helton et al. 2004; Holl et al. 1991). Optimal irradiation dose is 35–40 Gy to whole craniospinal axis plus 10–15 Gy boost to tumour bed. For age under 3 year-old dose reduced by 20–25% or chemotherapy is given instead. Chemotherapy with cisplatin, vincristine plus cyclophosphamide or lomustine; or neoadjuvant chemotherapy with cisplatin and etoposide were applied with little success (Er et al. 2008; Abenoza and Wick 1986). Patients frequently require permanent ventriculoperitoneal shunts following tumour resection. Younger age of the patient, especially under 3 age, disseminated disease, and inability to perform total resection are poor prognosticators for MMB.

Pathology

MMBs can be observed in a broad microscopic spectrum of cellular differentiation and varying anaplasia (Er et al. 2008). Light microscopic examination generally shows two distinct patterns in different areas. One area is seen as well-circumscribed, cellular small cell tumour with prominent stromal desmoplasia (Fig. 9.2). The tumour cells have small, ovoid nuclei with homogenous chromaffin and scanty amount of cytoplasm (Abenoza and Wick 1986). Mitoses are abundant and occasional Homer-Wright rosettes are observed. The other area consisted of interlacing bundles spindle cells, many of which are steplike with deeply eosinophilic cytoplasm (Chowdhury et al. 1985). Both striated and smooth muscle fibers can be found within MMB, and these muscular elements generally present a malignant appearance (Fig. 9.3), (Er et al. 2008). Glial fibrillary acidic protein (GFAP) stain may show scattered immunoreactive small cells in internal areas of the tumour. Neuron specific enolase (NSE) is present almost 70% of the neoplastic cells (Abenoza and Wick 1986). Tumour cells show strong synaptophysin positivity. Myogenic expression in muscular strands makes their rhabdomyoblastic character clear (Er et al. 2008).

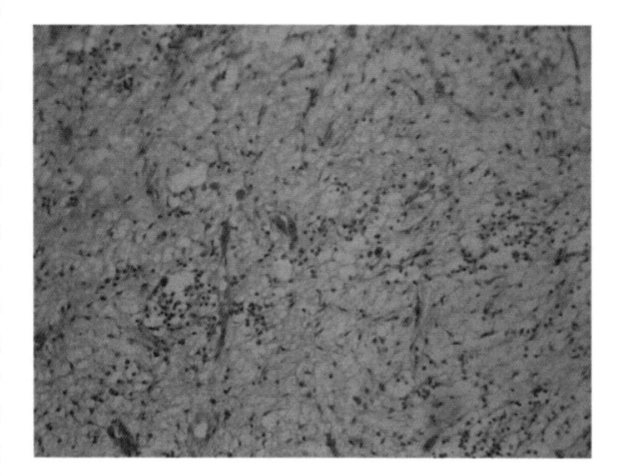

Fig. 9.2 The tumor composed of small, round, hyperchromatic cells with scant cytoplasm in hematoxylin and eosin (HE) stained sections is observed

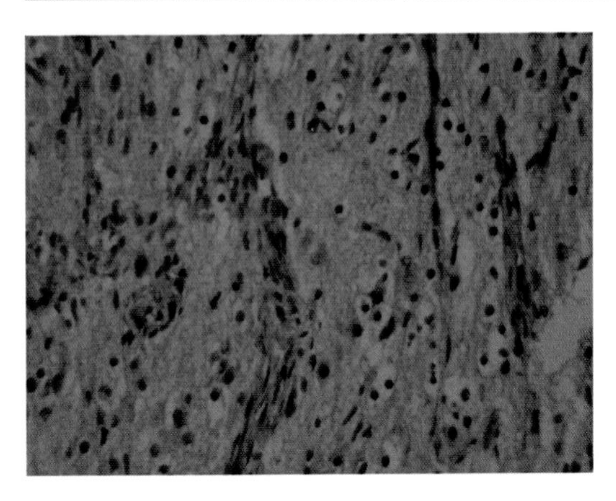

Fig. 9.3 Myogenin positivity in myoblastic cells is seen

Electron microscopy has confirmed the divergent neuroepithelial and rhabdomyoblastic differentiating features of the tumour cells. Both astrocytic and neuronal differentiation can be demonstrated in some cases, but in others only neuronal or neuroblastic differentiation is present. The cytoplasms of the cells are scanty with few organelles consisting mainly of mitochondria, ribosome and rough endoplasmic reticulum (Abenoza and Wick 1986). Distinct Z bands and mixture of thick and thin cytoplasmic filaments of rhabdomyoblasts can be seen ultrastructurally.

References

Abenoza P, Wick MR (1986) Primitive neuroectodermal tumor with rabdomyoblastic differentiation. Ultrastruct Pathol 10:347–354

Allen JC (1985) Childhood brain tumors: current status of clinical trials in newly diagnosed and recurrent disease. Pediatr Clin North Am 32:633–651

Cheema ZF, Cannon TC, Leech R, Brennan J, Adesina A, Brumback RA (2001) Medullomyoblastoma: case report. J Child Neurol 16(8):598–599

Chowdhury C, Roy S, Mahapatra AK, Bhatia R (1985) Medullomyoblastoma. A teratoma. Cancer 55:1495–1500

Er U, Yigitkanli K, Kazanci B, Ozturk E, Sorar M, Bavbek M (2008) Teratoid nature of a quite rare neoplasm. Surg Neurol 69:403–406

Helton KJ, Fouladi M, Boop PA, Perry A, Dalton J, Kun L, Fuller C (2004) Medullomyoblastoma: a radiographic and clinicopathologic analysis of six cases and review of the literature. Cancer 101:1445–1454

Holl T, Klehues P, Yaşargil MG, Wiestler OD (1991) Cerebellar medullomyoblastoma with advanced neuronal differentiation and hamartomatous component. Acta Neuropathol 82:408–413

Ingraham F, Bailey O (1946) Cystic teratomas and teratoid tumors of central nervous system in infancy and childhood. J Neurosurg 3:511–532

Laurent JP, Cheek WR (1985) Brain tumors in children. J Pediatr Neurosci 1:15–32

Lewis AJ (1973) Medulloblastoma with striated muscle fibers: case report. J Neurosurg 38:642–646

Marinesco G, Goldstein M (1933) Sur une forme anatomique non encore décrite, de médulloblastome: medullo-myo-blastome. Ann Anat Pathol 10:513–525

Rao C, Friedlander ME, Klein E, Anzil AP, Sher JH (1990) Medullomyoblastoma in an adult. Cancer 65:157–163

Smith TW, Davidson RI (1984) Medullomyoblastoma. A histologic, immunohistochemical and ultrastructural study. Cancer 54:323–332

Stahlberger R, Friede RL (1977) Fine structure of medulloblastoma. Acta Neuropathol (Berl) 37:43–48

Walter GF, Brucher JM (1979) Ultrastructural study of medullomyoblastoma. Acta Neuropathol (Berl) 48:211–214

Pediatric Medulloblastoma: Mechanisms of Initiation and Progression

10

Wayne D. Thomas and Jinbiao Chen

Contents

W.D. Thomas (✉)
Cell-Innovations Pty Limited, 21b Bathurst St, Liverpool, NSW 2071, Australia
e-mail: wthomas@cell-innovations.com.au

J. Chen
Centenary Institute of Cancer Medicine and Cell Biology, Bld 93, Royal Prince Alfred Hospital, Missenden Rd, Camperdown NSW 2050, Australia

Abstract

Medulloblastoma is the most common brain tumor in children. Despite multimodal therapy, survival is poor. In this review we highlight the pathogenesis of medulloblastoma, and the signalling pathways which may contribute to medulloblastoma tumorigenesis. Medulloblastoma is a neuro-embryonal tumor that presents many cellular characteristics similar to that of the precursor cells of the embryonic cerebellum. Clarification of the cells of origin, in addition, to the mechanisms of initiation, promotion, and progression of tumor are key steps that need to be unravelled to enable the identification of new therapeutic targets for medulloblastoma.

Introduction

It is now considered that tumorigenesis occurs in three phases initiation, promotion, and progression; with the transition from normal tissue to tumor being a multi-step process (Knudson 1971). Neuro-embryonal tumors (such as medulloblastoma), in comparison to adult tumors, have a shortened latency period, fewer genetic aberrations, and a reduced loss of apoptotic regulators. The rationale for this is that these cancers arise from embryonal cells that have persisted beyond birth, and may already be proliferating as part of a developmental process, to later undergo changes which result in clinical tumors.

M.A. Hayat (ed.), *Pediatric Cancer, Volume 3: Diagnosis, Therapy, and Prognosis*, Pediatric Cancer 3, DOI 10.1007/978-94-007-4528-5_10,

Neuro-development in the embryo and child requires the proliferation, migration, and maturation of neural crest cells. Neural crest cells are multipotent transient cells that give rise to diverse cell lineages during development. During neural development there is the requirement that cell numbers are greatly over-produced with only a minority (15–40%) of post-migratory cells surviving to form mature neural tissues. Those cells which have not differentiated or made appropriate connections are eliminated, suggestive of a selection process (Lossi and Merighi 2003). Over 100 years ago Durante (1874) and Cohnheim (1889) hypothesized that those cell remnants, or 'rests', that survive postnatal after normal neurodevelopment may later become tumorigenic. The embryonal cells, or 'rests', that persist and later go on to form tumors must have the capacity to resist cell death, and, undergo secondary changes which characterize later tumor promotion and progression. This review will focus on the molecular basis of medulloblastoma formation and progression. We also provide an overview of the signaling pathways involved in medulloblastoma tumorigenesis.

Development of the Human Cerebellum

Located near the base of the brain the cerebellum is divided into two lateral hemispheres connected by the median part, the cerebellar vermis. A set of large folds divide the structure into ten smaller lobules. Development of the human cerebellum is long and protracted, and occurs both in the embryonic period and postnatal over the first year. The complex neuronal arrangement in the cerebellum begins with two distinctive germinal layers; the ventricular and the external granule layer (EGL). The ventricular zone is active during embryonic development, and produces both Purkinje and deep cerebellar nuclear neurons. The EGL is a transient zone that forms the granule neuron precursors (GNPs).

Granule neuron precursors originate from the embryonic rhombic lip a specialized germinative epithelium. They migrate rostrally over the surface of the cerebellum to form the EGL, where once formed, a second wave of cell divisions within the EGL produces post-mitotic granule cells. This transient germinal zone of GNPs undergoes expansion during early postnatal life, and then either dies, or migrates inwards along the Bergmann glial fibers in the molecular layer. Once passed the molecular layer and in the internal granule layer (IGL) the GNPs further differentiate to become mature granule neurons. The EGL ceases to exist as cell proliferation ends, and post-mitotic neurons move to the internal granule layer (Fig. 10.1). The duration and intensity of the proliferation phase of the EGL is critical to enable the final shape and function of the cerebellum. The proliferation phase is regulated, in part, by the Purkinje cells that migrate radially towards the EGL and secrete the morphogen sonic hedgehog (Shh).

Once developed the cerebellum consists of three distinct cellular layers. The innermost layer being largely white matter that consist of myelinated nerve fibers which run to and from the cortex. The middle layer of densely packed granule cells along with Golgi cells, which are surrounded by Purkinje cell bodies. The third and outer layer is formed by the molecular layer (Fig. 10.1c, d). The complex developmental regime which enables the final development of the cerebellum requires a fine balance between proliferation, migration, differentiation, and death of cells. These intricate cellular programs, in addition, to the prolonged developmental time, may well make the cerebellum more susceptible to developmental errors.

Tumorigenesis of Medulloblastoma

Medulloblastoma often arise on the outside of the cerebellar, where the EGL is present during development, and often express GNP markers. It is postulated that persistent GNPs in the EGL during the final stages of cerebellar development may result in medulloblastoma (Kadin et al. 1970). The proliferation, differentiation and migration of GNPs is largely controlled by three distinct signalling pathways: the sonic hedgehog (Shh), Wnt and Notch. Mutations observed in these key pathways account for 25%, 15%, and 15%, respectively, of mutations

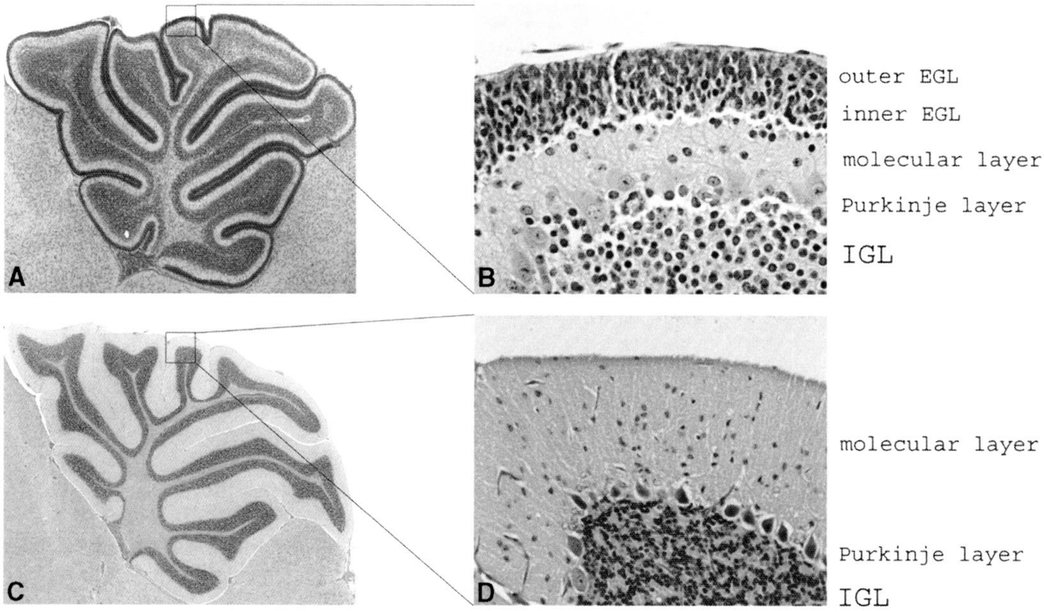

Fig. 10.1 Cerebellum development in the murine model. Photomicrographs of hematoxylin and eosin (H & E) staining of a murine cerebellum. (**a**) Staining of the developing cerebellum of postnatal day 7 (P7) wild-type mice. (**b**) Enlarged region of an EGL in a P7 cerebellum. (**c**) Adult wild-type mouse cerebellum. (**d**) Enlarged region of the surface of an adult mouse cerebellum

in medulloblastoma (Fan et al. 2004). These mutations are associated with less favorable clinical outcomes. Failure to regulate and switch off these developmental signaling pathways in the cerebellum is considered a pivotal event for medulloblastoma tumorigenesis, in addition to failure to die. Genes also noted to be associated with both proliferation of GNPs and medulloblastoma include: *Notch2*, *N-Myc*, *Mad3*, *Bmi1*, *cyclin D1*, *cyclin D2*, *Patched (Ptch)*, *Smoothened (Smo)*, *Gli1*, *Gli2*, *Wnt*, *β-catenin*, *Ren*, *Trp53*, *Insulin-like growth factor-2 (Igf-2)*, and *Math1* (reviewed in Behesti and Marino 2009). These genes are largely controlled by the developmental signaling pathways Shh, Wnt, and Notch.

Although persistent GNPs may result in medulloblastoma, histological variants and diverse genetic expressions suggest, however, that different cells of origin may also play a role. There are currently five histological variants of medulloblastoma that are recognized by the World Health Organization (2007) (Louis et al. 2007): (1) classical medulloblastoma (primarily undifferentiated cells with highly hyperchromatic nuclei, and little cytoplasm); (2) the large cell variant; (3) anaplastic tumors; (4) the desmoplastic variant and; (5) extensive nodularity. The desmoplastic variant is strongly associated with uncontrolled sonic hedgehog activation in both human and murine models. Eberhart (2007) has reported that medulloblastoma may also originate from stem/progenitor cells along the ventricles. Furthermore, Yang et al. (2008) demonstrated that hedgehog activated multipotent neural stem cells only formed medulloblastoma after they had committed to a neuronal lineage. Thus specific linage differentiation may be required for stem/progenitor cells to form medulloblastoma.

Sonic Hedgehog Pathway

The Shh signaling pathway is one of the central players in cerebellar development, regulating both expansion of the EGL and patterning. Granule neuron precursors proliferate rapidly under the paracrine influence of a Shh signal, originating from the Purkinje cell layer, to form

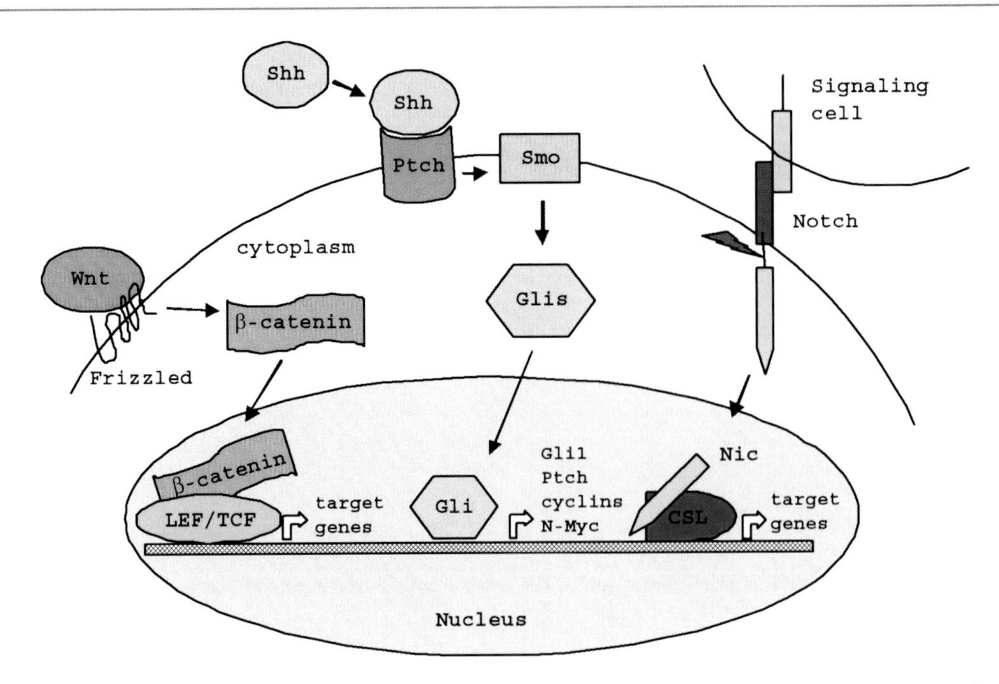

Fig. 10.2 A simplified schematic diagram of the three developmental signaling pathways: *Shh*, *Wnt*, and *Notch*, and their associations

the EGL before migrating and undergoing terminal differentiation in the IGL. The Shh protein is a member of the hedgehog family, and acts at the local level to drive GNP proliferation and cell fate through the Patched1 (Ptch1) and Smoothened (Smo) membrane proteins. In the absence of Shh, Ptch1 maintains Smo in an inactive state, thus silencing intracellular signaling. With the binding of Shh, Ptch1 inhibition of Smo is released, and the signal is transduced (Fig. 10.2).

Once activated the Shh-pathway mediates expression of downstream transcription factors including the Gli zinc-finger transcription factors (*Gli1*, *Gli2*, and *Gli3*) and *Bmi1*, *Smo*, and *N-Myc*. It is unclear whether the Gli proteins mediate all aspects of Shh-signaling. Pathway members that may act between Smo and Gli include negative regulators such as Suppressor of Fused (Sufu), Rab23, or Ren, as well as proteins exerting a positive effect on hedgehog signaling, such as intraflagellar transport proteins, tectonic, or Missing in Metastasis (MIM)/BEG4.

Sonic hedgehog-driven GNP proliferation is terminated in the EGL, with the EGL composed of two distinct layers: the outer EGL where GNPs actively proliferate, and the inner EGL which contain post-mitotic and pre-migratory GNPs. Several components have been shown to overcome Shh-induced proliferation and include: the extracellular matrix molecule vitronectin which is highly expressed within the inner EGL; forskolin which is activated by the pituitary adenylate cyclase activating peptide; basic fibroblast growth factor (bFGF); and bone morphogenic proteins (BMP's).

Sonic hedgehog-pathway dysregulation in medulloblastoma tumorigenesis was first suggested following the discovery that *Ptch1* is mutated in Gorlin's syndrome. Mutations in the *Ptch1* gene occur in ~8% of medulloblastoma, with aberrant regulation of the Shh signaling pathway noted in ~25% of medulloblastoma, including mutations in both *Smo* and *Sufu*. The second evidence for Shh-pathway involvement in tumorigenesis comes from murine models with knockout *Ptch* (Goodrich et al. 1997) or deregulated Shh signaling by either mutation or uncontrolled signaling. Dysregulation of the

Shh-pathway results in GNP overgrowth and transformation that faithfully recapitulates the biology of human medulloblastoma, in particular, desmoplastic medulloblastoma. This fundamental embryonic pathway is now believed to be a major driver of tumorigenesis in both child and adult, and may be prevalent in up to ~25% of all human cancers.

Gli Signaling and Medulloblastoma

The *Gli* transcription family consists of *Gli1*, *Gli2*, and *Gli3*; and is at the distal end of the Shh-pathway. *Gli1* is activated transcriptionally in the presence of Shh, possibly by pre-existing Gli2 or Gli3; Gli2 and Gli3 may act as both activators and repressors (Sasaki et al. 1999). A complex positive autoregulatory and negative feedback mechanism for the proto-oncogene *Gli1* regulates both the duration and strength of its signal.

Over expression of *Gli1* is present in approximately 30% of human medulloblastoma (Lee et al. 2003), with expression characterizing the desmoplastic subgroup of medulloblastoma. It has been proposed that sustained activation of Shh/Gli signaling during cerebellum development may disrupt the normal patterning of GNPs in the EGL, and initiate a persistent proliferative state of GNPs. These tumor initiating cells may then accrue enough oncogenic hits to drive tumor promotion and progression, in part, by progressively higher activating states of Gli1. This model provides an explanation for the observation that cerebellar tumor incidence is reduced in $Gli1^{-/-}/Ptch1^{+/-}$ mice, in comparison to $Ptch1^{+/-}$ mice (Kimura et al. 2005). The oncogenic function of *Gli1* is also supported by its ability *in vitro* to transform primary cells in co-operation with the E1A adenovirus.

Recently Yoon et al. (2009) identified 25 genes that are regulated by *Gli1* in medulloblastoma. The reactivation of these target genes were likely to drive developmental pathways that contribute to cell proliferation, survival, and genomic stability. It is proposed that these processes operate by the involvement of CXCR4, and by linking with p53, serum/glucocorticoid regulated kinase 1, O-6-methylguanine-DNA methyltransferase, and neurotrophic tyrosine kinase, receptor, type 2. Given the broad gamut of biological activities controlled by Shh/Gli signaling it is likely that there are additional routes which may initiate dysregulation of cellular processes when *Gli* signaling is reactivated or continues to be activated inappropriately.

N-Myc Signaling and Medulloblastoma

Cerebellar development requires only a brief transient expression of *N-Myc* to drive GNP proliferation, and provide mature granule neurons for a functional internal granule layer. In contrast, continued *N-Myc* expression in GNPs is a key factor contributing to Shh-driven medulloblastoma tumorigenesis (Hatton et al. 2006).

N-Myc is a member of the *Myc* transcription family, and has critical roles in cell cycle regulation (reviewed in Thomas et al. 2004). It is induced by both hedgehog and Wnt signaling pathways, and operates in a heterodimeric complex with Max to bind to E-Box motifs in DNA, thereby transcriptionally regulating hundreds to thousands of target genes. These target genes encode proteins with key roles in proliferation, cell cycle regulation, apoptosis, and genomic instability. *N-Myc* is essential for normal cerebellar growth (Kenney et al. 2003).

Physiological studies on *N-Myc* in GNPs report its involvement in mitosis, with its degradation crucial to cell cycle exit (Sjostrom et al. 2005). *N-Myc* transcription is increased during Shh-signaling with the Cdk1 complex reported to regulate the phosphorylation of serine-62-N-Myc (S62-N-Myc), priming N-Myc for degradation (Kenney et al. 2004; Sjostrom et al. 2005). Subsequently threnione-58-N-Myc (T58-N-Myc) is phosphorylated by glycogen synthase kinase (GSK-3β). Upon both sites being phosphorylated it is proposed, though debatable, that Pin1 and protein phosphatase (PP2A) interact to dephosphorylate $S62^{P}$-N-Myc. The ubiquitin ligase Fbxw7 is then able to target $T58^{P}$-N-Myc and permit proteasomal degradation.

Elevated *N-Myc* expression is present in medulloblastoma, particularly desmoplastic. In addition, other studies have reported up to ~68% of medulloblastoma having *N-Myc* mRNA present, although weakly expressed, indicative that perhaps it may have roles in other subtypes. It has been suggested that *Myc's* ability to induce genomic instability may increase the probability that tumors will escape from oncogene dependence. Studies on *N-Myc* oncogenesis have shown both epigenetic as well as genetic mechanisms including chromosomal translocations, genomic amplification, and transcription to be involved. Our studies have also recently demonstrated that protein stabilization of *N-Myc* by dysregulation of its degradation pathway may be one more mechanism, in the initiation and progression of tumor in the *Ptch1*$^{+/-}$ mouse model. Increased N-Myc protein typified the earliest selection of GNP focal hyperplasia destined for later tumor progression, rather than *N-Myc* mRNA, and effected enhanced proliferation and death resistance of GNPs. Increased expression of phosphorylated S62-N-Myc characterized this early stage of tumorigenesis (Thomas et al. 2009).

Wnt Pathway

Normal development of the cerebellum requires the activation of the Wnt-pathway. The Wnt-pathway is best known for its role in controlling early cell fate and differentiation of cells in the cerebellum. Wnt proteins exert their effects by binding to the ligand Frizzled and activating a cascade of downstream events, resulting in the destabilization of a stable multiprotein complex containing GSK-3β. The disruption of the multiprotein complex leads to nuclear accumulation of β-catenin, thereby activating Wnt target genes including *c-myc*, *cyclin D1*, and *Axin 2* (Fig. 10.2). GSK-3β is a multi-tasking kinase that has been shown to have critical roles in both Shh- and Wnt-signaling.

Approximately 15% of human medulloblastoma have genetic mutations impairing the Wnt signaling transduction pathway, with expression associated with classical medulloblastoma. Deregulation of the Wnt-pathway has been demonstrated to be present in both familial and sporadic medulloblastoma (Turcot et al. 1959). The significance of Wnt activation in medulloblastoma is still to be determined as pathogenic activation of Wnt appears to result in a less aggressive variant of medulloblastoma, and over expression of β-catenin is not sufficient to promote GNP proliferation or cerebellar tumors in postnatal transgenic mice (Fults et al. 2002). Although, mutations have been observed that affect the highly conserved β-catenin phosphorylation sites which are involved in protein stability. There is now sufficient evidence to indicate potential co-operation between the Shh and Wnt signaling pathways in medulloblastoma tumorigenesis, although, further studies are needed to clarify the role of the Wnt-pathway in the initiation and progression of tumor.

Notch Pathway

The Notch-pathway is physiologically important in the development of the EGL. Its role in cerebellum development, although, not implicated in the initial generation of progenitors *in vivo,* does influence both cell fate decision and induction of terminal differentiation of GNPs. The Notch family has several Notch receptors (Notch 1–4), and when cleaved the intracellular domain (Nic) is translocated to the nucleus where it forms a complex with a number of proteins including the CBF1/Suppressor of Hairless/Lag1 (CSL). This process results in the activation of target genes including: *Hairy-Enhancer of Split (Hes)1, Hes5, cyclin D1, p21, and NF-κB* (Fig. 10.2).

Notch 1 and *2* are expressed during cerebellar development. *Notch 1* is expressed primarily in post-mitotic differentiating cells, with loss of conditional *Notch 1* leading to incomplete differentiation and elimination of GNPs, and patterning of the cerebellar (Fan et al. 2004). *Notch 2* is predominately expressed in proliferating GNPs in the EGL. Analogous studies in medulloblastoma observed *Notch 1* expression to be scarce, in contrast, to *Notch 2* which is over expressed (Fan et al. 2004). Moreover, activation of *Notch 1* or *2* in medulloblastoma cell lines has antagonistic effects on medulloblastoma growth. Interestingly, recent studies have also demonstrated constitutive activation of the Shh-pathway in a SmoA1 murine model is sufficient to induce the Notch-pathway in GNPs, with *Notch 2* and the Notch target gene *Hes5* elevated. Dakubo et al. (2006) has reported the expression of several components of the Notch and Wnt signaling pathways in tumor from $Ptch^{+/-}$ mice. Indeed, medulloblastoma in both mice and humans have been found to have a concomitant increase in Shh- and Notch-pathway activities, both of which contributed to tumor survival.

MicroRNAs

MicroRNAs (miRNAs) a family of mature noncoding small RNAs ~19–23 regulate protein expression by targeting mRNA stability and translation. Recent data has provided evidence that miRNAs have a partiality for targeting developmental genes, play an extensive role in brain development, and in the development of brain cancers. Expression profiling has unveiled miRNA signatures that not only distinguish brain tumors from normal tissue, but can distinguish subtypes with altered genetic pathways. In human medulloblastoma currently 78 miRNAs have been identified as altered by expression profiling, in comparison, to normal cerebellar cells. Over 13 aberrantly expressed miRNA are demonstrated to be present in Shh-dependent anaplastic or desmoplastic medulloblastoma, with these linked to cell proliferation or apoptosis (reviewed in Turner et al. 2010). In particular, the miRNA-17~92 cluster has been recognized to be elevated in human medulloblastoma that have an activated Shh-signal (Uziel et al. 2009). Furthermore, the miRNA-17~92 cluster is observed to cooperate with the Shh-pathway in $Ptch1^{+/-}$ mice for the development of cerebellar tumor (Uziel et al. 2009). It has now become clear that miRNA are essential in the development of the cerebellum, with dysregulation contributing to the pathogenesis of medulloblastoma.

Cell Death Resistance

One of the initial stages necessary for embryonal tumor initiation is the survival or resistance to death of those cells that would normally be eliminated during neuro-development (Hansford et al. 2004). Little consideration until recently has been given to early cerebellar post-migratory cell death or mechanisms of resistance leading to tumor initiation. While apoptotic cells are present *in vivo* in the EGL during development, a quantitative estimate of cell death is not easy. The concurrent cell proliferation, differentiation, and rapid clearance of dead cells from this tissue, makes assessment difficult (Lossi and Merighi 2003).

It has been proposed that for neural progenitor cells to survive and permit rapid proliferation, the normal balance between apoptotic proteins are altered towards reduced proapoptotic proteins and increased antiapoptotic proteins (Johnsen et al. 2009). Other studies have indicated the existence of caspase-dependent and -independent apoptotic pathways that affect cerebellar granule cells at different stages of their life. Lossi et al. (2004) has reported that GNP apoptosis may occur in the absence of caspase-3 cleavage. The *Ptch* protein is also observed to have a role in mediating cell death through a smoothened-independent mechanism, and that Gli-3 may act as an inducer of apoptosis. In addition to those intrinsic factors, many extrinsic factors have been identified that may inhibit GNP death including: Igf, Shh, brain derived neurotrophic factor (BDNF), NT-4, and NT-5.

Neurotrophic factors such as BDNF are potent survival factors for cerebellar granule cells, as demonstrated by BDNF knockout mice having increased death of granule cells. Proliferation and survival of GNPs heavily depend on the presence of Shh, with a graded Shh signaling present in the EGL. The withdrawal of Shh *in vitro* from wild-type GNPs leads to cell death (Thomas et al. 2009). Moreover, postnatal $Ptch1^{+/-}$ mice GNPs exhibit increased survival when the Shh neurotrophic factor is withdrawn, in comparison, to wild-type GNPs. This survival is reversed when GNPs are transfected with siRNA for *N-Myc* (Calao et al. unpublished data). Another factor recognized as being mediated by the Shh/Gli1-pathway and inducing resistance to cell death in GNPs is *Bcl-2*. Over expression of *Bcl-2* in association with activation of the Shh-pathway induces a high frequency of medulloblastoma in mice.

Insulin-like growth factor is crucial for brain development and acts by regulating GSK-3β activity thru the PI3 kinase signaling cascade. Insulin-like growth factor-1 is thought to enable cell death resistance in trophic factor deprived GNPs by suppressing key elements of the mitochondrial death pathway including induction of *Bim* and *caspase-3*. Transgenic mice over-expressing Igf-1 have been observed to develop increased numbers of cerebellar granule neurons as a result of a decreased rate of apoptotic developmental elimination. The anti-apoptotic effect is related to an early over-expression of the antiapoptotic genes *Bcl-2* and *Bcl-X*, and a down regulation of the proapoptotic genes *Bax* and *Bad*. Reduced activity of *caspase-3* and cleavage substrates is also associated with over-expression of Igf-1.

While *N-Myc* over-expression *in vitro* induces an aggressive metastatic phenotype and increased proliferation rate, ironically *N-Myc* also suppresses Bcl-2, activates Bax, and sensitizes cells to genotoxicity-mediated apoptosis. Our studies and others suggest, however, that *N-Myc* could play an antiapoptotic role in embryonal cell types (Hansford et al. 2004; Thomas et al. 2009). Studies in murine models indicate that medulloblastoma tumorigenesis is advanced by inactivation of the Rb/p53/Bax pathway (Marino et al. 2000), however, mutations in these genes are uncommon in human medulloblastoma. Calao et al. (unpublished data) observed that overexpressed N-myc correlated with increased *Bim1* in *Ptch1*$^{+/-}$ GNPs which represses p53 following a stress response by serum withdrawal; inactivating p53-mediated apoptosis. Elucidation of the mechanisms repressing N-Myc-induced apoptosis in GNPs will be an important step toward understanding factors that collaborate with *N-Myc* to initiate medulloblastoma tumorigenesis.

Tumor Progression

Human clinical and epidemiological observations have noted the presence of postnatal 'hyperplasia' or 'rests', and that these hyperplasia frequently undergo spontaneous regression before progression to tumor. Acute lymphoblastic leukemia, neuroblastoma, and wilm's tumor, have all been observed to have spontaneous regression of hyperplasia, and that this proportion is greater than the clinical incidence (Beckwith and Perrin 1963).

Several groups have previously noted the presence of GNP focal hyperplasia on the edges of the molecular layer after EGL regression, as a pre-cancerous lesion in Shh-driven models of medulloblastoma, and as a first step in medulloblastoma tumorigenesis, and, that this was N-Myc-dependent (Goodrich et al. 1997). Whether these cells are partially transformed or essentially normal GNPs is unclear. The presence of focal hyperplasia has been observed to a limited extent in wild-type mice, but is more prevalent in medulloblastoma murine models such as *Ptch1*$^{+/-}$ (Kim et al. 2003; Thomas et al. 2009). However, studies by Oliver et al. (2005) suggest that these cells are not sufficient to progress to tumor, without undergoing further changes. The majority of these hyperplasias regress over time, with only a minority further proliferating and becoming tumors (Fig. 10.3).

Our recent studies in the perinatal period of *Ptch1*$^{+/-}$ mice have also demonstrated that a stepwise loss of *Ptch1* expression from tumor initiation to progression led to incremental increases in N-Myc expression. Moreover, this increase in N-Myc protein expression was required to progress from GNP hyperplasia to medulloblastoma, and was characterized by increased phosphorylation of S62- and T58-N-Myc protein. Increased N-Myc expression was associated as well with up regulated *N-Myc* transcriptional target genes: *Activin-A*, *Id2*, *Tert*, *MDM2*, and *Pax3*. Interestingly, up regulated N-Myc expression did not occur by transgene amplification or increased mRNA expression, but rather by stabilization and prevention of degradation of the protein.

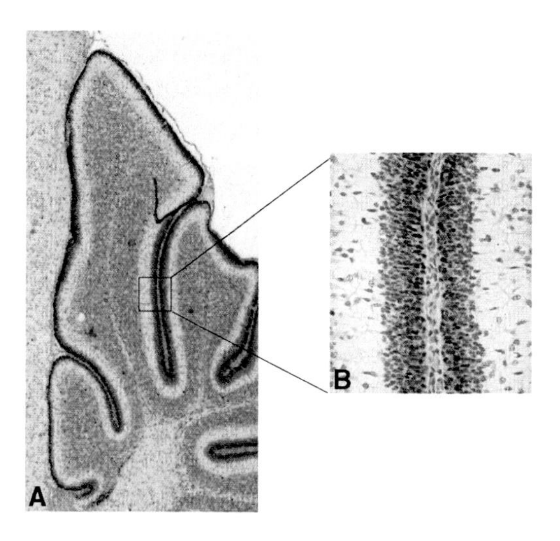

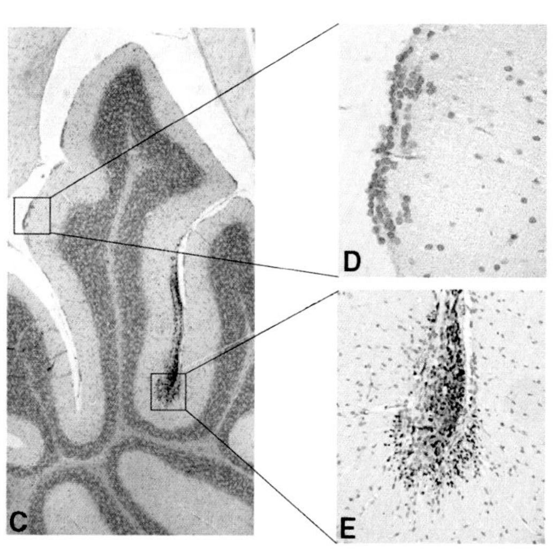

Fig. 10.3 (**a**, **b**) Photomicrographs of the EGL in P7 mice with H & E and proliferating cell nuclear antigen (PCNA) staining (*brown*). (**c**) Photomicrographs of lobules of the cerebellum in P21 mice with H & E and PCNA staining (*brown*). (**d**) A hyperplasia on the surface of the molecular layer negative for PCNA staining (*brown*). (**e**) A hyperplasia on the surface of the molecular layer positive for PCNA staining (*brown*)

This study is in agreement with emerging evidence indicating a permissive Myc expression threshold is required for tumor progression and tumor aggressiveness. Thus, the data indicates that one oncogenic event collaborating with the Shh signal in this model of medulloblastoma was a higher level of N-Myc expression promoting tumor progression.

Other pathways and molecules that have been demonstrated to promote and progress medulloblastoma include the: Notch-pathway, Igf-2, Bmi1, and inhibitors of apoptosis. An important role for tumor maintenance by the Notch pathway has been established by the observation that increased cell death occurs in Shh-pathway tumors when Notch is knocked out. Insulin-like growth factor -1 and -2 appear to have dissimilar roles in the GNP lifespan with Igf-1 effecting cell survival, and Igf-2 GNP expansion. Studies on Igf-2 have demonstrated that it may be necessary for GNP proliferation and medulloblastoma progression to advanced tumors, but not for early stages of tumor initiation (Hahn et al. 2000). Indeed, *Ptch*$^{+/-}$ mice with a constitutive activated Shh-pathway are found to have elevated levels of Igf-2, with Igf-2 activity necessary for medulloblastoma formation in these mice (Hahn et al. 2000). One mechanism of action may be insulin growth factor suppression of GSK-3β increases phosphorylation of S62-N-Myc during Shh-pathway activation in GNPs (Kenney et al. 2004).

Bmi1, a polycomb group gene, is essential for cerebellar development and repress the tumor suppressors *p16* and *p19*, and is likely to be involved in both pre- and post-natal GNP proliferation (Leung et al. 2004). Murine models with targeted deletion of *Bmi1* develop hypoplastic cerebella, and have been shown to have a reduced GNP population. *Bmi1* has also been identified as mediating the Shh signaling pathway for GNP proliferation (Michael et al. 2008). Up regulated *Bmi1* has been implicated in the pathogenesis of medulloblastoma, with expression correlated with *Ptch* expression (Leung et al. 2004). However, Michael et al. (2008) has also reported that transgenic mice that are heterozygous for *Bmi1* and have a constitutively activated Shh-pathway develop hyperplasia but do not progress to tumor, suggestive that *Bmi1* is essential for Shh-driven medulloblastoma expansion, but not initiation.

Despite the success of multi-agent, cytotoxic chemotherapy only 60% of patients survive longer than 5 years after diagnosis of medulloblastoma.

This therapeutic success has, however, been accompanied by severe short- and long-term side-effects in some patients, which reflect the unique susceptibility of the growing child. Many of the novel therapeutics now in use in adult cancer types have shown limited *in vitro* and *in vivo* efficacy in child cancer cells. Moreover, somatic mutations events such as p53 mutations, which are essential to the genesis of adult cancer types have been seen only rarely in child cancer. While these differences may have several explanations, taken together, they suggest different approaches are required for defining successful therapeutics for child cancer patients, compared to adult cancer patients. The elucidation of those factors which enable the initiation, persistence of hyperplasia, and progression to tumor, are vitally important and will impact on future therapeutic interventions for medulloblastoma.

Acknowledgements This work was supported by funds from the Cure For Life Foundation. In addition, the Children's Cancer Institute Australia for Medical Research provided funds and support (The Children's Cancer Institute Australia is affiliated with the University of New South Wales and Sydney Children's Hospital). We thank Prof. Glenn Marshall and Dr. Eric Sekyere, Children's Cancer Institute for Medical Research, for their support.

References

Beckwith JB, Perrin EV (1963) In situ neuroblastomas: a contribution to the natural history of neural crest tumors. Am J Pathol 43:1089–1104

Behesti H, Marino S (2009) Cerebellar granule cells: insights into proliferation, differentiation, and role in medulloblastoma pathogenesis. Int J Biochem Cell Biol 41(3):435–445

Calao M, Sekyere EO, Cui HJ, Cheung BB, Thomas WD, Keating J, Chen JB, Raif A, Jankowski K, Davies NP, Bekkum MV, Chen B, Tan O, Ellis T, Norris MD, Haber M, Kim ES, Shohet JM, Trahair TN, Liu T, Wainwright BJ, Ding HF, Marshall GM (2012) Direct effects of Bmi1 on p53 protein stability inactivates oncoprotein stress responses in embryonal cancer precursor cells at tumor initiation (unpublished manuscript)

Cohnheim J (ed) (1889) Lectures on general pathology: a handbook for practitioners and students (trans: McKee AB). New Sydneham Society, London

Dakubo GD, Mazerolle CJ, Wallace VA (2006) Expression of Notch and Wnt pathway components and activation of Notch signaling in medulloblastomas from heterozygous patched mice. J Neurooncol 79(3):221–227

Durante C (1874) Nesso fisio-patologico tra la struttura dei nei materni e la genesi di alcuni tumori maligni. Arch Memor Observ Chir Pract 11:217

Eberhart CG (2007) In search of the medulloblast: neural stem cells and embryonal brain tumors. Neurosurg Clin N Am 18(1):59–69, viii–ix

Fan X, Mikolaenko I, Elhassan I, Ni X, Wang Y, Ball D, Brat DJ, Perry A, Eberhart CG (2004) Notch1 and Notch2 have opposite effects on embryonal brain tumor growth. Cancer Res 64(21):7787–7793

Fults D, Pedone C, Dai C, Holland EC (2002) Myc expression promotes the proliferation of neural progenitor cells in culture and in vivo. Neoplasia 4(1):32–39

Goodrich LV, Milenkovic L, Higgins KM, Scott MP (1997) Altered neural cell fates and medulloblastoma in mouse patched mutants. Science 277(5329): 1109–1113

Hahn H, Wojnowski L, Specht K, Kappler R, Calzada-Wack J, Potter D, Zimmer A, Muller U, Samson E, Quintanilla-Martinez L, Zimmer A (2000) Patched target igf2 is indispensable for the formation of medulloblastoma and rhabdomyosarcoma. J Biol Chem 275(37):28341–28344

Hansford LM, Thomas WD, Keating JM, Burkhart CA, Peaston AE, Norris MD, Haber M, Armati PJ, Weiss WA, Marshall GM (2004) Mechanisms of embryonal tumor initiation: distinct roles for mycn expression and mycn amplification. Proc Natl Acad Sci U S A 101(34):12664–12669

Hatton BA, Knoepfler PS, Kenney AM, Rowitch DH, de Alboran IM, Olson JM, Eisenman RN (2006) N-myc is an essential downstream effector of shh signaling during both normal and neoplastic cerebellar growth. Cancer Res 66(17):8655–8661

Johnsen JI, Kogner P, Albihn A, Henriksson MA (2009) Embryonal neural tumours and cell death. Apoptosis 14(4):424–438

Kadin ME, Rubinstein LJ, Nelson JS (1970) Neonatal cerebellar medulloblastoma originating from the fetal external granular layer. J Neuropathol Exp Neurol 29(4):583–600

Kenney AM, Cole MD, Rowitch DH (2003) Nmyc upregulation by sonic hedgehog signaling promotes proliferation in developing cerebellar granule neuron precursors. Development 130(1):15–28

Kenney AM, Widlund HR, Rowitch DH (2004) Hedgehog and pi-3 kinase signaling converge on nmyc1 to promote cell cycle progression in cerebellar neuronal precursors. Development 131(1):217–228

Kim JY, Nelson AL, Algon SA, Graves O, Sturla LM, Goumnerova LC, Rowitch DH, Segal RA, Pomeroy SL (2003) Medulloblastoma tumorigenesis diverges from cerebellar granule cell differentiation in patched heterozygous mice. Dev Biol 263(1):50–66

Kimura H, Stephen D, Joyner A, Curran T (2005) Gli1 is important for medulloblastoma formation in ptc1+/– mice. Oncogene 24(25):4026–4036

Knudson AG Jr (1971) Mutation and cancer: statistical study of retinoblastoma. Proc Natl Acad Sci U S A 68(4):820–823

Lee Y, Miller HL, Jensen P, Hernan R, Connelly M, Wetmore C, Zindy F, Roussel MF, Curran T, Gilbertson RJ, McKinnon PJ (2003) A molecular fingerprint for medulloblastoma. Cancer Res 63(17):5428–5437

Leung C, Lingbeek M, Shakhova O, Liu J, Tanger E, Saremaslani P, Van Lohuizen M, Marino S (2004) Bmi1 is essential for cerebellar development and is overexpressed in human medulloblastomas. Nature 428(6980):337–341

Lossi L, Merighi A (2003) In vivo cellular and molecular mechanisms of neuronal apoptosis in the mammalian cns. Prog Neurobiol 69(5):287–312

Lossi L, Tamagno I, Merighi A (2004) Molecular morphology of neuronal apoptosis: analysis of caspase 3 activation during postnatal development of mouse cerebellar cortex. J Mol Histol 35(6):621–629

Louis DN, Ohgaki H, Wiestler OD, Cavenee WK (eds) (2007) WHO Classification of tumours of the central nervous system. IARC, Lyon

Marino S, Vooijs M, van Der Gulden H, Jonkers J, Berns A (2000) Induction of medulloblastomas in p53-null mutant mice by somatic inactivation of rb in the external granular layer cells of the cerebellum. Genes Dev 14(8):994–1004

Michael LE, Westerman BA, Ermilov AN, Wang A, Ferris J, Liu J, Blom M, Ellison DW, van Lohuizen M, Dlugosz AA (2008) Bmi1 is required for hedgehog pathway-driven medulloblastoma expansion. Neoplasia 10(12):1343–1349, 1345p following 1349

Oliver TG, Read TA, Kessler JD, Mehmeti A, Wells JF, Huynh TT, Lin SM, Wechsler-Reya RJ (2005) Loss of patched and disruption of granule cell development in a pre-neoplastic stage of medulloblastoma. Development 132(10):2425–2439

Sasaki H, Nishizaki Y, Hui C, Nakafuku M, Kondoh H (1999) Regulation of gli2 and gli3 activities by an amino-terminal repression domain: implication of gli2 and gli3 as primary mediators of shh signaling. Development 126(17):3915–3924

Sjostrom SK, Finn G, Hahn WC, Rowitch DH, Kenney AM (2005) The cdk1 complex plays a prime role in regulating n-myc phosphorylation and turnover in neural precursors. Dev Cell 9(3):327–338

Thomas WD, Raif A, Hansford L, Marshall G (2004) N-myc transcription molecule and oncoprotein. Int J Biochem Cell Biol 36(5):771–775

Thomas WD, Chen J, Gao YR, Cheung B, Koach J, Sekyere E, Norris MD, Haber M, Ellis T, Wainwright B, Marshall GM (2009) Patched1 deletion increases n-myc protein stability as a mechanism of medulloblastoma initiation and progression. Oncogene 28(13): 1605–1615

Turcot J, Despres JP, St Pierre F (1959) Malignant tumors of the central nervous system associated with familial polyposis of the colon: report of two cases. Dis Colon Rectum 2:465–468

Turner JD, Williamson R, Almefty KK, Nakaji P, Porter R, Tse V, Kalani MY (2010) The many roles of microRNAs in brain tumor biology. Neurosurg Focus 28(1):E3

Uziel T, Karginov FV, Xie S, Parker JS, Wang YD, Gajjar A, He L, Ellison D, Gilbertson RJ, Hannon G, Roussel MF (2009) The miR-17 92 cluster collaborates with the sonic hedgehog pathway in medulloblastoma. Proc Natl Acad Sci U S A 106(8): 2812–2817

Yang ZJ, Ellis T, Markant SL, Read TA, Kessler JD, Bourboulas M, Schuller U, Machold R, Fishell G, Rowitch DH, Wainwright BJ, Wechsler-Reya RJ (2008) Medulloblastoma can be initiated by deletion of patched in lineage-restricted progenitors or stem cells. Cancer Cell 14(2):135–145

Yoon JW, Gilbertson R, Iannaccone S, Iannaccone P, Walterhouse D (2009) Defining a role for sonic hedgehog pathway activation in desmoplastic medulloblastoma by identifying gli1 target genes. Int J Cancer 124(1): 109–119

Medulloblastoma Initiation and Growth: Role of Hepatocyte Growth Factor

11

Daniel W. Fults

Contents

Abstract

Hepatocyte growth factor/scatter factor (HGF/SF) is a polypeptide growth factor that drives cell cycle progression, blocks apoptosis, stimulates cell motility, and promotes angiogenesis in many tissues, especially during embryonic development. These diverse physiologic effects of HGF/SF are all mediated by a single cell surface receptor, the transmembrane tyrosine kinase encoded by the proto-oncogene *c-Met*. When pathologically overdriven, HGF/SF:c-Met signaling promotes tumor initiation and growth in many human cancers, including medulloblastoma, a pediatric brain tumor that originates from neural stem cells in the cerebellum. HGF/SF:c-Met signaling has emerged as a promising target for medulloblastoma therapy because the pathway is actively firing in tumor cells and because HGF/SF stimulates multiple oncogenic signaling molecules, against which specific molecular inhibitors have been designed.

Introduction

Medulloblastomas are malignant tumors that originate from neural stem cells in the cerebellum in children. Pediatric oncologists currently identify the tumor stage in medulloblastoma patients according to three clinical parameters: patient

D.W. Fults (✉)
Department of Neurosurgery,
University of Utah School of Medicine,
175 North Medical Drive East, Building 550,
Room 5228, Salt Lake City, UT 84132, USA
e-mail: daniel.fults@hsc.utah.edu

M.A. Hayat (ed.), *Pediatric Cancer, Volume 3: Diagnosis, Therapy, and Prognosis*, Pediatric Cancer 3,
DOI 10.1007/978-94-007-4528-5_11,

age, extent of surgical resection, and metastasis. These staging parameters define two patient groups, average risk and high risk, which correlate closely with prognosis. Short survival times are associated with age <4 years, incomplete resection, or dissemination of tumor cells to cerebrospinal fluid spaces or extraneural sites. Multimodality treatment regimens that combine surgery, craniospinal radiation, and chemotherapy result in 5-year survival rates approaching 90% in average-risk and 60–65% in high-risk patients, respectively (reviewed by Crawford et al. 2007). Although these long-term survival statistics are encouraging, the treatments necessary to achieve them are associated with significant neurotoxicity, which can be manifest by skeletal growth retardation, endocrine dysfunction, and progressive cognitive impairment in long-term survivors. These adverse effects have been attributed mainly to radiation-induced damage to the central nervous system during critical phases of development. Thus, a central objective of medulloblastoma research is to identify cell signaling molecules that can be targeted therapeutically to maximize tumor growth suppression and minimize collateral, treatment-related neurological injury.

Molecular genetic studies in large cohorts of medulloblastoma patients now strongly support the idea that medulloblastomas do not comprise a single nosological entity, but rather a diverse group of tumors, in which subgroups arise by transformation of different populations of neural stem cells in response to different molecular signals (Kool et al. 2008; Northcott et al. 2009; Thompson et al. 2006). According to this paradigm, treatment regimens will be more effective if they are designed to target those signaling molecules that are activated in each tumor subgroup. This chapter will review the important role of hepatocyte growth factor (HGF), also known as scatter factor (SF), in medulloblastoma initiation and growth and describe results of preclinical studies that support the idea that HGF/SF signaling is a feasible target for medulloblastoma therapy.

HGF/SF – A Multifunctional Oncoprotein

HGF/SF is a polypeptide growth factor that drives cell cycle progression, blocks apoptosis, stimulates cell motility, and promotes angiogenesis. These physiologic effects can be oncogenic when pathologically overdriven (reviewed by Abounader and Laterra 2005). The name "scatter factor" was derived from the ability of this growth factor to disrupt cell–cell junctions and cause epithelial cells to disperse. HGF/SF is synthesized as a single-chain precursor peptide, which is converted to an active, two-chain heterodimer via proteolytic cleavage. HGF/SF can be activated by any one of the following serine proteases: urokinase plasminogen activator; tissue-type plasminogen activator; coagulation factors X, XI, XII; and a close homolog of factor XII called hepatocyte growth factor activator (HGFA). These proteases cleave the HGF/SF precursor molecules into two fragments, which join via disulfide bonds to form the active heterodimer. All of the diverse physiologic effects of HGF/SF are mediated by a single cell surface receptor, the transmembrane tyrosine kinase encoded by the proto-oncogene *c-Met*. The complex structure/function relationships of HGF/SF and c-Met have been reviewed in detail previously (Birchmeier et al. 2003).

Considering the pleiotropic effects of HGF/SF, it is not surprising that engagement of c-Met by HGF/SF triggers multiple, intracellular, signaling pathways. A detailed description of the molecular responses that occur when cells are stimulated by HGF/SF is beyond the scope of this review. Nevertheless, it is important for oncologists to know that HGF/SF can activate three signal transduction pathways, which are actively firing in many types of cancer cells: the phosphatidylinositol 3-kinase (PI3K) pathway; the extracellular signal–regulated kinase/mitogen-activated protein kinase (ERK/MAPK) pathway; and the Jun amino-terminal kinase/signal transducer and activator of transcription (JAK/STAT) pathway.

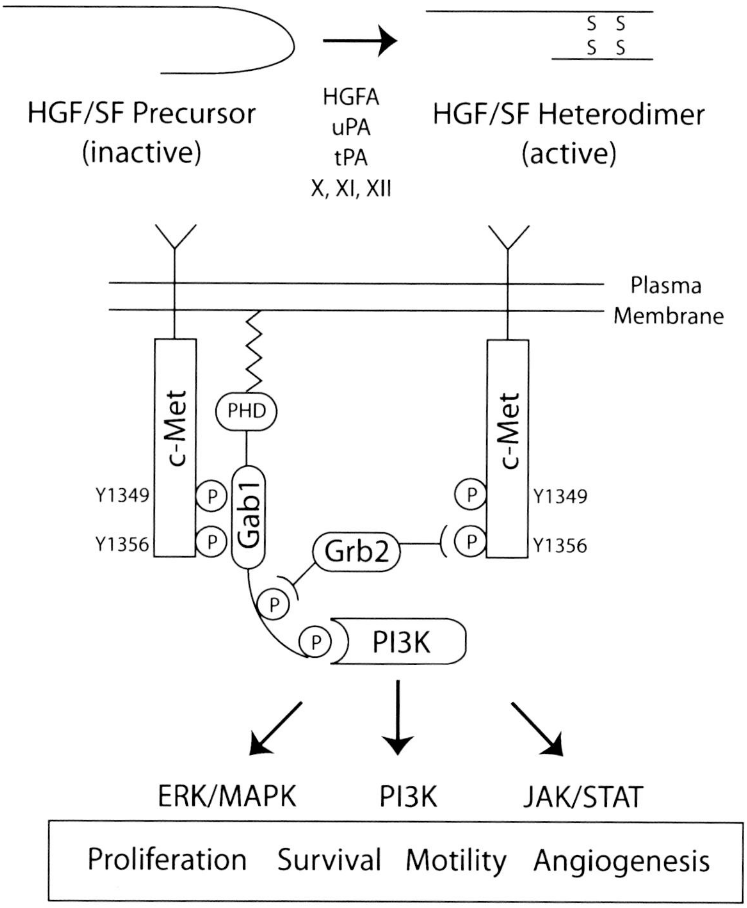

Fig. 11.1 The *HGF/SF*:c-Met signaling pathway. The inactive *HGF/SF* precursor is converted to an active heterodimer via cleavage by one of several serine proteases: hepatocyte growth factor activator (*HGFA*); urokinase plasminogen activator (*uPA*); tissue-type plasminogen activator (*tPA*); or coagulation factors *X*, *XI*, or *XII*. Engagement of c-Met by *HGF/SF* activates the c-Met tyrosine kinase, causing phosphorylation of tyrosine residues on the cytoplasmic domain of c-Met. Scaffold protein Gab1 binds to c-Met at a binding site containing phosphotyrosine residues *Y1349* and *Y1356*. Gab1 also binds phospholipids in the plasma membrane via a pleckstrin homology domain (*PHD*). Subsequent phosphorylation of Gab1 by unknown kinases creates a docking site for adaptor proteins like Grb2 and the enzyme phosphatidylinositol-3 kinase (*PI3K*). The assembly of intracellular signaling molecules at c-Met activates the downstream signaling pathways *ERK/MAPK*, *PI3K*, and *JAK/STAT*. These pathways mediate the *HGF/SF*:c-Met–induced physiologic responses proliferation, survival, motility, and angiogenesis

Understanding how these three oncogenic signaling pathways become activated by a single growth factor remains an important objective of cancer research. One protein that plays a key role is Gab1 (Grb2-associated binder 1). Gab1 was so named because of its ability to bind the important docking protein Grb2 (growth factor receptor–bound protein 2). When HGF/SF binds to c-Met, the cytoplasmic domain of c-Met becomes phosphorylated at multiple tyrosine residues, including Y1349 and Y1356 (Fig. 11.1). Gab1 binds specifically to an amino acid sequence in c-Met that contains these two phosphotyrosine residues. Moreover, Gab1 does not recognize this sequence on receptor tyrosine kinases other than c-Met. Once attached to c-Met on the cytoplasmic face of the plasma membrane, Gab1 becomes a scaffold on which other intracellular signaling molecules, like Grb2 and PI3K, can aggregate. Colocalization of these signal-relay molecules can thus trigger the firing of multiple downstream pathways.

Molecular biologists have tried to correlate the physiologic programs governed by HGF/SF (proliferation, survival, motility, angiogenesis) with signaling along individual pathways, but a coherent schema has not yet emerged. Nevertheless, some general themes are coming into focus. The fact that inhibition of either PI3K or ERK/MAPK signaling blocks HGF/SF-induced cell scattering indicates that both pathways mediate cell spreading and motility (Potempa and Ridley 1998). PI3K signaling, which potently inhibits apoptosis, appears to be the principal mechanism by which HGF/SF prolongs cell survival (Fan et al. 2001; Xiao et al. 2001). The ability of HGF/SF to drive proliferation and angiogenesis most likely involves cross-talk among multiple signaling pathways. JAK/STAT signaling mediates the ability of HGF/SF to induce formation of branched tubules, a process by which endothelial cells, for example, form blood vessels.

Studies in genetically engineered mice have shown that hyperactive HGF/SF:c-Met signaling can initiate tumor formation in a wide variety of tissues. Overexpression of HGF/SF in transgenic mice via the metallothionein gene promoter, which is constitutively active in many tissues, was shown to generate a diverse spectrum of tumor types (Takayama et al. 1997). Transgenic mice, in which mutant *c-Met* alleles encoding activated tyrosine kinase receptors were driven by the metallothionein promoter, developed mammary carcinomas (Jeffers et al. 1998; Liang et al. 1996). Furthermore, mice in which expression of wild-type *c-Met* was induced specifically in hepatocytes developed adenocarcinomas of the liver (Wang et al. 2001).

Activated HGF/SF Signaling Drives Medulloblastoma Growth

As mentioned previously, medulloblastomas probably originate from several different pools of neural stem cells in the cerebellum. Our understanding of the molecular events that initiate medulloblastoma formation is clearest for tumors arising from granule neuron precursors (GNPs). GNPs comprise a population of neural progenitor cells that make up the external granule layer, a germinal zone located on the cortical surface of the developing cerebellum. In mice and humans, GNPs proliferate rapidly during early postnatal development and subsequently differentiate to give rise to the abundant granule neurons, whose axons form the principal output circuits of the cerebellum in adults. The rapid postnatal expansion of GNPs is driven by Sonic Hedgehog (Shh), a protein that governs many cell fate decisions during embryonic development. In the cerebellum, Shh stimulates proliferation of GNPs and blocks their differentiation into postmitotic neurons (reviewed by Fogarty et al. 2005). This normal physiologic function of Shh inspired investigators to hypothesize that aberrant Shh signaling during cerebellar development, by stimulating GNP proliferation excessively, might initiate medulloblastoma formation. Indeed, several different methods of activating the Shh signaling pathway during cerebellar development in genetically engineered mice can induce tumors that closely resemble human medulloblastomas. These methods include (a) targeted deletion of the *Patched* gene, which encodes the inhibitory receptor for Shh (Goodrich and Scott 1998), (b) ectopic expression of Shh by retroviral transfer (Rao et al. 2003; Weiner et al. 2002), and (c) transgenic overexpression of Smoothened, a positive effector of Shh signaling (Hallahan et al. 2004).

Among the first clues that HGF/SF might play a role in medulloblastoma pathogenesis were the observations that (a) HGF/SF was neuroprotective for cerebellar granule neurons (Hossain et al. 2002), and (b) HGF/SF stimulated proliferation of GNPs during normal cerebellar development (Ieraci et al. 2002). A direct effect of HGF/SF on medulloblastoma cell growth was shown later in a report that overexpression of HGF/SF stimulated proliferation of human medulloblastoma cell lines and enhanced the growth of tumor xenografts implanted in mice (Li et al. 2005). An analysis of human medulloblastoma specimens showed that both *HGF* and *c-Met* were highly expressed and that elevated mRNA levels of these genes correlated with an unfavorable prognosis for patients (Li et al. 2005).

Further evidence that HGF/SF could increase the malignant behavior of medulloblastomas came from a report showing that forced overexpression of HGF/SF in the human medulloblastoma

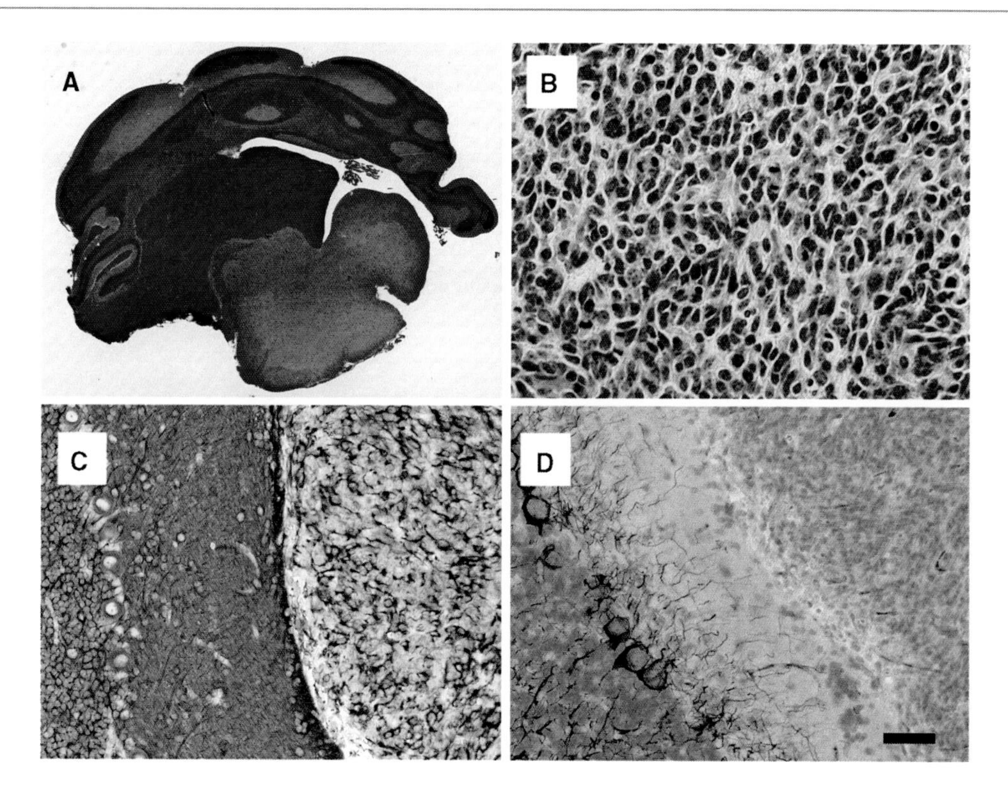

Fig. 11.2 Histopathology of medulloblastomas induced by RCAS transfer of Shh + HGF/SF to Nestin-expressing cerebellar progenitor cells. (**a**) Coronal brain section showing medulloblastoma in the cerebellum and fourth ventricle; (**b**) microscopic appearance of Shh + HGF/SF–induced medulloblastoma showing homogeneous sheets of tumor cells containing hyperchromatic nuclei (hematoxylin and eosin stain); (**c**–**d**) immunoperoxidase staining showing expression of βIII-tubulin, a marker of immature neurons (**c**), but no expression of neurofilament protein, a marker of terminally differentiated neurons (**d**), in tumor cells (*right*) adjacent to cerebellar cortex (*left*). Scale bar, 500 μm (**a**), 25 μm (**b**), 50 μm (**c**–**d**)

cell line DAOY caused a striking morphologic change when the cells were implanted as brain xenografts in mice (Li et al. 2008). Instead of the classic medulloblastoma cytoarchitecture, which is characterized by densely packed sheets of cells containing small, hyperchromatic nuclei, the HGF/SF-expressing tumor cells had large, irregularly shaped nuclei. These HGF/SF-expressing tumors resembled a human medulloblastoma variant called large-cell anaplastic medulloblastoma, which is a particularly aggressive subtype associated with poor patient prognosis. HGF/SF overexpression in DAOY cells secondarily induced the expression of the oncogenic transcription factor c-Myc. Interestingly, amplification of the *c-Myc* gene occurs frequently in human medulloblastomas of the large-cell anaplastic subtype.

These findings described above suggested to us that HGF/SF might be a potent growth factor for neural progenitor cells *in vivo* and that ectopic expression of HGF/SF in the developing cerebellum might initiate medulloblastoma formation or cooperate with Shh to promote tumor growth. We modeled the ability of HGF/SF to induce medulloblastomas in mice using a version of the RCAS/*tv-a* system that allowed retrovirus-mediated transfer of genes to Nestin^{+} neural progenitor cells in the cerebellum during their postnatal expansion phase, when these cells are highly susceptible to transformation. We found that retroviral transfer of HGF/SF and Shh in combination significantly increased the incidence of medulloblastoma formation compared with transfer of Shh alone (Binning et al. 2008). Figure 11.2 shows the histological features of medulloblastomas induced in mice by RCAS-mediated transfer of Shh + HGF/SF. In the absence of Shh, however, HGF/SF was not sufficient to initiate tumor formation. The tumors induced by Shh + HGF/SF showed increased tumor cell proliferation and decreased apoptosis compared with those induced by Shh alone, consistent with the dual role of HGF/SF as mitogen and survival factor. The addition of HGF/SF did not increase microvascular density in Shh-induced medulloblastomas in this mouse model. This was an unexpected finding because HGF/SF promoted angiogenesis in many other types of tumors.

Considering the potent effects of HGF/SF:c-Met signaling on cancer cell growth, it is not surprising that cells have evolved ways to inhibit this oncogenic pathway. Kongkham et al. (2008) carried out a genome-wide screen to identify gene promoters that were silenced by methylation in human medulloblastoma cell lines. Using this approach, the investigators discovered that expression of the *SPINT2* gene, which encodes serine protease inhibitor kunitz–type 2, was frequently suppressed by promoter methylation in the cell lines. Moreover, they found that *SPINT2* expression was significantly reduced in 73% of medulloblastoma specimens from patients compared with normal fetal cerebellum. The fact that these tumors often had focal hemizygous deletions of loci on chromosome 19q13.2, where *SPINT2* is located, further supported the idea that *SPINT2* was an important medulloblastoma suppressor gene. Of great functional relevance was that fact that the protein encoded by *SPINT2* was shown previously to inhibit the coagulation factor XII homolog HGFA, one of the serine proteases that can convert the inactive HGF/SF monomer to an active heterodimer (Miyazawa et al. 1993). Thus, loss of *SPINT2* function might promote medulloblastoma growth by removing a physiologic constraint to HGF/SF:c-Met signaling. We do not know whether loss of *SPINT2* plays a role in medulloblastoma initiation from cerebellar neural progenitor cells or progression of established tumors.

Molecular Therapy Targeting HGF/SF Signaling in Medulloblastoma

The enhancing effect of HGF/SF on Shh-induced medulloblastoma formation in mice indicated that HGF/SF or its downstream signaling molecules might be feasible targets for therapeutic intervention. The fact that kinase-activating mutations in the *c-Met* gene have not been reported in medulloblastomas – they occur in many other types of human tumors – suggested that HGF/SF:c-Met signaling in medulloblastoma was driven by ligand-dependent stimulation of c-Met, which could be blocked via the high specificity and avidity of monoclonal antibodies (mAbs). To explore this idea, we carried out a survival study in which we first induced medulloblastomas in mice via retroviral transfer of Shh + HGF/SF and subsequently treated the mice with an HGF/SF-neutralizing mAb L2G7. L2G7 had been shown previously to neutralize the ability of HGF/SF to stimulate proliferation, scattering, and survival of cells in culture (Kim et al. 2006). Moreover, in mice in which human glioblastoma cells expressing both HGF/SF and c-Met were implanted to form intracerebral xenografts, prolonged survival and tumor regression were observed after systemic administration of L2G7 (Kim et al. 2006). Our study showed that systemic administration of L2G7 significantly prolonged the survival of mice bearing Shh + HGF/SF-induced medulloblastomas and that L2G7 exerted its antitumor effect mainly by inducing apoptosis in tumor cells (Binning et al. 2008).

Despite the significant survival advantage conferred by L2G7 treatment, the cumulative survival of mice declined progressively during the observation period, throughout which the animals were treated with the drug. A possible explanation for sustained tumor growth despite HGF/SF blockade was that Shh stimulation remained unchecked. Consistent with this possibility, pharmacologic inhibition of Shh signaling by antagonists of Smoothened had been shown by other investigators to cause regression of medulloblastomas in *Patched*$^{+/-}$/*p53*$^{-/-}$ mice, in which hyperactive Shh signaling caused medulloblastomas to arise spontaneously (Romer et al. 2004; Sanchez and Ruiz i Altaba 2005). Therefore, we asked whether Shh+HGF–driven medulloblastomas were responsive to Shh signaling blockade and whether treatment response could be enhanced by combination therapy targeting both HGF/SF and Shh. To answer these questions, we carried out a survival study with mice in which we induced medulloblastoma by ectopic expression of Shh+HGF/SF. We treated these mice with agents that inhibit HGF/SF and Shh signaling, alone or in concert: (a) HGF/SF-neutralizing mAb L2G7; (b) cyclopamine, a small-molecular-weight compound that inhibits Shh signaling by binding and inactivating Smoothened; (c) Shh-neutralizing mAb 5E1; (d) L2G7+cyclopamine, or (e) L2G7+5E1 (Coon et al. 2010).

We found that monotherapy targeting either HGF/SF or Shh signaling prolonged survival and that anti-HGF/SF therapy had a more durable response than Shh-targeted therapy. The effect of L2G7+5E1 combination therapy on cumulative survival was equivalent to that of L2G7 monotherapy, and that of L2G7+cyclopamine therapy was worse. The observation that combination therapy either failed to improve or even reduced survival compared with monotherapy emphasized the need to test promising new molecular-targeted therapies in animal models of tumors in which the targeted pathways are known to be active.

The efficacy of HGF/SF-targeted therapy against medulloblastoma has not been tested in humans. A Phase I clinical trial is currently underway to test the safety of a humanized version of L2G7 (TAK-701) in adult patients with nonhematological malignancies. A Phase II clinical trial is now testing the efficacy of a different HGF/SF-neutralizing mAb (AMG102) when delivered systemically to patients with the malignant glial tumor glioblastoma (Toschi and Jänne 2008). Glioblastomas often show concurrent overexpression of HGF/SF and c-Met, a condition that sets up an autostimulatory feedback loop in which production of HGF/SF constantly stimulates its cognate receptor.

Perspectives

Hope for more effective and less toxic treatments for medulloblastoma patients lies in improving our understanding of the molecular signaling pathways, on which tumors cells have become dependent for their growth and survival. HGF/SF:c-Met signaling has emerged as an attractive target for therapeutic intervention because the pathway is actively firing in tumor cells and because HGF/SF:c-Met signaling potently inhibits apoptosis. Blockade of normal apoptotic programs is a well-known cause of cancer treatment resistance because radiation and chemotherapy, by inducing DNA damage, elicit an apoptotic death response in cancer cells. Furthermore, the fact that HGF/SF:c-Met engagement triggers multiple, downstream signaling pathways means that by interrupting this interaction and thus blocking the amplified signals downstream of c-Met, oncologists might be able to curb the numerous oncogenic effects of HGF/SF.

Investigators have designed many strategies for inhibiting HGF/SF:c-Met signaling in cancer cells, including blocking HGF/SF and c-Met using mAbs, antagonizing c-Met with truncated HGF/SF peptides, and inhibiting the tyrosine kinase activity of c-Met via small-molecular-weight compounds (reviewed by Toschi and Jänne 2008). We do not know which of these approaches will be the most effective for medulloblastoma patients or whether combining molecular-targeted therapies with conventional cytotoxic chemotherapy will enhance therapeutic efficacy. Although clues can be found in studies of other types of tumors, the response to therapeutic agents is likely to vary considerably among tumors derived from different tissues.

There is a pressing need to identify novel treatment targets for medulloblastomas, especially for children younger than 3 years of age, for whom the toxic effects of radiation on the developing nervous system are unacceptable. A special challenge for pediatric oncologists treating medulloblastomas in infants is to suppress tumor growth during critical stages of brain development, after which radiotherapy can be used with less risk of long-term neurotoxicity. Preirradiation chemotherapy is currently used for this purpose, but response rates are low. Novel therapies targeting HGF/SF:c-Met signaling, alone or in combination with conventional chemotherapy drugs, might be an effective tactic for delaying radiation therapy in these high-risk patients.

An important objective of future medulloblastoma research is to identify the molecular mechanisms by which medulloblastomas metastasize. Although medulloblastomas can metastasize outside the nervous system, their usual mode is to disseminate along cerebrospinal fluid channels to the spinal and intracranial leptomeninges. The molecular biology of cerebrospinal dissemination is likely to share important features with the invasion-metastasis cascade, by which carcinoma cells detach from solid tumors, enter the bloodstream, and travel to distant organs. The fact that HGF/SF:c-Met signaling plays a central role in cell migration and motility suggests that it might also mediate steps in medulloblastoma metastasis.

References

Abounader R, Laterra J (2005) Scatter factor/hepatocyte growth factor in brain tumor growth and angiogenesis. Neuro Oncol 7:436–451

Binning MJ, Niazi T, Pedone CA, Lal B, Eberhart CG, Kim KJ, Laterra J, Fults DW (2008) Hepatocyte growth factor and sonic hedgehog expression in cerebellar neural progenitor cells costimulate medulloblastoma initiation and growth. Cancer Res 68:7838–7845

Birchmeier C, Birchmeier W, Gherardi E, Vande Woude GF (2003) Met, metastasis, motility and more. Nat Rev Mol Cell Biol 4:915–925

Coon V, Laukert T, Pedone CA, Laterra J, Kim KJ, Fults DW (2010) Molecular therapy targeting Sonic hedghoe and hepatocyte growth factor signaling in a mouse model of medulloblastoma. Mol Cancer Ther 9:2627–2636

Crawford JR, MacDonald TJ, Packer RJ (2007) Medulloblastoma in childhood: new biological advances. Lancet Neurol 6:1073–1085

Fan S, Ma YX, Gao M, Yuan RQ, Meng Q, Goldberg ID, Rosen EM (2001) The multisubstrate adapter Gab1 regulates hepatocyte growth factor (scatter factor)-c-Met signaling for cell survival and DNA repair. Mol Cell Biol 21:4968–4984

Fogarty MP, Kessler JD, Wechsler-Reya RJ (2005) Morphing into cancer: the role of developmental signaling pathways in brain tumor formation. J Neurobiol 64:458–475

Goodrich LV, Scott MP (1998) Hedgehog and patched in neural development and disease. Neuron 21:1243–1257

Hallahan AR, Pritchard JI, Hansen S, Benson M, Stoeck J, Hatton BA, Russell TL, Ellenbogen RG, Bernstein ID, Beachy PA, Olson JM (2004) The SmoA1 mouse model reveals that notch signaling is critical for the growth and survival of sonic hedgehog-induced medulloblastomas. Cancer Res 64:7794–7800

Hossain MA, Russell JC, Gomez R, Laterra J (2002) Neuroprotection by scatter factor/hepatocyte growth factor and FGF-1 in cerebellar granule neurons is phosphatidylinositol 3-kinase/akt-dependent and MAPK/CREB-independent. J Neurochem 81:365–378

Ieraci A, Forni PE, Ponzetto C (2002) Viable hypomorphic signaling mutant of the Met receptor reveals a role for hepatocyte growth factor in postnatal cerebellar development. Proc Natl Acad Sci U S A 99:15200–15205

Jeffers M, Fiscella M, Webb CP, Anver M, Koochekpour S, Vande Woude GF (1998) The mutationally activated Met receptor mediates motility and metastasis. Proc Natl Acad Sci U S A 95:14417–14422

Kim KJ, Wang L, Su YC, Gillespie GY, Salhotra A, Lal B, Laterra J (2006) Systemic anti-hepatocyte growth factor monoclonal antibody therapy induces the regression of intracranial glioma xenografts. Clin Cancer Res 12:1292–1298

Kongkham PN, Northcott PA, Ra YS, Nakahara Y, Mainprize TG, Croul SE, Smith CA, Taylor MD, Rutka JT (2008) An epigenetic genome-wide screen identifies SPINT2 as a novel tumor suppressor gene in pediatric medulloblastoma. Cancer Res 68:9945–9953

Kool M, Koster J, Bunt J, Hasselt NE, Lakeman A, van Sluis P, Troost D, Meeteren NS, Caron HN, Cloos J, Mrsic A, Ylstra B, Grajkowska W, Hartmann W, Pietsch T, Ellison D, Clifford SC, Versteeg R (2008) Integrated genomics identifies five medulloblastoma subtypes with distinct genetic profiles, pathway signatures and clinicopathological features. PLoS One 3:e3088

Li Y, Lal B, Kwon S, Fan X, Saldanha U, Reznik TE, Kuchner EB, Eberhart C, Laterra J, Abounader R (2005) The scatter factor/hepatocyte growth factor: c-met pathway in human embryonal central nervous system tumor malignancy. Cancer Res 65:9355–9362

Li Y, Guessous F, Johnson EB, Eberhart CG, Li XN, Shu Q, Fan S, Lal B, Laterra J, Schiff D, Abounader R (2008) Functional and molecular interactions between the HGF/c-Met pathway and c-Myc in large-cell medulloblastoma. Lab Invest 88:98–111

Liang TJ, Reid AE, Xavier R, Cardiff RD, Wang TC (1996) Transgenic expression of tpr-met oncogene leads to development of mammary hyperplasia and tumors. J Clin Invest 97:2872–2877

Miyazawa K, Shimomura T, Kitamura A, Kondo J, Morimoto Y, Kitamura N (1993) Molecular cloning and sequence analysis of the cDNA for a human serine protease responsible for activation of hepatocyte growth factor. Structural similarity of the protease precursor to blood coagulation factor XII. J Biol Chem 268:10024–10028

Northcott PA, Fernandez LA, Hagan JP, Ellison DW, Grajkowska W, Gillespie Y, Grundy R, Van Meter T, Rutka JT, Croce CM, Kenney AM, Taylor MD (2009) The miR-17/92 polycistron is up-regulated in sonic hedgehog-driven medulloblastomas and induced by N-myc in sonic hedgehog-treated cerebellar neural precursors. Cancer Res 69:3249–3255

Potempa S, Ridley AJ (1998) Activation of both MAP kinase and phosphatidylinositide 3-kinase by Ras is required for hepatocyte growth factor/scatter factor-induced adherens junction disassembly. Mol Biol Cell 9:2185–2200

Rao G, Pedone CA, Coffin CM, Holland EC, Fults DW (2003) c-Myc enhances Sonic hedgehog-induced medulloblastoma formation from nestin-expressing neural progenitors in mice. Neoplasia 5:198–204

Romer JT, Kimura H, Magdaleno S, Sasai K, Fuller C, Baines H, Connelly M, Stewart CF, Gould S, Rubin LL, Curran T (2004) Suppression of the Shh pathway using a small molecule inhibitor eliminates medulloblastoma in Ptc1(+/−) p53(−/−) mice. Cancer Cell 6:229–240

Sanchez P, Ruiz i Altaba A (2005) In vivo inhibition of endogenous brain tumors through systemic interference of Hedgehog signaling in mice. Mech Dev 122:223–230

Takayama H, LaRochelle WJ, Sharp R, Otsuka T, Kriebel P, Anver M, Aaronson SA, Merlino G (1997) Diverse tumorigenesis associated with aberrant development in mice overexpressing hepatocyte growth factor/scatter factor. Proc Natl Acad Sci U S A 94:701–706

Thompson MC, Fuller C, Hogg TL, Dalton J, Finkelstein D, Lau CC, Chintagumpala M, Adesina A, Ashley DM, Kellie SJ, Taylor MD, Curran T, Gajjar A, Gilbertson RJ (2006) Genomics identifies medulloblastoma subgroups that are enriched for specific genetic alterations. J Clin Oncol 24:1924–1931

Toschi L, Jänne PA (2008) Single-agent and combination therapeutic strategies to inhibit hepatocyte growth factor/MET signaling in cancer. Clin Cancer Res 14:5941–5946

Wang R, Ferrell LD, Faouzi S, Maher JJ, Bishop JM (2001) Activation of the Met receptor by cell attachment induces and sustains hepatocellular carcinomas in transgenic mice. J Cell Biol 153:1023–1034

Weiner HL, Bakst R, Hurlbert MS, Ruggiero J, Ahn E, Lee WS, Stephen D, Zagzag D, Joyner AL, Turnbull DH (2002) Induction of medulloblastomas in mice by sonic hedgehog, independent of Gli1. Cancer Res 62:6385–6389

Xiao GH, Jeffers M, Bellacosa A, Mitsuuchi Y, Vande Woude GF, Testa JR (2001) Anti-apoptotic signaling by hepatocyte growth factor/Met via the phosphatidylinositol 3-kinase/Akt and mitogen-activated protein kinase pathways. Proc Natl Acad Sci U S A 98:247–252

Medulloblastoma – Molecular Genetics

12

Esther Manor and Lipa Bodner

Contents

E. Manor (✉)
Genetics, Laboratory, Institute of Human Genetics, Soroka University Medical Center, Ben Gurion University of the Negev, Beer Sheva 84101, Israel
e-mail: manore@bgu.ac.il

L. Bodner
Department of Oral and Maxillofacial Surgery, Soroka University Medical Center, Ben Gurion University of the Negev, Beer Sheva 84101, Israel
e-mail: lbodner@bgu.ac.il

Abstract

Medulloblastoma (MB) is an embryonal brain tumor of the cerebellum, it accounts for 4–6% of all primary intracranial tumors. It is the most common malignant brain tumor in children representing 15–30% of all pediatric brain tumors, with 85% of MB being diagnosed in patients younger than 18 years of age. MB is rare in adults and accounts for less than 1% of primary intracranial malignancies, thus most of the studies have been done on the MB of childhood. Histologically, MB is classified into five distinct subtypes: classic, desmoplastic, anaplastic, large cell and MB with extensive nodularity. These histological subtypes often are quite heterogeneous and exhibit highly variable clinical behavior, with anaplastic subtype typically associated with the worst prognosis, followed by classic and desmoplastic/nodular MB, which correlate with improved overall survival. Nowadays, there is a recognition that MB is a heterogeneous disease.

Looking for characteristic genetic features for each MB subtypes have focused in the last 20 years, on the chromosomal and the molecular levels. Presently, two new approaches are under study in MB: the role of epigenomic and the role of microRNA (miR) in MB's pathogenesis. The most common chromosomal finding in MB was i(17q) that appears in 30–50% of the pediatric MB. Consequently, a net loss of one 17p arm and a net gain of the 17q arm, can be seen. This aberration is in

M.A. Hayat (ed.), *Pediatric Cancer, Volume 3: Diagnosis, Therapy, and Prognosis*, Pediatric Cancer 3, DOI 10.1007/978-94-007-4528-5_12, © Springer Science+Business Media Dordrecht 2012

correlation with a poor clinical outcome. Other, less frequently found, aberrations are the gain of 1q7, 17q, 6q and loss of chromosomes 6, 6q, 8p, 9q, 10q 11, 16q, 17p and X chromosome in females. Loss of 6q mainly monosomy 6, is in correlation with improved outcome, while gain of 6q correlates with a considerably poor prognosis.

Until recently, the molecular research strategy in most of the studies has been focused on genes that are already known to be involved in other different tumors or syndromes. In general two subtypes were clearly identified in MB: those involved Wnt pathways (Turcot syndrome) and those involved SHH pathways (Gorlin syndrome), other non Wnt/SHH subtypes were less defined. Wnt subtype is found to be associated with the best prognosis while SHH subtype is found to be associated with the worst prognosis. Mutated CTNNB1 gene has been found in 10–15% of the MB cases with an activated Wnt pathway, while in about 25–30% of the MB cases, components of the SHH pathway: about 10% carrying the germ line mutation in the PTCH1 gene will develop MB, also SUFU and SMOH rarely found to be mutated.

Deregulation of the signaling cascade of p53 was also found to be implicated in pathogenesis of MB. P53 gene is the cause of Li-Fraumeni syndrome which occurs in 5–10% of the sporadic MB. In about 5–10% of the MB an amplification of the MYC family OTX2, PDGFRA, and CDK6 have been found. MYC1/MYCN amplification is in correlation with a poor outcome. The genes mentioned above are found in 5–30% of the MB, most probably point to the general pathway/s of tumors pathogenesis rather than MB specific pathway. However, recent advanced technologies enabled the finding of genes which are involved in chromatin modification particularly histone 3 lysine 9 (H3K9). Recurrent homozygous deletions of the H3K9 methyltransferase EHMT1; high level amplifications of JMJD2C, an H3K9 demethylase and a global reduction of H3K9 methylation levels have been found to be involved in MB.

Recently, microRNAs have been implicated in MB pathogenesis, mir17/19 has been found to be over expressed, and its over expression has been associated with SHH pathways.

The chapter will review the reported genetic alterations in MB and its correlation with the clinical and histopathological features.

Introduction

Medulloblastoma (MB) is an embryonal brain tumor of the cerebellum. MB accounts for 4–6% of all primary intracranial tumors. It is the most common malignant brain tumor in children, it represents 15–30% of all pediatric brain tumors, with 85% of MBs being diagnosed in patients younger than 18 years of age. The peak incidence occurs between the ages 3–9 years, with about 35% metastasis disease (Crawford et al. 2007; Rossi et al. 2008). In contrast, medulloblastoma is rare in adults and accounts for less than 1% of primary intracranial malignancies in this age group (Louis 2007).

Based on histopathological features, the 2007 WHO classification of CNS tumors (Gilbertson and Ellison 2008), has separated MB into five recognizable subtypes: the classic tumor which is the most common subtype of MB in general and in children in particular. The other four variants are: (1) desmoplastic/nodular which is the second most common (10–20% of the cases) in very young patients and adults, (2) MB with extensive nodularity is predominantly observed in infants (less than 3 years old), (3) anaplastic MB, (4) large cell MB is rare in infants, both of which account for 5–10% of the cases.

The histological classification and clinical staging have proven to be less than ideal methods for stratification. Histological subtypes are often quite heterogeneous and exhibit highly variable clinical behavior, with anaplastic subtype typically associated with the worst prognosis, followed by classic and desmoplastic/nodular MB, which correlate with improved overall survival. MB with extensive nodularity and desmoplastic/nodular MB in infants have a better outcome than the classic MB tumors, while large cell and anaplastic MB behave aggressively. Thus infants with desmoplastic MB should be stratified into a low risk therapeutic group while the large cell MB is rare but points to a poor prognosis that often presents with metastatic disease (Gilbertson and Ellison 2008). The increasing recognition of MB as a heterogeneous disease, with histological and molecular variants that have distinct biological behavior, affected the disease classification and treatment.

In spite of current aggressive therapies, approximately one third of the patients eventually succumb to the disease due to metastasis. Furthermore the post-treatment squeal, which includes neurological, vascular and long-term neurocognitive impairments, can be devastating for survivors of the disease (Ribi et al. 2005).

It is imperative to gain a better understanding of the molecular alterations and other biological squeal in MB for future targeted therapies that are more effective and less toxic.

A combination of clinicopathological evaluation and assays based on molecular subgroups of the disease allow stratification of patients into risk groups and more tailored approach to therapy which should prevent the significant adverse effects among survivors. Studies in the last 5 years have helped to build a consensus on the value and means of using molecular markers in the therapeutic stratification of childhood MB. These studies have revealed the genetic heterogeneity within MB including dysregulation of several signaling pathways. The genetic heterogeneity appears to be the basis for differential response to treatment and give a new impact to the traditional histological sub typing and improve to some extend the accuracy of diagnosis and prognosis and as a consequence the stratification to risk groups.

Although, adult MB is considered different from their childhood counterparts in terms of tumor biology and clinical variables, yet, because of the high incidence of MB in childhood and low incidence in adults most of the studies have been done on the MB of childhood. Some studies documented differences between childhood and adults tumors with regards to localization, cell of origin, histopathologic features, tumor cell differentiation, and treatment outcome. The adult's MB found to be also genetically distinct from the pediatric MB (Korshunov et al. 2010).

Here we focused on the genetic alteration reported so far in MB and their significance in sub-typing, stratification, and medical care.

Heritability of Medulloblastoma

Neither familial cases of MB, nor MB's cases affected by defined environmental factors have been described so far. Also, no specific chromosomal aberration has been described in more than about 40% of the MB cases. Unlike Ewing's sarcoma, where t(11;21) can be found in about 90% of the cases, in MB no main specific gene alteration can be detected. Yet, there is a wide basis to believe that inheritable factors play a significant role in MB pathogenesis and prevalence. Some of the evidence that support this point of view are:

Age of Onset

MB is most prevalent in childhood including about 3% in infancy, mainly MB with extensive nodularity, while it is rare in adults. MB is mostly a childhood brain tumor with a peak in 3–9 years age. Inheritable markers are most probably expressed phenotypically at the early ages of life. The younger the patient is, the higher chance that the genetic part is more pronounced, and so in the adults, the latter the age of tumor appearance the higher chance for multi-factorial environmental cause. About 85% of the primary intracranial tumors diagnosed as MB in patients younger than 18 years of age while in adults about 1% of the primary intracranial tumors diagnosed as MB. It is well known that infants are the more vulnerable group with 25–60% rate of cure, while the overall 5-year survival rate in childhood is about 80%. Although, the environmental factors could not be totally excluded, yet the younger age of MB appearance with 35% metastatic, points toward a more pronounced genetic background rather than environmental (Rossi et al. 2008).

Severity of the Disease

The most prevalent MB sub-type in infancy is the desmoplastic which is considered the most aggressive sub-type especially when it also appear with metastasis, 35% of the childhood MB are metastatic at presentation. Metastatic phenotype considered as a high risk group with the worst prognosis. Cure rates are lower for infants than for older children. This might point either to the more significant-effective role of the in heritage genetics predisposition in infants then in elderly or adults MB. Also most probably radiotherapy can be particularly more adverse in the immature infant brain (Rutkowski et al. 2009). The main consequence of carniospinal irradiation (CSI) is notably cognitive problems children's IQ can decrease by as much as 30 points in the standard risk group. The high risk group (metastasis, significant post operative residual tumor) remains poor 5-years event free survival (EFS) being 25–40% the worse prognosis is particularly in younger children.

Although 5-years overall survival rates have reached 60–80%, survivors often face a variety of long term neurological, neuroendocrine, and social squeal as a result of conventional treatment regimens, surgery, radiotherapy, and chemotherapy (Frange et al. 2009; Rossi et al. 2008). It is imperative to gain a better understanding of the molecular alterations in MB for future targeted therapies that are more effective and less toxic.

Predisposition

Predisposition to develop MB due to known genetic alterations- some MB cases are associated with known hereditary syndromes such as Gorlin, Turcot and Li-Fraumeni. (Reviewed by Ellison 2010; Northcott et al. 2010; Onvani et al. 2010) will be discussed in the gene alteration part. All the above points support the suggestion that genetic factors cause predisposition for MB's development.

Most studies on MB have focused on genes that are already known to be involved in the pathogenesis of tumors, such as Wnt, SHH, Notch TP53. The specific genetic pathway/s in MB is/are still unknown. Studying the different MB's subtypes with the most advanced technologies will significantly contribute to the overall understanding of MB pathogenesis in general and in particular in MB genetic knowledge.

Chromosomal Aberrations and Its Correlation to Clinicopathological Classification

Cytogenetics and molecular genetics are two different levels of genetic studies. Both of them are in use for characterization of tumors in general and MB in particular. Nowadays, these tests in combination with other standard methods such immunohistochemistry, significantly improved the diagnosis, prognosis and consequently the treatment modalities and survival of the patients with malignant diseases. Cytogenetics, molecular cytogenetics (FISH, CGH) and molecular genetics are three methods that supplement each other, and their combination leads to the identification of the genes that are involved in tumorigenesis (tumor suppressor genes and oncogenes) and thus can give complete information for prognostic and diagnostic purposes . Although, impressive progress has been achieved in the nano molecular genetics, next generation sequencing, proteomics and transcriptomics, in the last decade, yet, we can not give up the "macro-tests": the old gold standard methods such as cytogenetics and histology. The nano tests are still new and very expensive to implicate to routine work up, they are in a developing stage and the accumulated experience with their use is still limited. There is still missing information regarding the whole range of polymorphism and how to differentiate it from significant changes. Also the exact interactions between all the nano tests (molecular genetics, proteomics and transcriptomics) are only partially understood so far. Moreover the significance and the importance of the immerging field of epigenetics is still not clear. The field of epigenetics is dealing with changes that do not affect the molecular genetics itself but rather the changes in the expression of the gene/s by changing methylation, acetylation, phosphorylation and ubiquitination. Its effects include the most delicate interactions of all the living levels, starting from biochemical reaction and the interactions inside the cell compartments, cell to cell, in the organ, in the host and between the host and the environment.

Chromosome analysis of tumor cells plays an important role in the diagnosis, prognosis and follow up of many malignancies. It is a standard of care in hemato-oncology. Culturing solid tumor cells *in vitro* is essential for cytogenetic analysis. The success in getting specific chromosomal aberrations in solid tumors after in vitro culturing is limited because of technical problems such as: an overgrowth of cells from healthy part of the tissue mostly fibroblasts, limited growth of the abnormal tumor cells and low quality of the tumor cell metaphases and also the need for special and well trained cytogeneticists. These are probably the main reasons for the limited and what seems like a non specific chromosomal aberration in MB. Only about 40% of the MBs demonstrate chromosomal aberrations. Presently, advanced technologies such as microarray CGH and next generation sequencing enable us to better evaluate chromosomal aberrations in MB. It will take some time for the accumulation of new data regarding chromosomal aberrations using the new methods, mainly because reliable results should be done on a large cohort which include sufficient size group of all MB subtypes.

Copy number abnormalities of chromosome 17 isodicentric, isochromosome of chromosome 17q, loss of 17p, or gain of 17q are the most frequent chromosomal abnormality in MBs (Mitelman et al. 2011; McCabe et al. 2006) it is found in 30–50% of the studied cases. Isochromosome –isodicentric chromosome 17 is present in approximately one third of the tumors and in some cases is the only chromosomal aberration . It has been observed in 25–30% of childhood MB. In fact there is a loss of 17p and a gain of 17q which is the most common isochromosome in cancer in general. This might point toward the fact that i(17q) is a general marker of neoplastic process rather then a specific marker of MB. Its role as an indicator for a poor outcome in MB stratification is controversial. The controversial evidence based mainly on the findings of i(17q) also in Wnt pathway subgroup which in consensus considered as a favorable outcome. The question whether to consider copy number abnormality of chromosome 17 as a marker for poor prognosis and to exclude those found to be Wnt pathway, is still in debate (Mitelman et al. 2011; Pfister et al. 2009).

Using more sophisticated and advanced techniques such as CGH to profile a panel of 27 primary MB revealed frequent loss of 10q, 11, 16q, 17p, and 8p as well as recurrent gains of chromosomes 7, and 17q. These losses and gains were also confirmed by other techniques, such as G-banding, SKY and FISH. Array CGH of 47 MB showed gain of 17q, 7, and 1q and loss of 17p, 11p, 10q and 8.

There have also been reports, although less frequently of losses on chromosomes 10q, 11, 17p and 22 as well as gains on chromosomes 1q, 7 and 7q (Mitelman et al. 2011). SKY analysis of 19 primary MB revealed structural aberrations involving chromosomes 7, 17, 3, 14, 10 and 22. Monosomy 6 is strongly associated with Wnt profile in MB. Chromosomal abnormalities including loss of chromosome X in females and loss of chromosome 8, have been found mainly in non SHH/Wnt subgroups. (Reviewed by Ellison 2010; Northcott et al. 2010; Onvani et al. 2010.)

Genetic Alterations and Its Correlation to Clinicopathological Classification

Tumorigenesis is a process in which one of the pathways leading to normal cell development has lost its control and its normal function. In addition, the neovasculization, cell proliferation, differentiation, motility and apoptosis (death) are also altered. There are two possible categories in tumor specific genetic alteration; one is inheritable or germ cells mutation and the other is acquired alteration. Also there is a difference between general tumorigenesis pathways and tumor specific pathway and general chromosomal aberration and tumor specific chromosomal aberration. Usually, the tumor specific pathway is a part of the general tumorigenesis pathways but still it is predominant in one specific tumor subgroup, for example RB gene that causes mainly retinoblastoma, WT gene that causes mainly Willm's tumor, both are also causing predisposition to other tumors. Similarly, the acquired gene alteration occurring during the life time, such as BCR/ABL is causing chronic myeloid leukemia and EWSR1-FLI1 is causing Ewing sarcoma. Specific acquired aberration found in addition to the cancer they caused, also in other cancers, there its significance and its prognostic value is different, for instance BCR/ABL points to a favorable prognosis in CML and points to a poor prognosis in acute lymphocytic leukemia (ALL).

Among the life time acquired mutation, one should differentiate between the first event, such as alteration of a gene that causes the disease and has a diagnostic value and those mutations that are considered as the latter (the second or the third) events for example KRAS and TP53 mutation in adenomatose polyposis coli (APC) and MNP1 or FLT1 mutation in acute leukemia. Those gene alterations have mainly prognostic value and may play as a general event seen in other tumors as well.

Unfortunately, neither MB specific chromosomal changes nor MB specific gene were found to be a clear evidence for the possible pathogenesis of MB, neither in MB general nor in one of its subtypes. The understanding of MB pathogenesis is still limited, mainly because most of the MB studies are associated with genes that are already known to be involved in other tumors or syndromes, rather than studying the MB specific gene alterations as the first goal. Indeed, MB is associated with other (tumor's) syndromes such as Gorlin, Turcot and Li Fraumeni, in which several important developmental signal transduction pathways, including sonic hedgehog (SHH), Wingless (Wnt) and Notch signaling cascades. SHH, Wnt, TP53 and Notch signaling cascades are implicated in the cells migration and localization in the cerebrum, and their proliferation and differentiation. The alterations in these pathways by any component of each signaling pathway may lead to tumorigenesis (Ingham and Placzek 2006). For example, Gorlin's syndrome characterized by a germ line mutation in the patched homologue 1 (PTCH1) located on 9q22 that served as a negative regulator of SHH gene during normal cerebella development. Mutation in PTCH1 gene can cause predisposition to different tumor development including MB with incidence of 5–20%.

Turcot syndrome is characterized by the mutation in the APC a tumor suppressor gene that is predisposed mainly (about 90% during life time) to colon cancer adenomatous polyposis coli (APC), but also predisposed to a lesser extend to other tumors including MB. The APC gene regulates the Wnt signaling pathway.

Recent advances in gene expression profiling techniques have led to the generation of several molecular classification schemes in MB (Thompson et al. 2006; Kool et al. 2008; Northcott et al. 2010, 2011).

In general, based on the molecular studies done so far, three main subgroups were defined: SHH, Wnt and non SHH/Wnt pathways which include another two subgroups which are less distinct .SHH pathway subgroup accounts for 15–25% cases of MB and have a poor prognosis, Wnt pathway subgroup accounts for 15–20% cases of MB and mostly has favorable prognosis, and non SHH/Wnt subgroups account for 60% cases of MB (Thompson et al. 2006; Kool et al. 2008; Onvani et al. 2010; Ellison 2010; Northcott et al. 2010, 2011) (Table 12.1).

According to the Thompson's (2006) classification based on molecular and FISH examination 5 distinct subtypes identified (A to E) including subgroup B in which Wnt pathway and monosomy 6 have been found and subgroup D in which SHH pathway has been found. Kool et al. (2008) further corroborated Thompson's classification using CGH and defined five subgroups: (A)-Wnt signaling subgroup, (B)-SHH signaling pathway, C and D expression of neural differentiation genes, D and E expression of photoreceptor genes. Subgroups C, D and E are genetically closely related and most often associated with metastatic appearance mainly subgroup E.

SHH pathway MB associated with desmoplastic phenotype and also with large cell and anaplastic MB. They are both reported mainly in

Table 12.1 Medulloblastoma classification according to: Louis (2007), Thompson et al. (2006), Kool et al. (2008), Pfister et al. (2009), Northcott et al. (2011)

[a]Thompson's (2006) classification (46)	WHO classification	Prognosis	Molecular alteration	Chromosomal aberration	Age of onset
A				Gain: 17q Loss: 17p	
B	Classic MB	Favorable	Wnt- β catenin↑ CTNNB1-predominant, APC, AXIN! mutation	Monosomy 6	≥3 years
C			SHH PTCH, SUFU mutation	Gain: 17q Loss: 17p	
D	Desmoplastic		SHH, PTCH, SUFU mutation		≤3 years
E				Gain: 17q Loss: 17p	
[a]**Kool's** (2008) **classification (52)**	**WHO classification**	**Prognosis**	**Molecular alteration**	**Chromosomal aberration**	**Age of onset**
A	Classic		Wnt β-catenin mutation NOTCH, PDGF	Monosomy 6	Older children
B	Desmoplastic		SHH PTCH1 mutation NOTCH, PDGF	9q loss	Young children years and adults
C	Classic	Metastases	Neural differentiation genes	17 alteration, loss of X chromosome (females)	Children
D	Classic	Metastases	Neural differentiation genes Photoreceptor genes	17 alteration, loss of X chromosome (females)	Children
E	Classic	Metastases	Photoreceptor genes	Loss of X chromosome (females)	Young children
[a]**Pfister's** (2009) **classification (80/260)**	**WHO classification**	**Prognosis**	**Frequency**		**OS**
MYC/MYCN amplification + 10ch.aber./ MYC/MYCN amplification + 6q-gain + 17q gain + 10ch.aber.	Large cell/anaplastic	Poor prognosis metastases	6%/4%/10%		13%

(continued)

Table 12.1 (continued)

[a]Thompson's (2006) classification (46)	WHO classification	Prognosis	Molecular alteration	Chromosomal aberration	Age of onset
6q-gain + 10ch.aber.		Poor prognosis	8%		16%
17q-gain/17p-loss/ i(17q) + 7.5ch.aber.		Poor prognosis	48%/39%/30–48%		56%
6q, 17q balanced + 4ch.aber.					90%
6q deletion + 2ch.aber.		Favorable prognosis	12%		100%
[a]Northcott's (2010) classification (103)[b]	**WHO classification**	**Prognosis**	**Molecular alteration**	**Chromosomal aberration**	**Age of onset**
Wnt			MYC↑ Wnt-β catenin	Monosomy 6	Distributed age median 9–10 years, 3:1 F/M
SHH	Desmoplastic-predominant Anaplastic, large cell		MYCN↑ Wnt-β catenin	Del9q Isochromosome 9p Gain: 3q, 20q, 21q, 2 Loss: 10q, 14	Infants ≤3 years-most common, adults ≥ 16 years
C	Desmoplastic Anaplastic, large cell (23%)	Metastases (46.5%) Worst prognosis	OTX2↑, FOXG1B↑, MYC(8q24)↑, Wnt-β catenin Neural development[a]	Isochromosome(17q) Gain: 1q, 17q, 8 Loss: 10q, 5qdistal, 16q, 11p, 8p	Childhood peak 3–10 years
D	Desmoplastic Anaplastic, large cell (8%)	Metastases (29.7%)	OTX2↑, FOXG1B↑ Wnt-β catenin, Neural development[a]	Isochromosome (17q) Gain: 17q, 8 Loss: 11p, X (females), 8p, 8q	Distributed age median 9–10 years

WHO (2007): Classic, desmoplastic, MB with extensive nodularity, anaplastic, Large cell
[a]For more details see: Louis (2007), Thompson et al. (2006), Kool et al. (2008), Pfister et al. (2009), Northcott et al. (2011), Parenthesis-Year of publication
[b]See table 2 in Ellison (2010), Table 2 in Huse and Holland 2010, Table 1 in Northcott et al. (2011). Parenthesis – Number of samples

infancy and childhood. Metastatic disease at presentation characterizes some SHH pathway mostly large cells and anaplastic MB. Less than half of the SHH pathway MB have PTCH1 mutations or show copy number loss at the PTCH1 locus, 9q22, mutations in SMOH and SUFU are rare thus there must be other undiscovered SHH pathway/s (Thompson et al. 2006; Kool et al. 2008; Northcott et al. 2010, 2011).

In contrast Wnt pathway is mostly associated with classic MB (Fattet et al. 2009) it has a favorable outcome it tends to be present in childhood in the pre-teen years (6–13 years) but almost do not present in infancy. Most of the children with this tumor survived (Thompson et al. 2006). Metastatic disease at presentation is rare in Wnt pathway. There is no report on desmoplastic medulloblastoma with Wnt pathway and also large cell and anaplastic MB with Wnt is rare. The APC protein is a regulator of Wnt signaling that function in a complex with other components to regulate several important developmental processes, including proliferation and specification of neural progenitor cells during early cerebellar development. APC function as a tumor suppressor through CTNNB1 (β-catenin) of sporadic cases of MB, a downstream component of the Wnt signaling pathway this account for 15% of the cases. β-catenin by itself also activates transcription of several oncogenes such as MYC and CCND1 resulting in enhanced cell proliferation (Ellison et al. 2005).

Only a small part of the Wnt pathway MBs are found to be carrying mutations in CTNNB1 gene-captured by identification of the nuclear activity of β-catenin in the MB. Mutations in APC and AX1N1/2 are rare, thus there are still undiscovered components also in Wnt pathway (Ellison et al. 2005; Fattet et al. 2009; Northcott et al. 2010, 2011).

Most of non SHH/Wnt MBs have a classic pathology and present in infancy and childhood. About half of the large cell and anaplastic MBs are non SHH/Wnt. Metastatic disease at presentation also falls into the non SHH\Wnt tumor subgroup.

Other molecular markers beside the above three identified groups is the amplification or of MYC family (MYC and MYCN proto-oncogenes), that account for 4–15% of MBs (Rossi et al. 2008; McCabe et al. 2006). MYCN is an early transcriptional target of the SHH pathway and activation by SHH promotes the expression of the cell cycle proteins cyclinD1 and CyclinD2 leading to GCP proliferation. A high expression level of MYC is reported to cause progression of MB to an anaplastic phenotype and has been linked to a poor prognosis while even though MYCN shows some association with large cells and anaplastic MB yet it is less established as a marker for an adverse outcome (Aldosari et al. 2002; Pfister et al. 2009).

Both SHH and Wnt subgroups rarely show copy number abnormalities of chromosome 17, amplification of MYC and MYCN or any other widespread ploidy changes. MB occurred also in 5% of the Li Fraumeni syndrome's patients carrying mutation in the suppressor gene TP53 (Northcott et al. 2009). Other known pathways are involved in the normal cerebellar development found also to be aberrant in some of the MB. For example a disturbance of the RAS-MAP upregulation through downstream components such a MAP2K1, MAP2K2, and MAPK1/3. It is found to be correlated with metastatic behavior (Gilbertson and Clifford 2003). Also, over expression of the EGF receptor family member ERBB2 is linked to metastatic behavior. A number of proto-oncogenes in MB such as CDK6, PDGFRA, KIT and MYCL1 have been found to be amplified by array CGH. A single copy numbers gains of MET locus on chromosome 7q in 38.5% of the cases in 13 MBs (McCabe et al. 2006).

The Notch pathway was found to be implicated in MBs pathogenesis in a number of studies. Notch promote granule cell precursor (GCP) proliferation and prevents their differentiation. Increased copy number of Notch2 has been found in 15% of the studied MBs. Also, mutated Hes1 gene that unregulated the Notch pathway have been found in a small study group, although it has been associated with poor prognosis and outcome, its role and implication should be carefully considered and further examined (Thompson et al. 2006; Kool et al. 2008; Northcott et al. 2009).

Due to technology limitations and the availability research strategies most molecular studies of MBs, we are still missing the MB specific molecular markers. Hopefully, MB subtypes specific markers will be discovered by using the advanced technologies which enables us to study MB at different levels: DNA by next generation sequencing, gene expression by transcriptomic and proteomic, epigenomic and miRs.

An accurate classification and the stratification will implicate the medical care. An optimal classification will differentiate between MB in each age interval (infancy, childhood and adult) and between the subgroups in each age.

There is a general consensus that a better understanding of the disease biology should allow us to develop more effective and less harmful treatments of MB.

Northcott et al. (2010) generated a class prediction algorithm, an 8-gene classification model which successfully predicted the survival status for 47 out of the 60 patients profiled. The markers of the cerebellar differentiation (β-NAP, NSCLI, TRKC) and component of the extracellular matrix (lysyl hydroxylase[PLOD], collagen TypeVai and elastin) predict favorable prognosis. While genes involved in cell proliferation and metabolism (MYBL2, enolas 1, LDH, HMGI[y], and cytochrome C oxidase) as well as ribosomal protein coding genes predict poor prognosis.

Micro-RNA (miR) and Its Correlation to Clinicopathological Classification

The field on miRNA emerged in the last few years, concentrates on small non coding, single strand RNA molecules that are found to play a regulatory role on gene expression.

Differential microRNA (miR) expression analysis has also contributed to our knowledge on MB pathogenesis. The miRs are the short fragments of endogenous noncoding RNA that play an important role in the developmental processes by regulating gene expression (Fernandez et al. 2009). Target mRNAs are either degraded or translationed by specific miRNAs. Ferretti et al. (2008) performed one of the earliest expression profiles on MB. Northcott et al. (2009) identified amplification of miR17/92 polycistron proto-oncogen in 6% of pediatric MBs and showed upregulation of miR17/92 expression in a large percentage of primary cases. Similarly, Piterson et al. (2008) demonstrated decreased expression of miR-124a in primary MB as well as in MB cell line. Onvani et al. (2010) have reported that miR124a as a negative regulator of CDK6 which are found to be overexpressed in MB. Additional oncogenic targets, such as miR-30b and miR-30d have also been proposed through miRNA profiling (Lu et al. 2009)

Northcott et al. (2009) have described subgroup classification based on transcription profile, using mRNA and miRNA examination. They identified four distinct subgroups including the well known Wnt and SHH and another two independent subgroup C and D. It has been found that mir17/92, cluster of oncogenic miRNAs, was highly expressed in SHH tumors in association with MYCN expression, while group C was found to be correlated with MYC.

High–resolution SNP array profiling on a group of >200 MB revealed high–level amplification of miR-17/92 on 13q31 (Northcott et al. 2009). It has been found that miR-17/92 and related paralogs (miR-106a/363 and miR-106b/25) were identified as the most highly upregulated miRNAs in MB when compared with normal cerebellum in this analysis. The combination of miR 17/92 amplification and consistent overexpression suggested miR-17/92 as a key player in MB pathogenesis. There is evidence that miR17/92 might cooperate with SHH in MB, as it showed preferential upregulation in SHH subtype. Recently the role of miRNA in MB has been studied on 14 primary cases using profile of 248 miRNAs showing a general biased down regulation in MB cells as compared to the control cells. A subset of 86 miRNAs which were previously reported to be expressed in neuronal tissues and/or cancer studied in cohort of 34 among them two neuronal candidates miR-9 and miR-125a were chosen for functional analysis. Induction of their expression resulted in the decrease in tumorigenic features: promoted apoptosis, inhibited cell proliferation and impaired anchorage-independent growth. Moreover loss of miR9 and miR125a correlated well with upregulation of truncated trkC which was identified as a target for posttranscriptional repression (Northcott et al. 2009).

In order to discriminate between miRs deregulation in SHH–driven MB from non SHH-cases, 31 MBs studied using a set of 250 miRs. Two groups were defined GLI1-high and GIL1-low. A set of 34 miRs was found with a significant differential expression between the two classes. For functional analysis of the GLI1-high class three candidates (miR-125b, miR-324-5p, and miR-326) exhibiting reduced expression were chosen based on their predicted capacity to target the SHH family members, Smo and Gil1. They were proven to repress Smo mRNA level in the MB cell line (Ferretti et al. 2008).

SNPs array profiling of more than 200 MB revealed copy number aberration of multiple unreported regions including high level amplification of miR17/92.

Another miRNAome study of 90 MB revealed that four distinct molecular subgroups can be described. These subtypes include the well characterized Wnt and SHH subgroups and another two subgroup designated C and D (Northcott et al. 2009).

The miR-17/92 was the most highly expressed in SHH-driven MB but also in tumors exhibiting high MYCN (SHH) and MYC (group C, Wnt) expression. MiR-17/92 transcriptional upregulation by N-Myc and Myc and confirming miR-17/92 aberrancy in a large percentage of the MBs (about 60%). Based on experiments on mice it was suggested by Northcott et al. (2009) that miR 17/92 cooperate with SHH signaling to promote and/or enhance CGNP proliferation. The miRs studies are still in their initial stage and we are still far from understanding their exact role and how they affect processes in MB pathogenesis.

Epigenomic and Its Correlation to Clinicopathological Classification

Until recently the thought was that genetic alteration is the main cause of each tumor development and progress. Researchers invest their efforts in finding a tumor specific pattern of genetic alteration. Over the past few years another aspect has arisen which is the deregulation of epigenetics to malignancy (Bernstein et al. 2007).

Epigenetics involves nongenetic DNA modifications that result in changes in gene expression. These changes include gene promoter methylation on cytosine residues, most frequently of the CpG islands of the promoter, as well as their histone code. These changes are found to be involved in pathogenesis of tumors including MB, through hypermethylation of promoter of tumor suppressor genes and consequently silencing them.

Fruhwald et al. (2001) showed methylation of up to 1% of all CpG island in 17 primary medulloblastoms, it was linked to poor prognosis.

Epigenetics is defined as "mitotically heritable changes in gene expression that are not accompanied by modifications in primary DNA sequence". It is highly correlated with the MB class were ZIC and NSCL1, encoding transcription factors that are specific for cerebellar granule cells point to the MB arised from cerebellar granule cells.

Anderton et al. (2008) have identified tumor – specific methylation of COL1A2 in 77% of the studied primary MBs (46 out of 60) and showed an age-dependent methylation pattern for this gene in desmoplastic tumors, which presented COL1A2 as a potential MB subtype biomarker. Kongkham et al. (2008) identified serin protease inhibitor kuntiz-type2 (SPINT2/HAI-2), an HGF/cMET signaling inhibitor, as a novel tumor suppressor gene that is frequently silenced by promoter hypermethylation in MBs (Kongham et al. 2008). Also Waha et al. (2007) found promoter hypermethylation-induced reduction of SCG5 expression in primary 16 out of 23 primary cases compared to normal cerebellar controls, points to its possible role in pathogenesis of MB. Furthermore, promoter hypermethylation-mediated silencing of CASP8, HICI and RASSF1A tumor suppressor genes has also been discovered in more than 30% of MBs by various groups (Lindsey et al. 2004).

Pfister et al. (2007) showed a striking association between samples classified as either "low methylators" or "high methylators" and patient outcome, where the "high methylators" group exhibited reduced overall survival. Also the GLI C2H2-type zing-finger protein family member ZIC2 was identified as hypermethylated and thus it has been silenced.

It has been found that EHMTI function as part of a transcriptional repressor complex that mediates gene silencing by promoting dimethylation of H3K9 (Tachibana et al. 2005), a repressive epigenic modification (Bernstein et al. 2007) in the promoter regions of target genes. An obvious correlation between loss of EHMTI leads to H3K9 hypomethylation. Another study using microarray-based differential methylation hybridization (Waha et.al. 2007) identified hypermethylation of the SCG5 (secretory granule, neuroendocrine protein 1[7B2 protein] gene) in 16 out of 23 (70%) primary MB. Expression of SCG5 found to be downregulated in the MB in comparison with normal cerebral controls. Another gene that found to be down regulated is SPINT2 that was found in 41 out of 56 primary MBs. Stable expression of SPINT2 resulted in attenuation of the malignant phenotype: inhibiting cell proliferation, anchorage-independent growth in soft agar and cell motility, of cell lines (Kongham et al. 2008). This study suggested that SPINT2 is a suppressor gene. Treatment of MB cell lines suggesting that SCG5 is a suppressor gene (Fruhwald et al. 2001) or increased gene with demethylation agent (5-aza-2' deoxycytidine) reduced colony formation expression (Anderton et al. 2008).

The MB epigenomic studies demonstrate that not only the genetic alteration can cause loss of control in a cell and transformation to a malignant cell but also other mechanism can cause malignancy implicated epigenetic gene silencing as important mechanism of the tumor suppressor gene inactivation in MB.

Summary

The reported genetic alterations of MB, either chromosomal or molecular, are so far not specific. The main distinct subgroups are the Wnt and the SHH both account for 30–40% of MB. These pathways are common in many other tumors, suggesting they are not exclusive to MB. There are some other pathways involved in MB pathogenesis that might be more specific to MB. Similarly, the chromosomal aberration i(17q) which is found in about 40% of MBs, as well as in many other tumors including in chronic myelocytic leukemia (CML) can possibly be a secondary chromosomal aberration. Some of the features found in different subtypes but not in an equal distribution, for instance i(17q) were found in 34%, 36%, 12% in classic, large cell and desmoplastic MB respectively and are associate with poor prognosis (Gilbertson and Ellison 2008). Another example NOTCH and PDGF, they both have been found in A and B Kool's subtypes and also subtypes C, D and E share increased expression of neural differentiation genes. Another example is the Wnt-β catenin, found in all subtypes defined in Northcott's classification. This overlapping between the different subtypes, points toward the fact that some of the alterations are not, necessarily, a specific prognostic marker.

Studies have been done on a mice model and on cell lines in order to learn more about pathogenesis of MB are important; however the data learned from these experimental systems should be first corroborated with the data learned from human primary MBs, before going to conclusions on the pathogenesis of human MB. This is the reason for focusing in this chapter mainly on the studies done on primary human MBs studies.

Due to the variable results, the exact and specific chromosomal changes in MB which is a crucial event in pathogenesis, is still unknown.

Gilberston and Ellison (2008) wrote in their review: "Genomic-seeing the wood and the trees". The literature is full of studies (over 200 papers) on genetic alteration in MB trying to understand the MB pathogenesis, some of them corroborate with each other. Most of the studies have been done from different research points of view and emphasis, using different technologies. Presently, there are at least 5 different suggestions for classification and stratification of MB: Thompson's (2006), (Louis (2007), Kool's (2008), Pefister's (2009) and Northcott's (2010). It is very difficult to combine them to one clear cut classification (Table 12.1).

There is also early evidences that epigenetics and miRs might play a role in MB pathogenesis and can be used as a prognostic tool. However, the data regarded to epigenetics and miRs in MB is still limited and uncompleted, as part of the studies done on MB cell line which might point to a candidate involved genes with no assurance for their role in the MB tumor. There are few studies on primary MBs, thus any conclusion from this data is still immature. This emphasized the need for further studying the MB pathogenesis for either specific germ line mutation or other specific level of alteration (transcriptome, proteome, epigenome levels). These should be done as a multi-center study, on a large size of cohort including sufficient number of samples of each MB subtype including adult and childhood MBs. The study should be performed uniformly using different levels of examinations: histologic, cytogenetic, molecular, transcriptome, proteome, epigenetics, and miRs. Hopefully such a study will provide us with more personalized medical care with less adverse side effects.

References

Aldosari N, Bigner SH, Burger PC, Becker L, Kepner JL, Friedman HS, McLendon RE (2002) MYCC and MYCN oncogene amplification in medulloblastoma. A fluorescence in situ hybridization study on paraffin sections from the children's oncology group. Arch Pathol Lab Med 126:540–544

Anderton JA, Lindsey JC, Lusher ME, Gilbertson RJ, Bailey S, Ellison DW, Clifford SC (2008) Global analysis of the medulloblastoma epigenome identifies disease-subgroup-specific inactivation of COLIA2. Neuro Oncol 10:981–994

Bernstein BE, Meisner A, Lander ES (2007) The mammalian epigenome. Cell 128:669–681

Crawford JR, MacDonald TJ, Packer RJ (2007) Medullblastoma in childhood; new biological advances. Lancet Neurol 6:1073–1085

Ellison DW (2010) Childhood medulloblastoma: novel approaches to the classification of a heterogenous disease. Acta Neuropathol 120:305–316

Ellison DW, Onilude OE, Lindsey JC, Lusher ME, Weston CL, Taylor RE, Pearson AD, Clifford SC (2005) Beta-catenin status predicts a favorable outcome in childhood medulloblastoma: the United Kingdom Children's Cancer Study Group Brain Tumour Committee. J Clin Oncol 23:7951–7957

Fattet S, Haberler C, Legoix P, Varlet P, Lellouch-Tubiana A, Lair S, Manie E, Raquin MA, Bours D, Carpentier S, Barillot E, Grill J, Doz F, Puget S, Janoueix-Lerosey I, Delattre O (2009) Beta-catenin status in paediatric medulloblastoma: correlation of immunohistochemical expression with mutational status, genetic profiles and clinical characteristics. J Pathol 218:86–94

Fernandez LA, Northcott PA, Taylor MD, Kenney AM (2009) Normal and oncogenic roles of microRNAs in the developing brain. Cell Cycle 8:4049–4054

Ferretti E, De Smaele E, Miele E, Laneve P, Po A, Pelloni M, Paganelli A, Di Marcotulli L, Caffarelli E, Screpanti L, Bozzoni L, Gulino A (2008) Concerted microRNA control of Hedgehog signalling in cerebellar neuronal progenitor and tumor cells. EMBO J 27:2616–2627

Frange P, Alapetite C, Gaboriaud G, Bours D, Zucker JM, Zerah M, Brisse H, Chevignard M, Mosseri V, Bouffet E, Doz F (2009) From childhood to adulthood: long-term outcome of medulloblastoma patients. The Institut Curie experience. J Neurooncol 95:271–279

Fruhwald MC, O'Dorisio MS, Dai Z, Tanner SM, Balster DA, Gao X, Wright FA, Plass C (2001) Aberrant promoter methylation of previously unidentified target genes is a common abnormality in medulloblastomas-implications for tumor biology and potential clinical utility. Oncogene 16:5033–5042

Gilbertson RJ, Clifford SC (2003) PDGFRB is overexpressed in metastatic medulloblastoma. Nat Genet 35:197–198

Gilbertson RJ, Ellison DW (2008) The origins of medulloblastoma subtypes. Annu Rev Pathol 3:341–365

Huse JT, Holland EC (2010) Targeting brain cancer: advances in the molecular pathology of malignant glioma and medulloblastoma. Nat Rev Cancer 10:319–31

Ingham PW, Placzek M (2006) Orchestrating oncogenesis: variations on a theme by sonic hedgehog. Nat Rev Genet 7:841–850

Kongham PN, Northcott PA, Ra YS, Nakahara Y, Mainprize TG, Croul SE, Smith CA, Taylor MD, Rutka JT (2008) An epigenetic genome-wide screen identifies SPINT2 as a novel tumor suppressor gene in pediatric medulloblastoma. Cancer Res 68:9945–9953

Kool M, Koster J, Bunt J, Hasselt NE, Lakeman A, van Sluis P, Troost D, Meeteren NS, Caron HN, Cloos J, Mrsic A, Ylstra B, Grajkowska W, Hatmann W, Pietsch T, Ellison D, Clifford SC, Versteeg R (2008) Integrated genomics identifies five medulloblastoma subtypes with distinct genetic profiles, pathway signatures and clinicopathological features. PLoS One 3:e3088

Korshunov A, Remke M, Werft W, Benner A, Ryzhova M, Witt H, Sturm D, Wittman A, Scholter A, Felsberg J, Reifenberg G, Rutkowski S, Scheurlen W, Kulozik AE, von Deimling A, Lichter P, Pfister M (2010) Adult and pediatric medulloblastomas are genetically distinct and require different algorithms for molecular risk stratification. J Clin Oncol 28:3054–3060

Lindsey JC, Lusher ME, Anderton JA, Bailey S, Gilbertson RJ, Pearson AD, Ellison DW, Clifford SC (2004) Identification of tumour-specific epigenetic events in medulloblastoma development by hypermethylation profiling. Carcinogenesis 25:661–668

Louis DN (2007) WHO classification of tumors of the central nervous system. International Agency for Research on Cancer, Lyon

Lu Y, Ryan SL, Elliott D, Bingell GR, Futreal PA, Ellison DW, Bailey S, Clifford SC (2009) Amplification and overexpression of Hsa-miR-30b, Hsa-miR-30d and KHDRBS3 at 8q24.22-q24.23 in medulloblastoma. PLoS One 4:e6159

McCabe MG, Ichimura K, Liu L, Plant K, Backlund LM, Pearson DM, Collins VP (2006) High-resolution array-based comparative genomic hybridization of medulloblastomas and supratentorial primitive neuroectodermal tumors. J Neuropathol Exp Neurol 65:549–561

Mitelman F, Johansson B, Mertens F (eds) (2011) Mitelman database of chromosome aberrations in cancer. Retrieved from: http://cgap.nci.nih.gov/Chromosomes/Mitelman. Database last updated 10 Feb 2011

Northcott PA, Nakahara Y, Wu X, Feuk L, Ellison DW, Croul S, Mack S, Kongkham PN, Peacock J, Dubuc A, Ra YS, Zilberberg K, McLeod J, Scherer SW, Sunil Rao J, Eberhart CG, Grajkowska W, Gillespie Y, Lach B, Grundy R, Pollack IF, Hamilton RL, Van Meter T, Carlotti CG, Boop F, Binger D, Gilbertson RJ, Rutka JT, Taylor MD (2009) Multiple recurrent genetic events converge on control of histone lysine methylation in medulloblastoma. Nat Genet 41:465–472

Northcott PA, Rutka JT, Taylor MD (2010) Genomics of medulloblastoma: from Giesma-banding to next-generation sequencing in 20 years. Neurosurg Focus 28:E6

Northcott PA, Korshunov A, Witt H, Hielschner T, Eberhart CG, Mack S, Bouffet E, Clifford SC, Hawkins CE, French P, Rutka JT, Pfister S, Taylor MD (2011) Medulloblastoma comprises four distinct molecular variants. J Clin Oncol 29(11):1408–1414

Onvani S, Etame AB, Smith CA, Rutka JT (2010) Genetics of medulloblastoma: clues for novel therapies. Expert Rev Neurother 10:811–823

Pfister S, Schlaeger C, Mendrzyk F, Wittmann A, Benner A, Kulozik A, Scheurlen W, Radlwimmer B, Lichter P (2007) Array-based profiling of reference-independent methylation status (aPRIMES) identifies frequent promoter methylation and conservative downregulation of ZIC2 in pediatric medulloblastoma. Nucleic Acids Res 35:e51

Pfister S, Remke M, Benner A, Mendrzyk F, Toedt G, Felsberg J, Wittmann A, Devens F, Gerber NU, Joos S, Kulozik A, Reifenberger G, Rutkowsky S, Wiestler OD, Radlwimmer B, Scheurlen W, Lichter P, Korshunov A (2009) Outcome prediction in pediatric medulloblastoma based on DNA copy-number aberrations of chromosomes 6q and 17q and the MYC and MYCN loci. J Clin Oncol 27:1627–1636

Pierson J, Hostager B, Fan R, Vubhakar R (2008) Regulation of cyclin dependent kinase 6 by microRNA 124 in medulloblastoma. J Neurooncol 90:1–7

Ribi K, Relly C, Landolt MA, Allber FD, Boltshauser E, Grotzer MA (2005) Outcome of medulloblastoma in children: long-term complications and quality of life. Neuropediatrics 36:357–365

Rossi A, Caracciolo V, Russo G, Reiss K, Giordano A (2008) Medulloblastoma: from molecular pathology to therapy. Clin Cancer Res 14:971–976

Rutkowski S, Gerber NU, von Hoff K, Gnekow A, Bode U, Graf N, Emser A, Ottensmeiser H, Deinlein F, Schlegel PG, Kortmann RD, Pietsch T, Kuehl J (2009) Treatment of early childhood medulloblastoma by postoperative chemotherapy and deffered radiotherapy. Neuro Oncol 11:201–210

Tachibana M, Ueda J, Fukuda M, Takeda N, Ohta T, Iwanari H, Sakihama T, Kodama T, Hamakubo T, Shinkai Y (2005) Histone methyltransferases 69a and GLP from heterometric complexes and are both crucial for methylation of euchromatin at H3-K9. Genes Dev 19:815–826

Thompson MC, Fuller C, Hogg TL, Dalton J, Finkelstein D, Lau CC, Chintagumpala M, Adesina A, Ashley DM, Kellies SJ, Taylor MD, Curran T, Gajjar A, Gilbertson RJ (2006) Genomics identifies medulloblastoma subgroups that are enriched for specific genetic alterations. J Clin Oncol 24:1924–1931

Waha A, Koch A, Hartman W, Milde U, Felsberg J, Hubner A, Mikeska T, Goodyer CG, Sorensen N, Lindberg I, Wiestler OD, Pietsch T, Waha A (2007) SGNE1/7B2 is epigenetically altered and transcriptionally downregulated in human medulloblastomas. Oncogene 26:5662–5668

Pediatric Medulloblastoma: The Role of Heterozygous Germ-Line Mutations in the *NBN* Gene

13

Krystyna H. Chrzanowska, Joanna Trubicka, and Elżbieta Ciara

Contents

K.H. Chrzanowska (✉) • J. Trubicka • E. Ciara
Department of Medical Genetics, The Children's Memorial Health Institute, Al. Dzieci Polskich 20, 04-730 Warsaw, Poland
e-mail: k.chrzanowska@czd.pl

Abstract

Medulloblastoma is a highly invasive malignancy of the cerebellum (WHO grade IV) with a high tendency to metastasize via cerebrospinal fluid (CSF) pathways, and the most common malignant brain tumor in childhood. At present, multiple molecular dysfunctions are known to be responsible for medulloblastoma formation, including aberrant activation of the Sonic Hedgehog and Wingless signaling pathways. Nonetheless, recent observations that defects in DNA repair pathways can lead to genomic instability in neural progenitor cells and result in medulloblastoma development have underscored the importance of further genome surveillance. Moreover, recent studies evaluating the role of mutational inactivation of DNA repair genes in the development of medulloblastoma indicate that changes within genes coding such proteins as MRE11, RAD50, and NBN, forming the MRN protein complex, seem to be particularly important. Among these, the germ-line mutations detected in pediatric patients with medulloblastoma were found most frequently in the *NBN* gene, which codes for a protein that is an essential component of the MRN complex. All the mutations had a heterozygous status and were associated with the classic type of this tumor. Epidemiological data show that the *NBN* gene can be considered a susceptibility factor for cancer development. This is supported by both the fact that the NBN protein participates in the cellular response to DNA damage, and

M.A. Hayat (ed.), *Pediatric Cancer, Volume 3: Diagnosis, Therapy, and Prognosis*, Pediatric Cancer 3,
DOI 10.1007/978-94-007-4528-5_13,

that medulloblastoma is the most frequently reported solid tumor in Nijmegen breakage syndrome patients, who are at increased risk of developing different types of malignancies. This chapter will focus on new findings implicating *NBN* in medulloblastoma, which have given new insight into signaling pathways involved in the development of this disease.

Introduction

Medulloblastoma (MB) is an invasive embryonal tumor of the cerebellum (WHO grade IV) with a high tendency to metastasize via the cerebrospinal fluid (CSF) pathway and is the most common malignant brain tumor in childhood (Louis et al. 2007; Northcott et al. 2010). The annual incidence of medulloblastoma has been estimated at 1 per 200,000 children under 15 years of age with two peaks of incidence: between 3 and 4 years, and between 8 and 9 years of age (Crawford et al. 2007; Louis et al. 2007). Approximately 10–15% of medulloblastomas are diagnosed in infancy (Crawford et al. 2007). According to the current WHO classification of nervous system tumors, medulloblastoma is classified in five distinct subtypes: classic, desmoplastic/nodular, anaplastic, large cell, and medulloblastoma with extensive nodularity (Louis et al. 2007). The classic type comprises the vast majority of cases (75–80%). The worst prognosis, however, is associated with the anaplastic subtype, followed by classic and desmoplastic/nodular medulloblastoma (Dubuc et al. 2010). The standard multimodal therapy for medulloblastoma requires aggressive treatment, such as surgical resection combined with radiotherapy or chemotherapy. Although the cure rates are improving (5-year overall survival rates have reached 60–80%), survivors suffer from serious long-term neurological, neuroendocrine, and social side-effects of the therapy (Northcott et al. 2010). Hence, more effective and less toxic therapies are urgently needed, but the molecular defects underlying medulloblastoma must first be understood before such therapies can be successfully developed. To date, the aberrant activation of several cell-signaling pathways has been shown to be involved in medulloblastoma pathogenesis. Recent data indicate that defects in DNA repair signaling pathways also play an important role in the development and progression of medulloblastoma.

Genetic Factors in Medulloblastoma Pathogenesis

Genetic Abnormalities in Signaling Pathways in Medulloblastoma Tumorigenesis

Significant progress has been made in recent years in understanding the molecular genetic abnormalities that are responsible for the initiation and/or progression of embryonal tumors, including medulloblastoma. Early Giemsa banding studies first identified the loss of chromosome 17p, usually associated with gain of 17q, resulting in isochromosome 17 (i17q) as the most common genetic lesion in medulloblastoma, currently reported in approximately 30–50% of patients (Dubuc et al. 2010). Other abnormalities detected by early cytogenetic studies concerned chromosome 1q, 2p, 6, 7, 8p, 9q, 10q, 11p and 16q (Louis et al. 2007; Northcott et al. 2010).

Conventional methods have now been supplemented by highly advanced molecular cytogenetic techniques, such as comparative genomic hybridization (CGH) or DNA microarrays that have confirmed the previously observed abnormalities and identified new chromosomal aberrations across the entire genome (Ellison 2002; Northcott et al. 2010). The clinicopathological significance of most of these aberrations in the development of medulloblastoma has yet to be explored.

Another strategy used by researchers to explore genetic abnormalities in medulloblastoma relied on searching for mutations in the genetic background of rare familial tumor syndromes predisposing to medulloblastoma and looking for candidate genes, with focus on developmental signaling pathways.

Studies on the *PTCH1* gene associated with Gorlin syndrome pointed to the contribution of mutations within this gene to the etiopathogenesis

Table 13.1 Germ-line mutations in medulloblastoma – signaling pathways

Gene	Histopathology of tumor	Syndrome	Signal pathway	References
APC	No data	Turcot syndrome	Wnt	Brasseur et al. (2009)
AXIN2	Classical	–	Wnt	Koch et al. (2007)
CXCR4	Desmoplastic and classical	–	SHH	Schüller et al. (2005)
GLI3	Desmoplastic and classical	Greig Cephalopoly-syndactyly syndrome	SHH	Erez et al. (2002)
PTCH1	No data	Gorlin syndrome	SHH	Takahashi et al. (2009)
SUFU	Desmoplastic/nodular	Gorlin syndrome	SHH	Brugières et al. (2009)

of medulloblastoma and allowed the role of the aberrant Sonic hedgehog (SHH) signaling pathway to be established in 25–35% of cases (Dubuc et al. 2010). Similarly, detection of *APC* mutations associated with Turcot syndrome in patients with medulloblastoma have implicated the Wingless (Wnt) signaling cascade in 10–15% of cases (Dubuc et al. 2010). This was a starting point for evaluation of the role of other genes related to the SHH and Wnt signal pathways. Mutational screening has implicated participation of the *SUFU* and *SMO* genes (SHH pathway), and also of *CTNNB1*, *AXIN1*, and *AXIN2* (Wnt signal pathway) (Crawford et al. 2007; Northcott et al. 2010). Furthermore, a molecular defect in the *TP53* gene, resulting in Li-Fraumeni syndrome, has also been correlated with increased medulloblastoma incidence; mutations in *TP53* occur in 5–10% of patients with this type of cancer (Dubuc et al. 2010).

The vast majority of mutations detected in medulloblastoma are somatic events, however, germ-line mutations have also been described. The germ-line mutations in signal pathways genes determined as factors in elevated risk of developing medulloblastoma are presented in Table 13.1.

The APC (adenomatous polyposis coli) protein is a multifunctional regulator of colonic epithelial cell renewal as well as a tumor suppressor gene. Although the complete function of the APC gene product is not known, it has been shown that the APC protein plays a critical role in regulating cellular proliferation, differentiation, migration, and apoptosis, and also interacts with a multiprotein complex regulating the level of expression of ß-catenin (Guessous et al. 2008). Germ-line mutations in the *APC* gene have been implicated in colorectal neoplasia associated with the autosomal dominant inherited disorder, familial adenomatous polyposis (FAP), but also in Turcot syndrome type 2 characterized by an increased incidence of brain tumors. The most common type of brain tumor identified in patients with germ-line *APC* mutations is medulloblastoma (Taylor et al. 2000). Almost all mutations found in the *APC* gene are insertions, deletions, or nonsense mutations leading to a stop codon and resulting in the production of a truncated protein without the C-terminal end. The most widely accepted explanation of how APC contributes to the pathogenesis of medulloblastoma is that it acts as an antagonist of the Wnt signal pathway. APC forms a multiprotein complex with AXIN1, glycogen synthase kinase-3 β (GSK-3 β), and β-catenin that normally promotes the proteolytic degradation of β-catenin (Taylor et al. 2000). When Wnt, a secreted ligand, binds to the cell-surface receptor of the Frizzled family, it inhibits the complex and increases cytoplasmic levels of β-catenin, which translocates to the nucleus to activate the transcription of various genes, including known oncogens like c-*myc*, n-*myc*, and protoonkogene-like coded cyclin D1 (*CCND1*). This supports the idea that misregulation of the Wnt pathway through mutations in APC promotes tumorigenesis. Germ-line alterations of other members of the Wnt signaling pathway like the *AXIN2* (conductin) gene have also been shown in patients with medulloblastoma. *AXIN2* is a homologue of the *AXIN1* gene that interacts functionally with APC and the GSK-3 β complex. It acts like a negative controller of the Wnt pathway and as a tumor suppressor gene. The identified frameshift germ-line mutation within the *AXIN2* gene leads to the early termination of the coded protein in the domain that is crucial for the inhibitory effect in the Wnt pathway (Koch et al. 2007).

Another group of genes predisposing to medulloblastoma are the protein components of the Sonic Hedgehog signal pathway. The SHH pathway is vital during embryonic development for the formation of many vertebrate organ systems, in particular the central nervous system. The role of SHH in medulloblastoma was first discovered through the observation that germ-line mutations of the Patched1 (*PTCH1*) gene, which result in familial nervoid basal cell carcinoma (Gorlin syndrome), are also present in patients with medulloblastoma (Guessous et al. 2008; Northcott et al. 2010). The *PTCH1* gene encodes the Patched1 protein (PTCH) that is involved in cerebellar development and is a cell surface receptor for the ligand secreted by Purkinje cells, Shh. In the absence of Shh receptors, PTCH acts as an inhibitor of the expression and activity of a transmembrane protein called Smothened (SMO). Binding of Shh to the PTCH receptor causes, however, dissociation of PTCH from SMO, which then acts as a positive signal transducer on downstream pathways (Ellison 2002; Takahashi et al. 2009). Therefore, loss of function of PTCH is thought to be functionally similar to excessive Shh, pointing to *PTCH* as a tumor suppressor gene.

Release of the SMO protein leads to activation of GLI transcription factors such as activators GLI1 and GLI2 and the repressor GLI3. Mutational activation of GLI3 has also been indicated as a cause of enhanced incidence of medulloblastoma. The *GLI3* gene, located on chromosome 7p13, codes one of the three zinc-finger GLI family proteins. Changes in this gene are a molecular cause of several rare genetic diseases including Pallister-Hall syndrome, postaxial polysyndactyly type A, and Greig syndrome. The germ-line mutations observed in patients with medulloblastoma introduce a stop codon in the crucial domain for the function of GLI3 and generate severely truncated proteins with diminished repressor activity that are predicted to result in over-activation of SHH pathways (Erez et al. 2002).

The hedgehog pathway can be also activated by another mechanism – loss of SUFU protein expression. In normal cerebral development, SUFU is a negative regulator of the pathway, acting as an inhibitor of the function of GLI molecules. Germ-line mutations of *SUFU* are also reported in patients with medulloblastoma. The vast majority of these mutations encode truncated proteins that are unable to export the GLI transcription factor from the nucleus to the cytoplasm, resulting in activation of SHH signaling (Erez et al. 2002).

Another effect of signaling pathway activation is increased expression of chemokine (C-X-C motif) receptor 4 (CXCR4) that plays a role in the proliferation and migration of granule neuron cell precursors during development. A high level of CXCR4 expression has been reported in a wide spectrum of cancers, including medulloblastoma. CXCR4 is probably a direct target of transcriptional factor GLI1. The germ-line mutations of *CXCR4* observed in patients with medulloblastoma were substitutions within the first transmembrane region of the CXCR4 receptor, a domain that is highly conserved in evolution (Schüller et al. 2005).

The correlations and roles of particular components in upregulation of the SHH and Wnt signal pathways in the pathogenesis of medulloblastoma still remain uncertain, although it has been suggested that their aberrant activation may reinitiate the developmental programs that control proliferation of external granule cells in the cerebellum and, therefore, is crucially involved in the tumorigenesis of medulloblastoma.

Although significant progress has been made in understanding of pathogenesis of medulloblastoma through the study of rare familial tumor syndromes and developmental signal pathways, the molecular background of medulloblastoma has been determined in only a small proportion (<20%) of cases (Saran 2009). This fact strongly suggests that an additional genetic defect(s) must be involved. The most recent studies suggest that defects in DNA repair signaling, in addition to deregulation of developmental pathways, play a crucial role in the pathogenesis of medulloblastoma.

Table 13.2 Germ-line mutations in medulloblastoma – DNA repair genes

Gene	Histopathology of tumor	Syndrome	References
PMS2	No data	Lynch syndrome	Roy et al. (2009)
BRCA2	No data	Li-Fraumeni syndrome	Offit et al. (2003)
TP53	No data	Li-Frameni syndrome	Rieber et al. (2009), Taylor et al. (2000)
NBN	Classical	Nijmegen breakage syndrome	Ciara et al. (2010)

The Role of Genes Involved in DNA Damage Signaling and Repair Pathways in Medulloblastoma Development – The MRN Complex Enters the Game

During embryonic and early postnatal life the nervous system undergoes rapid proliferation and differentiation of neural cells. Thus, maintenance of genomic integrity is critical during nervous system development, and essential for prevention of disease, including cancer.

Within the nervous system, all of the eukaryotic DNA repair systems cooperate, i.e.: nucleotide excision repair (NER), base excision repair (BER), mismatch repair (MMR), homologous recombination (HR) and nonhomologous end joining (NHEJ) pathways. The developing nervous system is particularly sensitive to DSBs (double-strand breaks) which are repaired via HR and NHEJ. HR is required to prevent genomic instability in proliferative progenitor cells, whereas NHEJ is critical in post-mitotic neurons. The central component of the HR pathway is MRE11-RAD50-NBN (MRN), a complex cooperating with BRCA2 and other proteins such as the RAD52 family, RPA, XCC2, XRCC3, DNA polymerase, and DNA ligase. NHEJ also involves DNA ligase-IV, a critical component of this system, as well as KU heterodimers (KU 70 and KU 80), DNA-PK$_{cs}$, XRCC4, and Artemis. Inactivation of proteins required for HR or NHEJ leads to defects in nervous system development, indicating that both these pathways can also play a crucial role in development and progression of various neurological diseases, including medulloblastoma. The essential evidence for this association comes from knockout mouse models. Lee and McKinnon (2002) observed that all double mutant DNA ligase-IV and p53 mice developed medulloblastoma (Lee and McKinnon 2002). Interestingly, other neural tumor types were not found, indicating that the cerebellum is particularly sensitive to DSBs repair system dysfunctions. In addition, targeted deletion of important genes that regulate DNA repair, such as poly (ADP-ribose) polymerase (*Parp-1*), *XRCCA*, and *Brca2* in combination with *p53* loss, also resulted in murine medulloblastoma (Saran 2009). Simultaneously, studies evaluating a role of mutational inactivation of DNA repair genes in human medulloblastoma development indicate that changes within genes coding proteins involved in the MRN complex and cooperative proteins seems to be particularly important. Germ-line mutations in medulloblastoma were found in the *NBN* gene, a part of the MRN complex, as well as in the *BRCA2* gene, which is closely related to this complex (Ciara et al. 2010; Offit et al. 2003). In addition, germ-line mutations were found in the *PMS2* gene belonging to the mismatch repair genes group (MMR) that shares the responsibility for DNA repair with the MRN complex, as well as in the *TP53* gene, a tumor suppressor indirectly activated by the MRE11-RAD50-NBN complex (Mirzoeva et al. 2006) (Table 13.2). Among all germ-line mutations detected in medulloblastoma, the most frequent are changes within the *NBN* gene (6.7%). Additionally, the results of several studies indicate that both reduced and increased levels of the NBN protein may play a role in carcinogenesis. While reduced levels of NBN can promote cancer development through deficiency in DSBs recognition and repair together with disturbance of cell cycle checkpoints, the activation of tumorigenesis via overexpression of NBN has still not been demonstrated (Dzikiewicz-Krawczyk 2008). Furthermore Frappart et al. (2005) reported that deficiency of *Nbn* in murine neuron cells leads to genomic instability and activation of the ATM/p53-mediated DNA damage response, as well as proliferation defects of granule cell progenitors and apoptosis of postmitotic neurons in the cerebellum. Disruption of proliferation and/or uncontrolled apoptosis were the cause of the extensive cell loss and abnormal development observed in the cerebellum. All these facts suggest that the *NBN* gene plays a crucial role in cerebellar development and that mutations within this gene can predispose to medulloblastoma.

Mutations in the *NBN* gene when it is in homozygous status are responsible for a rare autosomal recessive genetic disorder, Nijmegen breakage syndrome (NBS), characterized by severe microcephaly, dysmorphic facial appearance, short stature, premature ovarian failure, and immunodeficiency. NBS belongs to the chromosome instability syndromes associated with a high risk of malignancy (van der Burgt et al. 1996). Cultured NBS cells display spontaneous chromosomal aberrations and are hypersensitive to DNA double-strand break (DSB)-inducing agents, such as ionizing radiation and radiomimetic chemicals (Antoccia et al. 2006). The disease occurs mainly in Slavic populations, in which more than 90% of NBS patients are homozygous for the founder mutation, c.657del5 (p.K219fsX234), in exon 6 of the *NBN* gene (Varon et al. 1998). The protein product of the *NBN* gene is nibrin (also referred to as p95), which consists of 754 amino acids and has a molecular weight of 95 kDa. The encoded protein is composed of three regions: the N-terminal region contains a forkhead-associated domain (FHA) and two breast cancer carboxy-terminal domains (BRCT1 and BRCT2); the central region includes sequences phosphorylated by ATM or ATR kinases; the C-terminal region contains binding domains for binding proteins MRE11 and ATM. The ability to interact with these and other crucial proteins enables NBN to participate in cellular responses to DNA damage. Nibrin forms a multimeric, nuclear complex with proteins MRE11 and RAD50 (the MRN complex) which is considered to play a key role in the detection of DNA DSBs and initiation of DNA end processing (Antoccia et al. 2006). Upon exposure to ionizing radiation, this complex forms nuclear foci by a direct binding to histone H2AX at sites where DNA repair has taken place and, together with ATM kinase, is required for activation of cell cycle control and DNA repair pathways, as well as for regulation of chromatin remodeling and enzymatic repair. The MRN complex is also involved in DNA replication, recombination during meiosis, telomere maintenance, control of S and G2/M cell cycle checkpoints, as well as induction of apoptosis. The involvement of the MRN complex in DNA repair and cell cycle checkpoint signaling suggests that mutations disrupting the function of constitutive proteins of the complex may lead to genome instability and carcinogenesis.

The Contribution of *NBN* Gene Germ-Line Mutations in the Molecular Background of Medulloblastoma

To date, seven germ-line mutations identified within the *NBN* gene have been found in the heterozygous state in patients with different types of cancer: c.448C>T (p.L150F), c.511A>G (p.I171V), c.643C>T (p.R215W), c.657_661del5 (p.Lys219fsX19), c.742insGG, c.1142delC, and c.1397+2insT (http://www.nijmegenbreakage-syndrome.net; Bakhshi et al. 2003). Among them the most common are c.657_661del5 (50.1%), c.511A>G (32.2%), c.643C>T (21%) and c.1397+2insT (4.3%), respectively (di Masi and Antoccia 2008). All of these mutations cause dysfunction of a coded protein.

The c.657_661del5 mutation, also reported as the founder mutation, results in a 5 bp deletion in position 657 that splits the region connecting two BRCT domains within the NBN protein. The consequence of this mutation is two truncated proteins with molecular weights of 26 and 70 kDa. The 26 kDa protein consists of FHA and the first BRCT domain, while the 70 kDa protein is produced by alternative initiation of translation and includes the second BRCT domain and the C-terminal region of NBN. There is some evidence that disruptions within the region connecting two BRCT domains may alter the selectivity of target recognition by NBN, therefore may affect the signaling network required for efficient DNA damage response (di Masi and Antoccia 2008).

The next two mutations, p.I171V and p.R215W, occur within the first BRCT domain of the NBN protein. p.I171V determines the substitution of isoleucine with valine at position 171, while p. R215W leads to substitution of an arginine by a tryptophan at the 215 position. Functional analysis of these mutations indicates that substitutions may alter the relative geometry of the tandem BRCT domains, which impairs binding of H2AX, hence disturb the correct rejoining of DBS in DNA. The c.1397+2insT mutation also is a profoundly defective mutation. The insertion determines the synthesis of an 80 kDa protein lacking the MRE11- and ATM-binding domain at the C-terminal region of the NBN protein, resulting in defective interaction between other components of the MRN complex (di Masi and Antoccia 2008).

The first evidence of a possible correlation between *NBN* heterozygous carriership and cancer risk came from family data studies indicating that relatives of NBS patients are predisposed to develop cancer (Seemanova 1990). Additionally, studies of knockout $Nbn^{+/-}$ mice demonstrated that loss of one *Nbn* allele significantly increased the occurrence of lymphoma and solid tumors (Dumon-Jones et al. 2003). Furthermore, successive experiments with treatment of $Nbn^{+/-}$ mice with γ-rays showed that irradiation dramatically increased cancer occurrence. These data provide evidence for a strong association between *NBN* heterozygosity and increased cancer risk.

The precise mechanism of this association is still unclear, but the high incidence of malignances in NBS patients together with increased cancer risk of heterozygous carriers of the *NBN* mutation suggest that *NBN* may be a tumor suppressor gene. Loss of heterozygosity (LOH) analysis performed in breast, prostate and ovarian tumors, as well as lymphoid malignances in *NBN* mutation carriers were ambiguous, however, suggesting that haploinsufficiency may be the presumed pathogenic mechanism (reviewed by Dzikiewicz-Krawczyk 2008). Support for the haploinsufficiency hypothesis comes from the presence of a remaining wild-type allele and nibrin expression in $Nbn^{+/-}$ tumor cells (Dumon-Jones et al. 2003). Furthermore, cytogenetic analysis of tumor cells in $Nbn^{+/-}$ mice demonstrated an increased chromosomal aberration rate, including DNA breaks and fusions, providing experimental evidence that *Nbn* heterozygosity predisposes to malignant cell transformation due to chromosomal instability.

In contrast, there is evidence that the founder mutation within the *NBN* gene results in two alternative forms of the NBN protein with an altered molecular function that are still able to interact with other components of the MRN complex, and therefore may disturb the function of the wide allele. This phenomenon, called the dominant negative effect, can also be one of the hypotheses explaining the participation of heterozygous *NBN* mutations in carcinogenesis (di Masi and Antoccia 2008).

Inherited alterations in the *NBN* gene have been shown to be associated with a wide spectrum of malignances, including breast, prostate, colorectal, malignant melanoma, head and neck cancers (reviewed by di Masi and Antoccia 2008). In children, the vast of majority of cancers observed in *NBN* carriers are lymphoid malignancy (Chrzanowska et al. 2006; Mosor et al. 2006). There is also evidence that *NBN* mutations predispose to childhood medulloblastoma (Ciara et al. 2010).

The authors know of five NBS children who have developed medulloblastoma, three of whom were reported in the literature (Bakhshi et al. 2003; Chrzanowska et al. 1997; Distel et al. 2003; E. Seemanová, personal communication, 2002; F. Tzortzatou-Stathopoulou, personal communication, 2002). In four of these five children, the founder mutation, c.657del5, was identified on both alleles (Chrzanowska et al. 1997; Distel et al. 2003; and two further cases of Slavic origin, unpublished), and one patient was a compound heterozygote of the mutation c.657del5 in exon 6 and the mutation c.1142delC in exon 10 (Distel et al. 2003). Radiotherapy-related death was documented in three children. One patient was treated only with chemotherapy and died due to tumor relapse and progression (Chrzanowska, personal communication).

These observations underlie the study of the role of the *NBN* gene in medulloblastoma pathogenesis. To date, the occurrence of *NBN* mutations in non-NBS patients with this type of cancer has been demonstrated in two communications. Huang et al. (2008) indicated 15 miscoding *NBN* mutations in 7 of 42 cases of medulloblastoma (Huang et al. 2008). All of them were somatic mutations located in the crucial domains of the NBN protein that are essential for the DNA damage response (exons 2, 4 and 14) or close to them (exons 8 and 10 as well as introns 2, 6, 7 and 9). The mutational screening was performed on two different histopathological types of tumor: desmoplastic/nodular and classic medulloblastomas. Although the age of the entire study group ranged from 1 to 60 years old, all identified carriers of *NBN* mutations were children aged less than 14 years at first diagnosis. The study also notably showed the functional interactions between the *NBN* gene and the TP53 pathway by the co-presence of the mutations in both genes in medulloblastoma tumor tissue. The statistical significance of these associations was confirmed. The authors suggest that either simultaneous or sequential occurrence of *NBN* and *TP53* mutations may contribute to the pathogenesis of medulloblastoma.

To the best of our knowledge, only one paper reports germ-line mutations in the *NBN* gene in children with medulloblastoma. Ciara et al. (2010) screened a total of 104 patients (age range 1.69–18 years) with medulloblastoma and identified seven heterozygous carriers of two different germ-line mutations, c.511A>G (p.I171V in exon 5) and c.657_661del5 (p.Lys219fsX19 in exon 6) localized in the highly conserved BRCT tandem domains. The c.511A>G mutation was present in 3.85% (1/26) of the medulloblastoma cases, which was three times higher (OR = 3.00; 95% CI: 2.94–3.06) than calculated for the control group, 1.28% (1/78); the difference was statistically significant (*p = 0.0241*). A lower carrier frequency of 2.88% (1/35) was estimated for medulloblastoma patients with the c.657del5 mutation. Nevertheless, this was much higher than the control value 0.59% (1/169) and was associated with a significant increase (*p = 0.0028*) in medulloblastoma risk (OR = 4.86; 95% CI: 4.42–5.3). As many as 7 heterozygous carriers were identified among 74 patients with the classic type of medulloblastoma (9.5%), while only 1.38 were expected. Four carriers of the c.511A>G mutation and three carriers of the c.657_661del5 deletion were found vs. 0.94 and 0.44 expected, respectively. Thus, the frequencies of each mutation, c.511A>G and c.657_661del5, were significantly higher in the classic type of medulloblastoma than in controls (OR = 4.23; 95% CI: 4.16–4.29; *p = 0.0023* and OR = 6.83, 95% CI: 5.69–7.97; *p = 0.0001*, respectively).

To analyze whether the wild-type *NBN* allele is lost, the authors also performed LOH analysis. Interestingly, examination of the tumor samples from five heterozygous carriers of *NBN* mutations gave no evidence for loss or mutation of the wild-type allele, suggesting that another pathogenic mechanism was responsible for the carcinogenesis (Ciara et al. 2010).

The clinical features of seven *NBN* mutation carriers were as follows. Only one patient fulfilled the criteria of standard risk disease defined as minimal postoperative residual disease and no evidence of neuroaxis or extracranial disease. In three patients, the tumor occurred early (under 3 years of age). Four patients presented with disseminated disease at diagnosis and in five patients the tumor was large (T3-T4 according to the Chang staging system) (Chang et al. 1969). None of the four patients who underwent irradiation experienced radiotherapy-related serious adverse events, suggesting that irradiation in *NBN* heterozygotes is well tolerated, in contrast to the biallelic mutation carriers (Bakhshi et al. 2003; Chrzanowska et al. 1997; Distel et al. 2003). One patient was retreated at relapse with radiotherapy with no unexpected reactions. In general, the chemotherapy-related complications encountered by the seven reported patients were within acceptable limits (during 87 chemotherapy courses there were 33 grade 3 and 4 WHO toxic episodes; all hematological and infectious complications). One patient experienced gastrointestinal bleeding requiring 30 cm of small intestine resection after chemotherapy with carboplatin. Five out of seven patients are alive with a follow-up from 14 to 50 months: three are disease free, one with stable changes on MRI, and one with disease (Ciara et al. 2010).

A comparison of clinical features between medulloblastoma patients with heterozygous *NBN* mutations and without the mutation within the *NBN* gene indicated that the median age at diagnosis was 5 years and 2 months in *NBN* mutation carriers versus 8 years and 10 months in non-carriers (M. Perek-Polnik, personal communication, 2010). In respect to symptom duration, no significant differences were observed (10.9 versus 10.4 weeks). A more aggressive course of disease (dissemination) and residual tumors were observed in 43% of heterozygotes and in 30% of non-carriers. Event-free survival at 5 years was 57.1% and 72.4%, respectively. The overall survival rate at 5 years was 71% for the *NBN* mutation carriers and 83% for the other patients.

The report by Ciara et al. (2010) is the first to document the role of the heterozygous *NBN* germ-line mutations in the etiology of pediatric medulloblastoma. The presence of two germ-line mutations known as particularly pathogenic, as well as clinical features like younger than average age at diagnosis and more aggressive course of the disease suggest that heterozygous *NBN* mutations increase the risk of developing childhood medulloblastoma and, probably, also have an impact on the clinical course and outcome of this cancer. While these mutations may explain the molecular background of approximately 6% of medulloblastomas cases, the findings are nevertheless important and meritorious, especially in respect to other Central and Eastern European populations with a high frequency of heterozygous carriers of the germ-line founder mutation of the *NBN* gene.

Conclusion

Our understanding of the molecular genetics underlying pediatric brain tumors has improved significantly over the past few years. Several signaling pathways are known to contribute, individually and in cooperation, to medulloblastoma pathogenesis. Their interaction is apparently required for DNA damage processing and repair, as well as influencing proliferation and survival. Deregulation of these pathways, which take part in normal embryonic and postnatal nervous system development, seems to be sufficient for initiation of carcinogenesis. Identification of a new genetic marker for medulloblastoma, i.e., heterozygous mutations in the *NBN* gene, points to a new group of candidate genes as targets for future studies evaluating the molecular aspects of medulloblastoma development. Despite these recent advances, the identified gene(s) alteration(s) have been found in less than 30% of all studied medulloblastomas, therefore, other potential mechanisms responsible for the development of this tumor should be explored. In fact, better understanding of the genetic events underlying the pathology of these neoplasms may contribute to the development of new, more effective and less harmful treatments. Much of the evidence suggests that response to treatment is not determined by chance, but rather by the biology of the tumor. It can be hoped that improved therapeutic approaches will lead to decreased mortality and improved quality of life of patients with this aggressive disease.

References

Antoccia A, Kobayashi J, Tauchi H, Matsuura S, Komatsu K (2006) Nijmegen breakage syndrome and functions of the responsible protein, NBS1. Genome Dyn 1:191–205

Bakhshi S, Cerosaletti KM, Concannon P, Bawle EV, Fontanesi J, Gatti RA, Bhambhani K (2003) Medulloblastoma with adverse reaction to radiation therapy in Nijmegen breakage syndrome. J Pediatr Hematol Oncol 25(3):248–251

Brasseur B, Dahan K, Beauloye V, Blétard N, Chantrain C, Dupont S, Guarin JL, Vermylen C, Brichard B (2009) Multiple neoplasia in a 15-year-old girl with familial adenomatous polyposis. J Pediatr Hematol Oncol 31(7):530–532

Brugières L, Pierron G, Chompret A, Paillerets BB, Di Rocco F, Varlet P, Pierre-Kahn A, Caron O, Grill J, Delattre O (2009) Incomplete penetrance of the predisposition to medulloblastoma associated with germ-line SUFU mutations. J Med Genet 47(2):142–144

Chang CH, Housepian EM, Herbert C (1969) An operative staging system and a megavoltage radiotherapeutic technique for cerebellar medulloblastomas. Radiology 93:1351–1359

Chrzanowska KH, Stumm M, Bialecka M, Saar K, Bernatowska-Matuszkiewicz E, Michalkiewicz J, Barszcz S, Reis A, Wegner RD (1997) Linkage studies exclude the AT-V gene(s) from the translocation breakpoints in an AT-V patient. Clin Genet 51(5):309–313

Chrzanowska KH, Piekutowska-Abramczuk D, Popowska E, Gładkowska-Dura M, Małdyk J, Syczewska M, Krajewska-Walasek M, Goryluk-Kozakiewicz B, Bubała H, Gadomski A, Gaworczyk A, Kazanowska B, Kołtan A, Kuźmicz M, Luszawska-Kutrzeba T, Maciejka-Kapuścińska L, Stolarska M, Stefańska K, Sznurkowska K, Wakulińska A, Wieczorek M, Szczepański T, Kowalczyk J (2006) Carrier frequency of mutation 657del5 in the NBS1 gene in a population of Polish pediatric patients with sporadic lymphoid malignancies. Int J Cancer 118(5):1269–1274

Ciara E, Piekutowska-Abramczuk D, Popowska E, Grajkowska W, Barszcz S, Perek D, Dembowska-Bagińska B, Perek-Polnik M, Kowalewska E, Czajńska A, Syczewska M, Czornak K, Krajewska-Walasek M, Roszkowski M, Chrzanowska KH (2010) Heterozygous germ-line mutations in the NBN gene predispose to medulloblastoma in pediatric patients. Acta Neuropathol 119(3):325–334

Crawford JR, MacDonald TJ, Packer RJ (2007) Medulloblastoma in childhood: new biological advances. Lancet Neurol 6(12):1073–1085

di Masi A, Antoccia A (2008) NBS1 heterozygosity and cancer risk. Curr Genomics 9(4):275–281

Distel L, Neubauer S, Varon R, Holter W, Grabenbauer G (2003) Fatal toxicity following radio- and chemotherapy of medulloblastoma in a child with unrecognized Nijmegen breakage syndrome. Med Pediatr Oncol 41(1):44–48

Dubuc AM, Northcott PA, Mack S, Witt H, Pfister S, Taylor MD (2010) The genetics of pediatric brain tumors. Curr Neurol Neurosci Rep 10(3):215–223

Dumon-Jones V, Frappart PO, Tong WM, Sajithlal G, Hulla W, Schmid G, Herceg Z, Digweed M, Wang ZQ (2003) Nbn heterozygosity renders mice susceptible to tumor formation and ionizing radiation-induced tumorigenesis. Cancer Res 63(21):7263–7269

Dzikiewicz-Krawczyk A (2008) The importance of making ends meet: mutations in genes and altered expression of proteins of the MRN complex and cancer. Mutat Res 659(3):262–273

Ellison D (2002) Classifying the medulloblastoma: insights from morphology and molecular genetics. Neuropathol Appl Neurobiol 28(4):257–282

Erez A, Ilan T, Amariglio N, Muler I, Brok-Simoni F, Rechavi G, Izraeli S (2002) GLI3 is not mutated commonly in sporadic medulloblastomas. Cancer 95(1):28–31

Frappart PO, Tong WM, Demuth I, Radovanovic I, Herceg Z, Aguzzi A, Digweed M, Wang ZQ (2005) An essential function for NBS1 in the prevention of ataxia and cerebellar defects. Nat Med 11(5):538–544

Guessous F, Li Y, Abounader R (2008) Signaling pathways in medulloblastoma. J Cell Physiol 217(3): 577–583

Huang J, Grotzer MA, Watanabe T, Hewer E, Pietsch T, Rutkowski S, Ohgaki H (2008) Mutations in the Nijmegen breakage syndrome gene in medulloblastomas. Clin Cancer Res 14(13):4053–4058

Koch A, Hrychyk A, Hartmann W, Waha A, Mikeska T, Waha A, Schüller U, Sörensen N, Berthold F, Goodyer CG, Wiestler OD, Birchmeier W, Behrens J, Pietsch T (2007) Mutations of the Wnt antagonist AXIN2 (Conductin) result in TCF-dependent transcription in medulloblastomas. Int J Cancer 121(2): 284–291

Lee Y, McKinnon PJ (2002) DNA ligase IV suppresses medulloblastoma formation. Cancer Res 62(22): 6395–6399

Louis DN, Ohgaki H, Wiestler OD, Cavenee WK, Burger PC, Jouvet A, Scheithauer BW, Kleihues P (2007) The 2007 WHO classification of tumours of the central nervous system. Acta Neuropathol 114(2): 97–109

Mirzoeva OK, Kawaguchi T, Pieper RO (2006) The Mre11/Rad50/Nbs1 complex interacts with the mismatch repair system and contributes to temozolomide-induced G2 arrest and cytotoxicity. Mol Cancer Ther 5(11):2757–2766

Mosor M, Mosor M, Ziółkowska I, Pernak-Schwarz M, Januszkiewicz-Lewandowska D, Nowak J (2006) Association of the heterozygous germline I171V mutation of the NBS1 gene with childhood acute lymphoblastic leukemia. Leukemia 20(8):1454–1456

Northcott PA, Rutka JT, Taylor MD (2010) Genomics of medulloblastoma: from Giemsa-banding to next-generation sequencing in 20 years. Neurosurg Focus 28(1):1–20

Offit K, Levran O, Mullaney B, Mah K, Nafa K, Batish SD, Diotti R, Schneider H, Deffenbaugh A, Scholl T, Proud VK, Robson M, Norton L, Ellis N, Hanenberg H, Auerbach AD (2003) Shared genetic susceptibility to breast cancer, brain tumors, and Fanconi anemia. J Natl Cancer Inst 95(20):1548–1551

Rieber J, Remke M, Hartmann C, Korshunov A, Burkhardt B, Sturm D, Mechtersheimer G, Wittmann A, Greil J, Blattmann C, Witt O, Behnisch W, Halatsch ME, Orakcioglu B, von Deimling A, Lichter P, Kulozik A, Pfister S (2009) Novel oncogene amplifications in tumors from a family with Li-Fraumeni syndrome. Genes Chromosomes Cancer 48(7):558–568

Roy S, Raskin L, Raymond VM, Thibodeau SN, Mody RJ, Gruber SB (2009) Pediatric duodenal cancer and biallelic mismatch repair gene mutations. Pediatr Blood Cancer 53(1):116–120

Saran A (2009) Medulloblastoma: role of developmental pathways, DNA repair signaling, and other players. Curr Mol Med 9(9):1046–1057

Schüller U, Koch A, Hartmann W, Garrè ML, Goodyer CG, Cama A, Sörensen N, Wiestler OD, Pietsch T (2005) Subtype-specific expression and genetic alterations of the chemokinereceptor gene CXCR4 in medulloblastomas. Int J Cancer 117(1):82–89

Seemanova E (1990) An increased risk for malignant neoplasms in heterozygotes for a syndrome of microcephaly, normal intelligence, growth retardation, remarkable facies, immunodeficiency and chromosomal instability. Mutat Res 238(3):321–324

Takahashi C, Kanazawa N, Yoshikawa Y, Yoshikawa R, Saitoh Y, Chiyo H, Tanizawa T, Hashimoto-Tamaoki T, Nakano Y (2009) Germline PTCH1 mutations in Japanese basal cell nevus syndrome patients. J Hum Genet 54(7):403–408

Taylor MD, Mainprize TG, Rutka JT (2000) Molecular insight into medulloblastoma and central nervous system primitive neuroectodermal tumor biology from hereditary syndromes: a review. Neurosurgery 47(4): 888–901

van der Burgt I, Chrzanowska KH, Smeets D, Weemaes C (1996) Nijmegen breakage syndrome. J Med Genet 33(2):153–156

Varon R, Vissinga C, Platzer M, Cerosaletti KM, Chrzanowska KH, Saar K, Beckmann G, Seemanová E, Cooper PR, Nowak NJ, Stumm M, Weemaes CM, Gatti RA, Wilson RK, Digweed M, Rosenthal A, Sperling K, Concannon P, Reis A (1998) Nibrin, a novel DNA double-strand break repair protein, is mutated in Nijmegen breakage syndrome. Cell 93(3):467–476

Pediatric Medulloblastoma: Pituitary Adenylyl Cyclase Activating Peptide/Protein Kinase A Antagonism of Hedgehog Signaling

14

Joseph R. Cohen, Linda M. Liau, and James A. Waschek

Contents

J.R. Cohen, Ph.D. (✉) • J.A. Waschek, Ph.D.
Semel Institute, Department of Psychiatry and Biobehavioural Sciences, David Geffen School of Medicine, University of California Los Angeles, CA 90095, USA
e-mail: cohenjr@mail.nih.gov; jwaschek@mednet.ucla.edu

L.M. Liau, Ph.D.
Jonsson Comprehensive Cancer Center, David Geffen School of Medicine, University of California Los Angeles, CA 90095, USA

Abstract

Medulloblastoma is a highly malignant pediatric brain tumor thought to commonly arise from cerebellar precursor cells that exhibit increased hedgehog signaling. Several treatment modalities, including surgical resection, radio- and chemo-therapy have enhanced the survival rates of individuals with medulloblastoma. However, significant adverse effects from some of these approaches in the developing brain necessitate the development of targeted molecular therapeutics that will minimize toxicity while maximizing tumor regression and eradication. Recent evidence suggests that the neuropeptide pituitary adenylyl cyclase activating polypeptide (PACAP) – a neuropeptide highly expressed and implicated in the development of the cerebellum and other neural structures – may play an important role in the development of medulloblastoma. Via activation of cAMP-dependent protein kinase A (PKA), PACAP negatively regulates the hedgehog pathway both in cerebellar development and medulloblastoma pathogenesis. The PACAP/PKA signaling pathway may therefore offer a novel therapeutic target to minimize the tumor burden in the pediatric population suffering from medulloblastoma.

M.A. Hayat (ed.), *Pediatric Cancer, Volume 3: Diagnosis, Therapy, and Prognosis*, Pediatric Cancer 3,
DOI 10.1007/978-94-007-4528-5_14,

Introduction

Medulloblastoma (MB), initially described by Wright in 1910 and subsequently identified by Bailey and Cushing in 1925, is a malignant pediatric brain tumor arising in the cerebellum (Dhall 2009). Occurring in 20% of pediatric central nervous system (CNS) tumor cases, MB is considered to be the most prevalent pediatric brain tumor (Dhall 2009). The majority of MB cases are diagnosed between the first and tenth year of life (Dhall 2009). Headaches, vomiting, ataxia and papilledema are some of the clinical symptoms of MB caused by CNS tissue invasion and hydrocephalus due to tumor growth (Dhall 2009). While the 5-year survival rate for children ages 0–19 years with MB is about 53%, higher survival rates are observed post-treatment (which may include surgical removal, radiotherapy and/or chemotherapy) (Dhall 2009). Clinical decision-making regarding treatment depends on prior risk stratification after initial diagnosis, based on age, class of MB, and degree of metastasis (Dhall 2009). However, in younger children, chemotherapy is preferred over radiotherapy due to the adverse side effects of radiation, which include growth retardation and significant neurocognitive deficiencies (Ris et al. 2001).

Histopathologically, MB may be classified into several types: (1) classical MB, (2) desmoplastic MB, and (3) large cell/anaplastic MB. Classic MB is characterized by round cells that have a large nucleus-to-cytoplasm ratio. Reticular networks and densely packed tumor cells characterizes desmoplastic MB – typically found in individuals with basal cell nevus syndrome (Gorlin's syndrome) (Dhall 2009). Lastly, the large cell/anaplastic class of MB possess nuclei with several shapes, as well as large nucleoli (Ellison 2002; Dhall 2009). Genetic stratification – based on the expression of several genes – has also been used to predict treatment outcome in patients with desmoplastic and classic MB (Ellison 2002), and to develop models that accurately predict MB patient relapse (Tamayo et al. 2011). In addition to histological aberrations, MB is characterized by the presence of chromosomal abnormalities (Ellison 2002). High-resolution array comparative genomic hybridization (ACGH) revealed losses in chromosomes 8p, 10q, 13q, 16q, 17p, and 20p and gain in chromosomes 4p, 7, 8q, 9, 12, 17q, 18, and 19 (Ellison 2002). Furthermore, a significant number of studies, including those discussed in more detail below, indicate that MB is associated with mutations in, or disregulation of, hedgehog (Hh) signaling molecules (Wechsler-Reya and Scott 2001; Dhall 2009; Teglund and Toftgård 2010).

Alterations in molecules of the Hh pathway have been associated with a variety of cancers, including Gorlin's syndrome, prostate cancer, glioma, digestive tract tumors, pancreatic cancer and medulloblastoma (Teglund and Toftgård 2010). Further evidence that the Hh molecular machinery contributes to MB has been demonstrated through the development of genetic mouse models that overexpress this pathway and recapitulate the human MB phenotype (Huse and Holland 2009). Moreover, evidence indicates that small molecule antagonism of the Hh pathway inhibits tumor growth in these mouse models (Berman et al. 2002; Sanchez and Ruiz i Altaba 2005) and has led to testing of a variety of Hh pathway antagonists in clinical trials (Mas and Ruiz i Altaba 2010; Ng and Curran 2011). On the other hand, recent evidence indicates that pituitary adenylyl cyclase activating polypeptide (PACAP) plays a role in the pathogenesis of MB of mice (Lelievre et al. 2008), and is capable of antagonizing Hh signaling in both cerebellar granule neurons progenitors (Vaudry et al. 2009; Nicot et al. 2002) and cells derived from primary tumors (Cohen et al. 2010).

PACAP and Its Biology

Pituitary adenylyl cyclase activating polypeptide (PACAP) is a 38-amino-acid peptide identified on the basis of its ability to induce production of cyclic adenosine monophosphate (cAMP) in the pituitary cells of rats (Vaudry et al. 2009). Belonging to the secretin/glucagon family of peptides, PACAP exists in two isoforms, PACAP-38 and PACAP-27 – the latter a truncated form of

PACAP-38 (Arimura 1998; Vaudry et al. 2009). A similar peptide, vasoactive intestinal peptide (VIP), isolated from the pig small intestine (Fahrenkrug 2010), shares 68% homology with PACAP (Vaudry et al. 2009; Fahrenkrug 2010). In humans, the PACAP gene (Adcyap1) is located on chromosome 18 region 11p, while in mice it is located on chromosome 17 (Vaudry et al. 2009). The product of the human *Adcyap1* gene is a 176 amino acid precursor called prepro-PACAP (Vaudry et al. 2009), which is cleaved into: PACAP-27, PACAP-38, the PACAP related peptide (PRP), and other peptide fragments (Vaudry et al. 2009).

Expression of PACAP is observed in neurons throughout the CNS including neocortex, the amygdala and hippocampus, the thalamus (Köves et al. 1991), the hypothalamus and the cerebellum (Vaudry et al. 2009). Furthermore, PACAP expression is detected in the peripheral nervous system, the retina, a variety of neuroendocrine cells, the pancreas (Hannibal and Fahrenkrug 2000), the digestive system, and the immune system (Vaudry et al. 2009). Additionally, receptors for PACAP are expressed in many tissues and throughout the brain, including the cerebellum. Thus, it is not surprising that a large number of biological functions are regulated by PACAP. Growth factor-like actions of PACAP regulate neuroblast proliferation and survival, and promote neuroprotection and nerve regeneration (Vaudry et al. 2009).

The expression of PACAP and its receptors has been demonstrated in the developing brains at embryonic day (E)9.5 and E10.5 in mice and rats, respectively (Vaudry et al. 2009), suggesting that PACAP may play a vital role in the patterning and development of the CNS. In 1996, Sheward and colleagues demonstrated gene expression of the PACAP receptor PAC1 in the rhombic lip, which gives rise to the external granule layer providing support of PACAP's role in early cerebellar development (Vaudry et al. 2009). The expression of PACAP within the Purkinje and granule cells of the cerebellum, as well as expression of PAC1R in the external granular layer (EGL) of the cerebellum (Vaudry et al. 2009), further implicate PACAP in regulating cerebellar development.

PACAP Receptors and Signaling Pathways

PACAP binds and interacts with high affinity to three members of the B1 family of G-protein coupled receptors (GPCRs): VPAC1R, VPAC2R and PAC1R (Vaudry et al. 2009). The human, rat and mouse versions of each of these receptors have been cloned. Both PACAP and VIP bind VPAC1R and VPAC2R with high affinity, whereas PAC1R binds only PACAP with high affinity (Vaudry et al. 2009). VPAC1R, VPAC2R and PAC1R are all strong inducers of cAMP production (Vaudry et al. 2009). While all three receptors are known to mediate neurotransmitter and immunomodulatory actions of PACAP, PAC1R seems to be the primary receptor involved in its growth factor-like actions.

The human PAC1R gene has been cloned and is located on chromosome 7 region p15, and has 16 exons (Vaudry et al. 2009). The mouse PAC1R gene, cloned by Hashimoto et al. (1996) and located on chromosome 6, is about 50 kb in length and has 18 exons (Vaudry et al. 2009). It is now well known that there are a variety of alternatively spliced variants of PAC1R, including, null, hip, hop1, hop2 and hiphop (Vaudry et al. 2009). Concentrations of PACAP between 0.1and 10 nM seemed to predominantly stimulate cAMP production via the PAC1R-hop1 and the -hiphop1 variants, while PACAP concentrations ranging from 100 to 1,000 nM stimulated cAMP production via all variants. PACAP is also known to induce phospholipase C (PLC) through the PAC1R-hop1 isoform. The null and the hop1 isoforms of PAC1R seem to be the most predominant forms in the brain (Vaudry et al. 2009). PACAP stimulation of the PAC1R-hop variant is known to elevate Ca^{+2} levels (Mustafa et al. 2007), while the PAC1R-hop1 variants are known to activate phospholipase D (PLD) (Vaudry et al. 2009).

Additionally, the activation of PAC1R by PACAP induces the hydrolysis of phosphatidylinositol 4,5-bisphosphate (PIP_2) (Vaudry et al. 2009). Furthermore, PACAP activates the mitogen-activated protein (MAP) kinases preventing apoptosis in granule cells. The protective action by PACAP has also been observed in granule cells treated with hydrogen peroxide and ethanol (Vaudry et al. 2009). The neuroprotective mechanism of PACAP is thought to occur via the upregulation of the expression of the B-cell lymphoma-2 (Bcl-2) and of c-fos – a transcription factor that regulates Bcl-2 expression (Vaudry et al. 2009). The protein Bcl-2 is known to prevent mitochondrial release of cytochrome C and subsequent apoptosis. Furthermore, the neuroprotection of granule cells induced by the activation of ERK in a cAMP-dependent manner (Vaudry et al. 2009), and by PKA mediated CREB phosphorylation. PACAP also promoted cerebellar cortical cell migration by cAMP-dependent and PLC-dependent mechanisms. Finally, PACAP antagonized Hh induction of granule cell proliferation in a PKA-dependent manner (Vaudry et al. 2009; Nicot et al. 2002).

Hedgehog Signaling, Origins and Developmental Actions

Groundbreaking work on genetic mechanisms regulating animal development, including the discovery of the "Hedgehog" (Hh) gene, was performed by Nusslein-Volhard and Wieschaus in 1980 through their genetic screen to understand larval body segmentation Drosophila melanogaster (Hooper and Scott 2005). Hedgehog (Hh), a secreted peptide, was later shown to be expressed in the posterior portions of each segment, as well as, the wing and leg imaginal discs – indicating its importance in development (Huangfu and Anderson 2006). Since those seminal studies in flies, Hh signaling has been determined to be critical for normal development of the vertebrate CNS and hematopoiesis, and for the development of the gastrointestinal tract, prostate, and many other organs (McMahon et al. 2003; Hooper and Scott 2005).

Hedgehog (Hh) signaling is activated by binding of the ligand Sonic hedgehog (Shh) to its receptor Patched1 (Ptch1) (Cohen 2003). Drosophila has one Hh gene, while mammals, including mice and humans have three forms of hedgehog: sonic hedgehog (Shh), Indian hedgehog (Ihh) and desert hedgehog (Dhh) (Huangfu and Anderson 2006). In the absence of Hh ligand, Ptch1 inhibits smoothened (SMO) activity, consequently preventing SMO interaction with a protein complex (consisting of SuFu, PKA, Fu, and the Gli transcription factors) which promotes the proteolytic processing of the Gli into the repressor form – thus preventing the transcription and expression of Hh target genes. In the presence of Hh ligand, SMO is disinhibited and free to interact with this protein complex, inhibiting the formation of the Gli repressor form, and promoting the translocation of the activator form of Gli – which leads to the transcription of Hh target genes and the activation of molecular developmental programs (Ruiz i Altaba et al. 2002). As for the receptor, Drosophila has one Ptch1 gene, while vertebrates such as mice and humans (Huangfu and Anderson 2006; Teglund and Toftgård 2010) have two similar proteins: Ptch1 and Ptch2. The mutations in Ptch1 are associated with Basal Cell Nevus (Gorlin's) Syndrome (BCNS) and medulloblastoma (MB) in both mice and humans (Dhall 2009).

In vertebrates, specifically in mammals, the axial mesoderm and notochord are two sites where Shh is produced (Martí et al. 1995). The expression and release of Shh from the notochord ultimately leads to the induction of Shh from the floor plate and the formation of a Shh gradient that patterns the ventral portions of the developing CNS (Huangfu and Anderson 2006). Patterning of the ventral forebrain from the developing telencephalon is dependent on Shh (Fuccillo et al. 2004). Furthermore, studies also indicate that Shh (in combination with Fibroblast Growth Factor signaling) is crucial for the development of the midbrain (Ishibashi and McMahon 2002; Kiecker and Lumsden 2004) and rhombomere 1 (the area that gives rise to the cerebellum) (Teglund and Toftgård 2010).

Regulation of Hedgehog Signaling by Protein Kinase A (PKA)

Research in both invertebrates (Jiang and Struhl 1995) and vertebrates (Huangfu and Anderson 2006) implicates a role for cAMP dependent protein kinase A (PKA) in the regulation of Hh signaling. Jiang and Struhl (1995) as well as other groups have demonstrated that that PKA may antagonize Hh signaling. In Drosophila, ectopic furrows and wing duplications (resulting from increased Hh signaling) have been observed in flies with cells lacking PKA activity in the anterior margins of wing or leg disks indicating that PKA may indeed antagonize Hh signaling (Huangfu and Anderson 2006; Teglund and Toftgård 2010). Similar observations of PKA mediated Hh pathway antagonism have been made in zebrafish and mice (Huangfu and Anderson 2006; Teglund and Toftgård 2010). Expression of a constitutively active subunit of PKA suppressed the expression of Hh target genes, while suppression of PKA induced the activation of Hh target genes (Huangfu and Anderson 2006; Teglund and Toftgård 2010).

Before activation, PKA is in an inactive state as part of a heterotetrameric protein complex consisting of two catalytic (C) subunits and two regulatory (R) subunits – thus forming the R2C2 complex (Taylor et al. 1990). The R subunits prevent the catalytic activity of the substrate binding domains of PKA (Taylor et al. 1990). Canonical PKA signaling is initiated by binding of an extracellular ligand to a G-protein coupled receptor (which is usually a seven transmembrane domain protein) (reviewed extensively in Gilman 1987). Upon ligand binding the receptor undergoes a conformational change that activates the associated heterotrimeric G-protein, inducing the dissociation of the stimulatory-G-protein (Gs) (Gilman 1987). The Gs complex allows Gsα to associate with membrane bound adenylyl cyclase (AC), catalyzing the conversion of ATP to cAMP, and allowing cAMP binding to the regulatory subunits of PKA and their subsequent dissociation (Gilman 1987). PKA is known to phosphorylate a variety of intracellular substrates (Gao et al. 2008) including the transcription factor cAMP response element binding protein (CREB) which plays a role in development and tumorigenesis (Rosenberg et al. 2002).

In Drosophila, PKA has been shown to be crucial for the proteolytic processing of cubitus interruptus (Ci) – a transcription factor homologous to the Gli transcription factors in vertebrates. In 1999, Wang and Holmgren (1999) showed that PKA targets Ci-155 for proteosomal degradation and blocks its activity (Huangfu and Anderson 2006). Furthermore, PKA is can regulate the cleavage of Ci-155 into Ci-75 which acts as a transcriptional inhibitor (Huangfu and Anderson 2006). Interestingly, PKA phosphorylation of SMO promotes Hh signaling in Drosophila (Hooper and Scott 2005). Similarly, in vertebrates both the proteosomal processing of Gli3 into a smaller repressor form, and eventual proteosomal-mediated degradation of Gli2 and Gli3, are dependent on phosphorylation by PKA (Teglund and Toftgård 2010). Recent work by our laboratory has demonstrated that antagonism of Hh signaling and cellular proliferation in primary medulloblastoma derived cells (tumorspheres) may occur in a manner that relies on cAMP-dependent PKA (Cohen et al. 2010). These findings, along with other lines of investigation highlight the regulation of Hh signaling by PKA. As a negative regulator of Hh signaling, PKA may have implications for developmental and tumor biology.

PACAP and Hedgehog Interactions in Cerebellar and Medulloblastoma Development

Both Shh and PACAP seem to play crucial roles in the development of the cerebellum. Purkinje cells of mice and chicks express Shh (Wechsler-Reya and Scott 2001). The secreted Shh ligand of Purkinje cells acts as a potent mitogen in the granule cell precursors of the EGL, the cells believed to give rise to MB (Wechsler-Reya and Scott 2001). The Hh receptor Ptch1, along with the Gli transcription factors are expressed in the EGL of the developing cerebellum (Wechsler-Reya and Scott 2001). Additionally, the level of Shh affects the foliation of the cerebellum (Corrales et al. 2006), and blocking this action of Shh inhibits the migration of granule neurons and leads to abnormal cerebellar development (Wechsler-Reya and Scott 2001). The effects induced by Shh on GNPs may be counteracted by cAMP, PKA or PACAP (Huangfu and Anderson 2006; Ruiz i Altaba et al. 2002; Vaudry et al. 2009).

Within the rat cerebellum, fibers around granule cells, as well as, Purkinje cells express PACAP, and PACAP expression reaches adult levels by postnatal day (P) 7 (Vaudry et al. 2009). Additionally, autoradiographic studies in the developing rat cerebellum indicate that the EGL expresses binding sites for PACAP from P8 to P25 (Vaudry et al. 2009). In cultured GNPs and mature granule cells PACAP has been shown to prevent apoptosis from oxidative stress and ethanol-induced apoptosis, and to promote their survival. Falluel-Morel and colleagues showed that PAC1$^{-/-}$ mice exhibited decreased granule cell survival. Furthermore, PACAP$^{-/-}$ mice exhibited significant decreases in the EGL and IGL thickness, along with increased apoptosis within the developing cerebellum (Vaudry et al. 2009). Injection of PACAP into the subarachnoid space above the cerebellum of rats results in an increase in cerebellar cortical volume (Vaudry et al. 2009), and PACAP prevented the migration of granule neurons (Vaudry et al. 2009).

As mentioned previously, PACAP antagonizes the proliferative action of Shh on granule cells in rats and mice (Vaudry et al. 2009; Nicot et al. 2002). Moreover, loss of a single copy of the PACAP gene in *ptch1* mutant mice increased the incidence of MB when compared to *ptch1* mutant mice alone (Lelievre et al. 2008). Recently, our laboratory found that Hh signaling and proliferation in mouse MB tumorsphere cultures was antagonized by PACAP, and that this action of PACAP was blocked in a PKA dependent manner (Cohen et al. 2010). PACAP is a neuropeptide that is important for the proper development of the cerebellum and medulloblastoma tumors in mice. Further research is needed to understand the *in vivo* effect of PACAP administration on human MB. Either PACAP, or the small molecule agonists of PACAP receptors (PAC1R), may provide novel alternative strategies to reverse the increased Hh signaling thought to drive the growth of many cases of MBs.

In conclusion, the neuropeptide PACAP is a molecule with a variety of important biological actions in the CNS, and in cerebellar and MB development. Several findings, including the ability of PACAP to regulate PKA and hedgehog signaling in both cerebellar granule neuron precursors and primary MB-derived tumorsphere cells, and the increased MB tumor incidence in *patched-1* mutant mice bearing a mutation of a single PACAP allele, suggests that the PACAP pathway is a promising target for the treatment MB through the attenuation of excessive hedgehog signaling.

References

Arimura A (1998) Perspectives on pituitary adeylate cyclase activating polypeptide (PACAP) in the neuroendocrine, endocrine and nervous systems. Jpn J Physiol 48:301–331

Berman DM, Karhadkar SS, Hallahan AR, Pritchard JI, Eberhart CG, Watkins DN, Chen JK, Cooper MK, Taipale J, Olson JM, Beachy PA (2002) Medulloblastoma growth inhibition by Hedgehog pathway blockade. Science 297(5586):1559–1561

Cohen MM Jr (2003) The Hedgehog signaling network. Am J Med Genet A 123A(1):5–28

Cohen JR, Resnick DZ, Niewiadomski P, Dong H, Liau LM, Waschek JA (2010) Pituitary adenylyl cyclase activating polypeptide inhibits gli1 gene expression and proliferation in primary medulloblastoma derived tumorsphere cultures. BMC Cancer 10:676

Corrales JD, Blaess S, Mahoney EM, Joyner AL (2006) The level of sonic Hedgehog signaling regulates the complexity of cerebellar foliation. Development 133:1811–1821

Dhall G (2009) Medulloblastoma. J Child Neurol 24(11): 1418–1430

Ellison D (2002) Classifying the medulloblastoma: insights from morphology and molecular genetics. Neuropathol Appl Neurobiol 28:257–282

Fahrenkrug J (2010) VIP and PACAP. Results Probl Cell Differ 50:221–234

Fuccillo M, Rallu M, McMahon AP, Fishell G (2004) Temporal requirement for Hedgehog signaling in ventral telencephalic patterning. Development 131:5031–5040

Gao X, Jin C, Ren J, Yao X, Xue Y (2008) Proteome-wide prediction of PKA phosphorylation sites in eukaryotic kingdom. Genomics 92:457–463

Gilman AG (1987) G proteins: transducers of receptor-generated signals. Annu Rev Biochem 56:615–649

Hannibal J, Fahrenkrug J (2000) Pituitary adenylate cyclase-activating polypeptide in intrinsic and extrinsic nerves of the rat pancreas. Cell Tissue Res 299(1):59–70

Hashimoto H, Yamamoto K, Hagigara N, Ogawa N, Nishino A, Aino H, Nogi H, Imanishi K, Matsuda T, Baba A (1996) cDNA cloning of a mouse pituitary adenylate cyclase-activating polypeptide receptor. Biochim Biophys Acta 281(2):129–133

Hooper JE, Scott MP (2005) Communicating with Hedgehogs. Nat Rev Mol Cell Biol 6:306–317

Huangfu D, Anderson KV (2006) Signaling from Smo to Ci/Gli: conservation and divergence of Hedgehog pathways from Drosophila to vertebrates. Development 133(1):3–14

Huse JT, Holland EC (2009) Genetically engineered mouse models of brain cancer and the promise of preclinical testing. Brain Pathol 19(1):132–143

Ishibashi M, McMahon AP (2002) A sonic Hedgehog-dependent signaling relay regulates growth of diencephalic and mesencephalic primordia in the early mouse embryo. Development 129:4807–4819

Jiang J, Struhl G (1995) Protein Kinase A and Hedgehog signaling in Drosophila limb development. Cell 80:563–572

Kiecker C, Lumsden A (2004) Hedgehog signaling from the ZLI regulates diencephalic regional identity. Nat Neurosci 7:1242–1249

Köves K, Arimura A, Görcs TG, Somogyvári-Vigh A (1991) Comparative distribution of immunoreactive pituitary adenylate cyclase activating polypeptide and vasoactive intestinal polypeptide in rat forebrain. Neuroendocrinology 54(2):159–169

Lelievre V, Seksenyan A, Nobuta H, Yong WH, Chhith S, Niewiadomski P, Cohen JR, Dong H, Flores A, Liau LM, Kornblum HI, Scott MP, Waschek JA (2008) Disruption of the PACAP gene promotes medulloblastoma in ptc1 mutant mice. Dev Biol 313(1):359–370

Martí E, Takada R, Bumcrot DA, Sasaki H, McMahon AP (1995) Distribution of Sonic Hedgehog peptides in the developing chick and mouse embryo. Development 121(8):2537–2547

Mas C, Ruiz i Altaba A (2010) Small molecule modulation of HH-GLI signaling: current leads, trials and tribulations. Biochem Pharmacol 80(5):712–723

McMahon AP, Ingham PW, Tabin CJ (2003) Developmental roles and clinical significance of Hedgehog signaling. Curr Top Dev Biol 53:1–114

Mustafa T, Grimaldi M, Eiden LE (2007) The hop cassette of the PAC1 receptor confers coupling to Ca2+ elevation required for pituitary adenylate cyclase-activating polypeptide-evoked neurosecretion. J Biol Chem 282(11):8079–8091

Ng JM, Curran T (2011) The Hedgehog's tale: developing strategies for targeting cancer. Nat Rev Cancer 11(7):493–501

Nicot A, Lelièvre V, Tam J, Waschek JA, DiCicco-Bloom E (2002) Pituitary adenylate cyclase-activating polypeptide and sonic hedgehog interact to control cerebellar granuale precursor cell proliferation. J Neurosci 22(21):9244–9254

Ris MD, Packer R, Goldwein J, Jones-Wallace D, Boyett JM (2001) Intellectual outcome after reduced-dose radiation therapy plus adjuvant chemotherapy for medulloblastoma: a Children's Cancer Group study. J Clin Oncol 19(15):3470–3476

Rosenberg D, Groussin L, Jullian E, Perlemoine K, Bertagna X, Bertherat J (2002) Role of the PKA-regulated transcription factor CREB in development and tumorigenesis of endocrine tissues. Ann N Y Acad Sci 968:65–74

Ruiz i Altaba A, Palma V, Dahmane N (2002) Hedgehog-GLI signaling and the growth of the brain. Nat Rev Neurosci 3(1):24–33

Sanchez P, Ruiz i Altaba A (2005) In vivo inhibition of endogenous brain tumors through systemic interference of Hedgehog signaling in mice. Mech Dev 122(2):223–230

Tamayo P, Cho YJ, Tsherniak A, Greulich H, Ambrogio L, Schouten-van Meeteren N, Zhou T, Buxton A, Kool M, Meyerson M, Pomeroy SL, Mesirov JP (2011) Predicting relapse in patients with medulloblastoma by integrating evidence from clinical and genomic features. J Clin Oncol 29(11):1415–1423

Taylor SS, Buechler JA, Yonemoto W (1990) cAMP-dependent protein kinase: framework for a diverse family of regulatory enzymes. Annu Rev Biochem 59:971–1005

Teglund S, Toftgård R (2010) Hedgehog beyond medulloblastoma and basal cell carcinoma. Biochim Biophys Acta 1805(2):181–208

Vaudry D, Falluel-Morel A, Bourgault S, Basille M, Burel D, Wurtz O, Fournier A, Chow BK, Hashimoto H, Galas L, Vaudry H (2009) Pituitary adenylate cyclase-activating polypeptide and its receptors: 20 years after the discovery. Pharmacol Rev 61(3):283–357

Wang QT, Holmgren RA (1999) The subcellular localization and activity of Drosophila cubitus interruptus are regulated at multiple levels. Development 126:5097–5106

Wechsler-Reya R, Scott MP (2001) The developmental biology of brain tumors. Annu Rev Neurosci 24:385–428

Medulloblastoma: Role of *MYCN* Gene Amplification Using Fluorescence *In Situ* Hybridization and Real Time Quantitative PCR Methods

15

Cecilia Surace

Contents

C. Surace (✉)
Cytogenetics and Molecular Genetics, Children's Hospital "Bambino Gesú", Piazza S. Onofrio 4, 00165 Rome, Italy
e-mail: cecilia.surace@opbg.net

Abstract

Gene amplification is a mechanism that can activate cellular oncogenes to express abnormal levels of protein. The *MYCN* (v-myc myelocytomatosis viral-related oncogene) gene was the first amplified oncogene that was demonstrated to have a clinical significance in neuroblastoma. Moreover, it has also been reported in medulloblastoma, a malignant and invasive embryonal tumor of the central nervous system. In recent years, the improvement of cytomolecular techniques, such as fluorescence *in situ* hybridization (FISH) and real time quantitative polymerase chain reaction (RQ-PCR), has supplemented the classical cytogenetic analysis for diagnosis and prognosis of medulloblastoma. FISH has advanced the detection of gene amplification revealing episomes, not visible at the karyotype level and it has represented a powerful tool for investigating gene amplification on archival material. RQ-PCR analysis has been used for detecting *MYCN* copy number alterations and refining the breakpoints of the amplicon containing *MYCN* at higher resolution. Thus, these techniques investigating the *MYCN* amplification, have helped to identify a trend towards poorer outcomes in patients and, in combination with histo-pathological assessment, in the next future hopefully will assist a refined classification of medulloblastoma.

M.A. Hayat (ed.), *Pediatric Cancer, Volume 3: Diagnosis, Therapy, and Prognosis*, Pediatric Cancer 3,
DOI 10.1007/978-94-007-4528-5_15,

Introduction

Gene amplification is a mechanism that can activate cellular oncogenes to express abnormal levels of protein. The amplified elements are usually tandemly duplicated to form double minutes (dmin) and/or homogeneously staining regions (hsr) that are visible at the karyotype level. Recently, episomes, an additional form of gene amplification remaining undetectable by conventional cytogenetics, have been reported both in haematologic and in solid tumors (Graux et al. 2004; Surace et al. 2008). Episomes may result from a double-strand DNA break, followed by the end-fusion through the non-homologous end joining mechanism, and may represent the initial step of gene amplification. In the majority of cases, it is immediately followed by concatenation, leading to double minutes formation and/or subsequent integration into chromosomal sites in the form of homogenously staining regions (Savelyeva and Schwab 2001).

The amplicon size is usually larger than the transcriptional unit of a single oncogene and includes several coamplified genes. However, this situation complicates the identification of the target gene (Frühwald et al. 2000). The *MYCN* (v-myc myelocytomatosis viral-related oncogene) gene, located at 2p24, was the first amplified oncogene that was demonstrated to have a clinical significance due to its association with aggressively growing tumor phenotypes as brain tumors (Schwab and Amler 1990). It plays an important role in neurogenesis, being essential for rapid expansion of neural progenitor cells during central nervous system (CNS) development, and for inhibition of neuronal differentiation (Knoepfler et al. 2002). The most consistent association between *MYCN* amplification and tumor development is shown in human neuroblastoma, where this gene is amplified in both primary tumors and established cell lines (Corvi et al. 1994). It has also been reported in medulloblastoma (MB) that, as neuroblastoma, is a malignant and invasive embryonal tumor of the CNS (Bayani et al. 2000; Surace et al. 2008).

Medulloblastoma: An Overview

Medulloblastoma is a neuro-epithelial tumor formed from poorly differentiated cells at a very early stage of their life. It is a fast-growing tumor that usually origins in the cerebellum, but may spread to other parts of the brain. Although MB represents the most common malignant tumor of CNS among children, a significant proportion (30%) occurs in adults (Ellison 2002). The name MB appeared for the first time in the classification of CNS tumors created by Bailey and Cushing (1925), where they recognized similarities between its cytological features and those of the embryonic medullary velum. Four histological variants of classic MB have been reported by the 2007 World Health Organization (WHO) classification: desmoplastic/nodular medulloblastoma (DM), medulloblastoma with extensive nodularity (N), large cell medulloblastoma (LC), and anaplastic medulloblastoma (A) (Louis et al. 2007).

In the past, two additional rare variants were reported, medullomyoblastoma and melanocytic medulloblastoma, but now these lesions are no longer considered distinct entities. The former, currently termed "MB with myogenic differentiation", may be used to designate any histological MB subtype containing focal rhabdomyoblastic features with immunoreactivity to desmin, myoglobin and fast myosin, but not smooth muscle α-actin alone. The latter, now named "MB with melanotic differentiation" is distinguished by the presence of melanin in cell clusters which may occasionally have an epithelioid appearance and tubular or papillary architecture that can occur in any variant of medulloblastoma (Louis et al. 2007).

Regarding the prognosis, the LC variant appears to be aggressive and highly malignant (Brown et al. 2000); in contrast, the DM and N variants show a more favorable clinical course as compared to the large group of classic MB (Korshunov et al. 2008); instead, the A variant partly shares the poor prognosis of the LC variant (Giangaspero et al. 2006), and partly shows similar survival of DM and N (Min et al. 2006). However, the predictive performance of current risk stratification, which is entirely based on clinical variables, needs to be improved because of the bad prognosis of children with tumor relapse, and because of therapy-related long-term effects of survivors (Polkinghorn and Tarbell 2007). An increased understanding of the biology of MB to determine the cell of origin of the MB and the mechanisms in which it is involved, together with the identification of cytomolecular markers, could be used alongside histological diagnosis to refine tumor classification and direct existing therapies.

Chromosome and Gene Abnormalities in Medulloblastoma

For many years, the efforts of several authors focused on correlating the chromosome anomalies with particular tumors in order to identify molecular markers useful in diagnosis and in monitoring the progression of the tumor. Extensive cytogenetic characterization of MB has occurred during the last two decades (Bigner et al. 1988), revealing consistent genetic events. The most common cytogenetic abnormality is the isochromosome 17q. The breakpoint is in the proximal portion of the p arm at 17p11.2, resulting in an abnormal dicentric chromosome constituted by two copies of the long q arm, that is present in ~50% of the cases. In a few cases, partial or complete loss of the short arm of chromosome 17 occurs through interstitial deletion, unbalanced translocation or monosomy 17 (Capodano 2000). Studies on the loss of heterozygosity (LOH) confirmed loss of genomic segments of 17p in 30–45% of cases and showed a correlation between LOH for 17p and a poor response to therapy and shortened survival. Mutations of *p53* gene located on 17p13 have been found in only 5–10% of these tumors (Capodano 2000).

Chromosome 1 is also involved in MB. Rearrangements of chromosome 1 often result in trisomy 1q without loss of the p-arm (Lo et al. 2007). Other less common chromosomal changes are: deletions of 6q, 8p, 10q, 11p and 16q, and gain involving chromosome 7 (Lo et al. 2007). The most commonly reported amplified and overexpressed genes in MB are *cMYC* (myelocytomatosis viral oncogene homolog, 8q24) and *MYCN*, found in ~6–8% of cases (Bayani et al. 2000; Lamont et al. 2004; Surace et al. 2008).

Several other less known candidate genes have been found overexpressed in regions of gains/amplifications. For example, ribosomal protein S9 (*RPS9*, 19q13) has been shown to play an antiapoptotic role that protects neuronal cells from reactive oxygen species (Kim et al. 2003), although how its overexpression contributes to MB pathogenesis is not clear, because some reports have shown that *RPS9* is downregulated in pancreatic cancer (Crnogorac-Jurcevic et al. 2001).

Overexpression of *ErbB2* (*HER2*) (erythroblastic leukemia viral oncogene homolog 2, 17q21) has been found in aggressive variant of MB, while high *TrkC* (neurotrophic tyrosine kinase receptor type3, 15q25) expression indicates a favourable outcome. Instead, associations between abnormalities in the shh/PTCH pathway and the desmoplastic variant are more controversial (Ellison 2002).

Cytomolecular Tools in Revealing *MYCN* Gene Amplification

The cytogenetic and molecular analyses represent an important part of the assessment of several solid tumors. The methods for revealing chromosome abnormalities have been supplemented in recent years by the improvement of cytomolecular techniques, such as, classic and array comparative genomic hybridization (CGH), fluorescence *in situ* hybridization (FISH), and real time quantitative polymerase chain reaction (RQ-PCR). A brief overview of the CGH will be reported in this paragraph, while in the next sections FISH and Real Time Quantitative PCR methods (RQ-PCR) will be examined in detail. These approaches precisely define the level of amplification, the size of the amplified genomic segment, and the location of both proximal and distal breakpoints. CGH is one of the main approaches for the identification of losses, gains, and amplifications of chromosome regions in cancer cells, with the advantage that the analysis can be performed using relatively small amounts of DNA, without the need of tumor chromosomes. This approach has been extended to microarray platforms, which provide an increased resolution for the definition of small cytogenetic events and the positions of the breakpoints involved in abnormalities (Lo et al. 2007).

Although the resolution to study the copy number changes has improved considerably with the transition to a microarray platform, the cytogenetic landscape of MB has not changed significantly (Rossi et al. 2006). One advantage provided by array-CGH combined with high density gene expression studies from the same tumor, is the possibility to associate copy number changes with specific genes that show concordant changes in expression profiles. Lo et al. (2007) correlated the losses and gains observed in a group of 26 MB by means of array-CGH with increased and decreased expression of genes at those loci studied using gene expression array and they revealed *MYCN* amplification and overexpression.

Moreover, they studied the amplification on chromosome 2 involving the *MYCN* locus in two tumors. In one of these tumors the amplicon was largely confined to a 1.3 Mb region including the *MYCN* locus, as well as the *DDX1* and *NAG* genes. In the other tumor, there were several amplification events along the length of the chromosome, including a 2p amplicon that spanned the *NAG-DDX1-MYCN* interval. Although array-CGH allows detection of single copy number changes, it is more expensive, time consuming, and requires special equipments.

MYCN Gene Amplification Detected with FISH

Gene amplification in MB, both in primary tumors and in cell lines, is usually observed at karyotype level as double minutes and homogeneously staining regions. The FISH technique has improved the detection of gene amplification revealing episomes, not visible at the karyotype level. It represents a powerful tool for investigating gene amplification on archival material. The major advantage of FISH analysis on paraffin sections is its ability to identify clusters of cells in order to evaluate intra-tumoral heterogeneity. Korshunov et al. (2008) investigated a cohort of 28 of MB samples obtained from primary tumors finding *MYCN* amplification in three samples. Interphase FISH analysis of 5 μm paraffin sections was performed using a dual-color commercial probe set containing a centromere 2p11-q11 probe and a locus-specific 2p24/*MYCN* probe. All FISH experiments were performed in duplicate. Samples showing >90% of nuclei with signals were evaluated by two independent investigators, and signals were scored in at least 200 non-overlapping, intact nuclei. Ten non-neoplastic cerebellar specimens were used as a control for each probe set. Specimens were considered amplified for *MYCN*, when >10% of tumor cells exhibited either more than 8 signals of the oncogene probe with the reference/control ratio >2.0 or innumerable tight clusters of signals of the locus specific probe.

Different patterns of *MYCN* amplification can be recognized in tumor nuclei, ranging from spots of fluorescent signals (episome/double-minute pattern) to clumps of different sizes (pattern of homogeneously staining region). High-level amplification, defined as large masses of amplified signal occupying much of the nucleus, tended to occur in tumors with a high proportion of amplification-positive nuclei (high-frequency amplification). Amplification of *MYCN* gene in MB is highly variable, both in terms of the pattern of FISH signals in individual nuclei and in the proportion of nuclei that demonstrates amplification signals. Lamont et al. (2004) described these parameters, respectively, as level and frequency of amplification.

Other authors (Aldosari et al. 2002) investigated the frequency and prognostic significance of *MYCN* amplification in 77 MB samples using a dual-color FISH, displaying the centromere of chromosome 9 in green and *MYCN* gene in red. The number of signals for the chromosome 9 centromere, compared with the number of *MYCN*

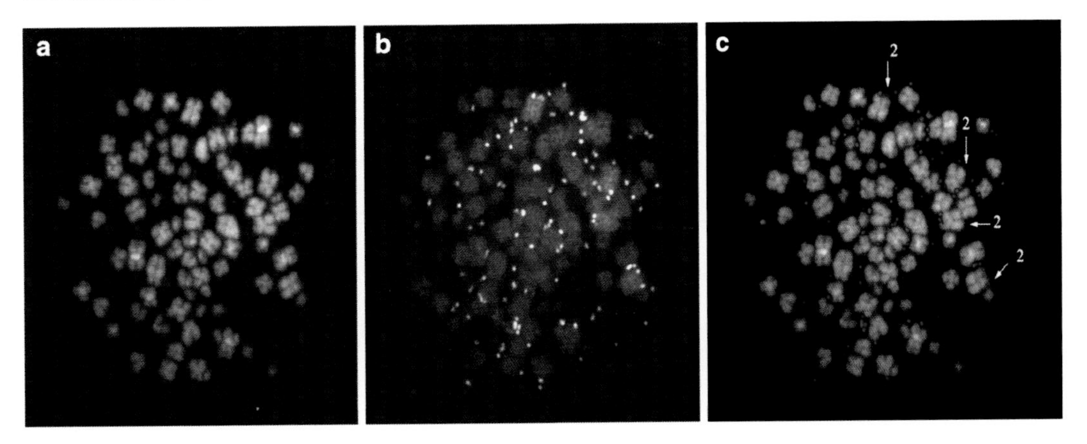

Fig. 15.1 Result of FISH experiment performed using a probe containing *MYCN* gene. (**a**) Metaphase DAPI-stained of a patient; (**b**) signals of the probe labeled with Cy3; (**c**) merge of the two previous pictures showing signals both on the normal chromosomes 2 and on the episomes

signals, revealed amplification. The presence of three or more signals for the centromere of chromosome 9 reflected changes in ploidy, a status that was found in 6/77 cases. The only case reported in the literature showing *MYCN* amplification in the form of episomes (Surace et al. 2008) also indicates that FISH analysis can disclose *MYCN* amplification in MB (Fig. 15.1) in the absence of detectable chromosome 2p24 abnormalities with Giemsa analysis, suggesting that amplification may be more frequent than expected by conventional cytogenetics. Reiterative FISH experiments using a panel of appropriate BAC clones located proximally and distally to the boundaries of the amplified segment revealed the location of both proximal and distal breakpoints defining the size of the amplified segment at FISH resolution level. Co-hybridization experiments did neither detect deletions internal to the episomes nor deletions at the normal chromosomes 2.

MYCN Gene Amplification Detected with RQ-PCR

RQ-PCR analysis has been used for detecting the *MYCN* copy number alterations and refining the breakpoints at higher resolution. Compared to endpoint quantitation methods, RQ-PCR offers precise and reproducible results relying on threshold cycle (C_T) values determined during the exponential phase of PCR rather than at the endpoint. Thus, the higher the starting copy number of the DNA target sequence is, the sooner a significant increase in fluorescence occurs and the lower the C_T values are observed.

Malakho et al. (2008) quantified the *MYCN* gene copy number, including low-level gain, in 22 MBs for designing a primer set for rapid and accurate measurement of *MYCN* gene dosage based on the RQ-PCR method. The absolute content of *MYCN* and the control gene *TBP* (TATA box binding protein) in tumor samples was obtained in one plate by extrapolation on calibration curves generated with reference DNA and subsequent comparison of copy numbers. The reverse primer and the probe were located in the exon 3 of the *MYCN* gene sequence and in the exon 6 of the *TBP* gene sequence, while the forward primer was positioned in the close upstream intron. Efficiency and sensitivity of selected primers and probes were preliminary validated on 4 MB DNA samples and a control. The authors detected an extra *MYCN* gene copy in 8 out of 22 samples showing a normalized copy number (*MYCN* copy number/*TBP* copy number) more than 1.3 times of the cut-off based on control DNA samples distribution in all RQ-PCR experiment sets. Low-level gain was

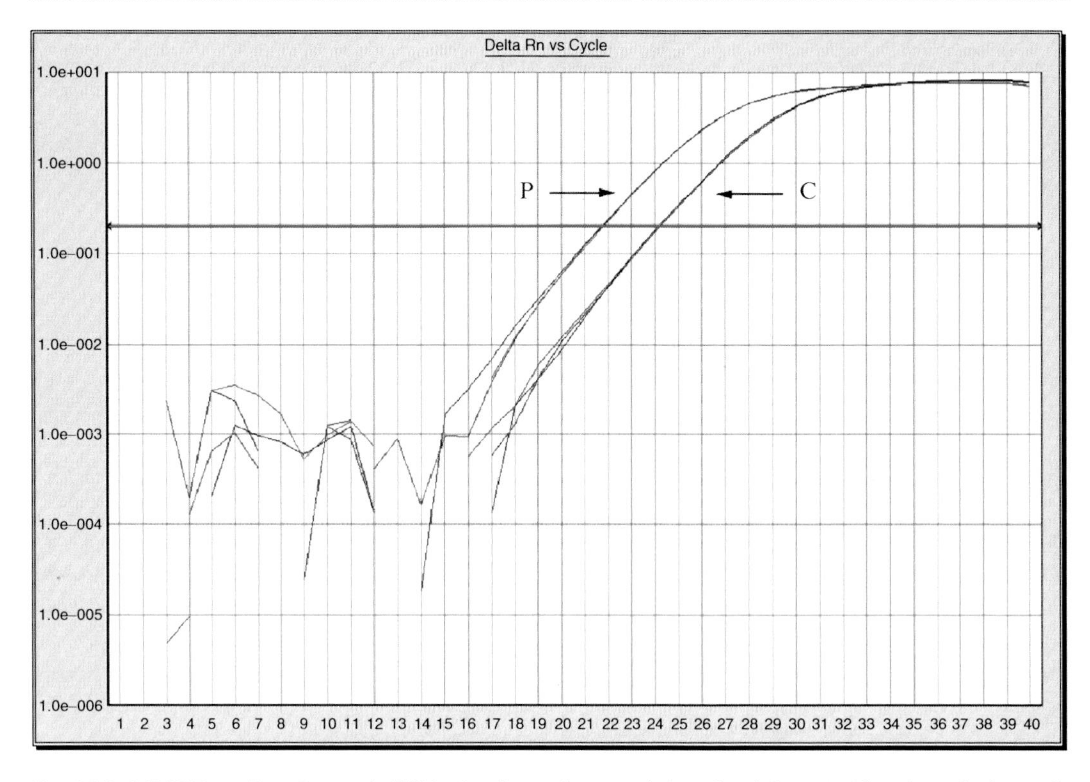

Fig. 15.2 RQ-PCR profiles of genomic DNA of patient (*P*) and healthy control (*C*) obtained using a primer pair included in the amplified region. Each experiment has been carried out in triplicate and has showed a lower C_T value for (*P*) than control (*C*), indicating a higher starting copy number of the DNA target sequence

observed in 5 out of 8 samples, whereas the remaining 3 out of 8 cases showed that *MYCN* was highly amplified.

Raggi et al. (1999) preferred to use *ACTB* (β-actin) as control gene, but it would have been best to choose two or more single copy genes on different chromosomes with the same amplification efficiency value as that of *MYCN* gene. Regarding the refining of the breakpoints at higher resolution, multiple primer pairs were designed on the sequence of the BAC clones encompassing, respectively, the distal and the proximal breakpoint of the amplified genomic segment in episomes, for identifying regions of switch between amplified and non-amplified sequences (Surace et al. 2008) (Fig. 15.2). RQ-PCR experiments using primers located within the *MYCN* gene yielded 30-fold copy number increase, resulting in a very clear-cut distinction between amplified/non-amplified sequences.

Association Between *MYCN* Amplification and Medulloblastoma Histologic Variants

Molecular markers that are strongly associated with particular histo-pathological variants help to promote diagnostic accuracy. A strong association has been reported between *MYCN* amplification and loss of 17p/presence of i(17q) in the large cell/anaplastic phenotype (Eberhart et al. 2002; Lamont et al. 2004). Patients with this MB variant show a shorter median survival, suggesting that tumor cells with these chromosomal abnormalities represent cytological sources for selective growth advantage, which may underlie further clinical progression.

The current concept of the molecular pathogenesis of MB suggests that these tumors have the ability to undergo stepwise progression, as it has been demonstrated for other tumors, including colocarcinoma. The hypothetic model of MB pathogenesis includes primary "initiation events" (i.e., Hedgehog, NOTCH, and WNT activation) and subsequent "progression events" (i.e., chromosome 17 aberrations, *cMYC/MYCN* amplifications, and others). Nevertheless, this is only a hypothesis, since conclusive evidence of temporal molecular MB progression has not been presented yet (Korshunov et al. 2008). Intriguingly, 2 MB cases showed unexpected loss of cells bearing *MYCN* amplification within their intracranial metastatic deposits. Metastatic lesions have been widely thought to arise from a small selected fraction of cells in the primary tumor, which share molecular alterations associated with loss of cell adhesion and increased cell motility. Perhaps, *MYCN* amplification has no effects on the capability of MB cells to disseminate throughout the CNS. However, this alteration seems to induce locally aggressive behavior (Korshunov et al. 2008).

In conclusion, some authors have examined in detail the prognostic importance of *MYCN* expression in medulloblastoma, identifying a trend towards poorer outcomes in patients whose tumors have detectable levels of *MYCN* mRNA (Eberhart et al. 2004). In the near future, a combined evaluation of histo-pathological and molecular assessments of MB, hopefully will evolve into a refined classification, as a result of efforts to understand the molecular basis of the biological diversity shown by individual neoplasms. It will advance the risk stratification of patients, improving existing therapies and suggesting novel treatments.

References

Aldosari N, Bigner SH, Burger PC, Becker L, Kepner JL, Friedman HS, McLendon RE (2002) MYCC and MYCN oncogene amplification in medulloblastoma. Arch Pathol Lab Med 126:540–544

Bailey P, Cushing H (1925) Medulloblastoma cerebelli. Arch Neurol Psychiatry 14:192–223

Bayani J, Zielenska M, Marrano P, Ng YK, Taylor MD, Jay V, Rutka JT, Squire JA (2000) Molecular cytogenetic analysis of medulloblastomas and supratentorial primitive neuroectodermal tumors by using conventional banding, comparative genomic hybridization, and spectral karyotyping. J Neurosurg 93:437–448

Bigner SH, Mark J, Friedman HS, Biegel JA, Bigner DD (1988) Structural chromosomal abnormalities in human medulloblastoma. Cancer Genet Cytogenet 30:91–101

Brown HG, Kepner JL, Perlman EJ, Friedman HS, Strother DR, Duffner PK, Kun LE, Goldthwaite PT, Burger PC (2000) Large cell/anaplastic medulloblastomas: a Pediatric Oncology Group Study. J Neuropathol Exp Neurol 59:857–865

Capodano AM (2000) Nervous system tumors: medulloblastoma. Atlas Genet Cytogenet Oncol Hematol. http://AtlasGeneticsOncology.org/Genes/MedulloblastomaID5065.html

Corvi R, Amler LC, Savelyeva L, Gehring M, Schwab M (1994) MYCN is retained in single copy at chromosome 2 band p23–24 during amplification in human neuroblastoma cells. Proc Natl Acad Sci U S A 91:5523–5527

Crnogorac-Jurcevic T, Efthimiou E, Capelli P, Blaveri E, Baron A, Terris B, Jones M, Tyson K, Bassi C, Scarpa A, Lemoine NR (2001) Gene expression profiles of pancreatic cancer and stromal desmoplasia. Oncogene 20:7437–7446

Eberhart CG, Kratz JE, Schuster A, Goldthwaite P, Cohen KJ, Perlman EJ, Burger PC (2002) Comparative genomic hybridization detects an increased number of chromosomal alterations in large cell/anaplastic medulloblastomas. Brain Pathol 12:36–44

Eberhart CG, Kratz JE, Wang Y, Summers K, Stearns D, Cohen K, Dang CV, Burger PC (2004) Histopathological and molecular prognostic markers in medulloblastoma: c-myc, N-myc, TrkC, and anaplasia. J Neuropathol Exp Neurol 63:441–449

Ellison D (2002) Classifying the medulloblastoma: insights from morphology and molecular genetics. Neuropathol Appl Neurobiol 28:257–282

Frühwald MC, O'Dorisio MS, Rush LJ, Reiter JL, Smiraglia DJ, Wenger G, Costello JF, White PS, Krahe R, Brodeur GM, Plass C (2000) Gene amplification in PNETs/medulloblastomas: mapping of a novel amplified gene within the MYCN amplicon. J Med Genet 37:501–509

Giangaspero F, Wellek S, Masuoka J, Gessi M, Kleihues P, Ohgaki H (2006) Stratification of medulloblastoma on the basis of histopathological grading. Acta Neuropathol 112:5–12

Graux C, Cools J, Melotte C, Quentmeier H, Ferrando A, Levine R, Vermeesch JR, Stul M, Dutta B, Boeckx N, Bosly A, Heimann P, Uyttebroeck A, Mentens N, Somers R, MavLeod RAF, Drexler HG, Look AT, Gilliland DG, Michaux L, Vandenberghe P, Wlodarska I, Marynen P, Hagemejijer A (2004) Fusion of NUP214 to ABL on amplified episomes in T-cell acute lymphoblastic leukemia. Nat Genet 36:1084–1089

Kim SY, Lee MJ, Cho KC, Choi YS, Choi JS, Sung KW, Kwon OJ, Kim HS, Kim IK, Jeong SW (2003) Alterations in mRNA expression of ribosomal protein S9 in hydrogen peroxide-treated neurotumor cells and

in rat hippocampus after transient ischemia. Neurochem Res 28:925–931
Knoepfler PS, Cheng PF, Eisenman RN (2002) N-MYC is essential during neurogenesis for the rapid expansion of progenitor cell populations and inhibition of neuronal differentiation. Genes Dev 16:2699–2712
Korshunov A, Benner A, Remke M, Lichter P, von Deimling A, Pfister S (2008) Accumulation of genomic aberrations during clinical progression of medulloblastoma. Acta Neuropathol 116:383–390
Lamont JM, McManamy CS, Pearson AD, Clifford SC, Ellison DW (2004) Combined histopathological and molecular cytogenetic stratification of medulloblastoma patients. Clin Cancer Res 10:5482–5493
Lo KC, Rossi MR, Eberhart CG, Cowell JK (2007) Genome wide copy number abnormalities in pediatric medulloblastomas as assessed by array comparative genome hybridization. Brain Pathol 17:282–296
Louis DN, Ohgaki H, Wiestler OD, Cavenee WK, Burger PC, Jouvet A, Scheithauer BW, Kleihues P (2007) The 2007 WHO classification of tumours of the central nervous system. Acta Neuropathol 114:97–109
Malakho SG, Korshunov A, Stroganova AM, Poltaraus AB (2008) Fast detection of MYCN copy number alterations in brain neuronal tumors by real-time PCR. J Clin Lab Anal 22:123–130
Min HS, Lee YJ, Park K, Cho BK, Park SH (2006) Medulloblastoma: histopathologic and molecular markers of anaplasia and biologic behavior. Acta Neuropathol 112:13–20
Polkinghorn W, Tarbell N (2007) Medulloblastoma: tumorigenesis, current clinical paradigm, and efforts to improve risk stratification. Nat Clin Pract Oncol 4:295–304
Raggi CC, Bagnoni ML, Tonini GP, Maggi M, Vona G, Pinzani P, Mazzocco K, De Bernardi B, Pazzagli M, Orlando C (1999) Real-time quantitative PCR for the measurement of MYCN amplification in human neuroblastoma with the TaqMan detection system. Clin Chem 45:1918–1924
Rossi MR, Conroy J, McQuaid D, Nowak NJ, Rutka JT, Cowell JK (2006) Array CGH analysis of pediatric medulloblastomas. Genes Chromosomes Cancer 45:290–303
Savelyeva L, Schwab M (2001) Amplification of oncogenes revisited: from expression profiling to clinical application. Cancer Lett 167:115–123
Schwab M, Amler L (1990) Amplification of cellular oncogenes: a predictor of clinical outcome in human cancer. Genes Chromosomes Cancer 1:181–193
Surace C, Pedeutour F, Trombetta D, Burel-Vandenbos F, Rocchi M, Storlazzi CT (2008) Episomal amplification of MYCN in a case of medulloblastoma. Virchows Arch 425:491–497

Pediatric Medulloblastoma: Ultrastructure

16

Gerhard Franz Walter and Douglas A. Weeks

Contents

G.F. Walter (✉)
Department of Neuropathology, Klinikum Kassel, Mönchebergstr. 41-43, D-34125 Kassel, Germany
e-mail: gerhard-franz.walter@klinikum-kassel.de

D.A. Weeks
Department of Pathology, Oregon Health and Science University, 3181 SW Sam Jackson Park Road, Portland, OR, USA
e-mail: weeksd@ohsu.edu

Abstract

In this chapter we explore the ultrastructural spectrum of medulloblastoma, the most common malignant tumor of the central nervous system in childhood. All medulloblastomas display morphologic evidence of neuronal differentiation by electron microscopy, ranging from minimal to quite prominent. A semi-quantitative classification scheme for this feature is provided and illustrated. A lesser known quality of some cases of medulloblastoma is their capacity to undergo divergent differentiation. We describe and illustrate three forms of this, including astrocytic, myogenic and melanotic. Recognition of such divergent differentiation in the neoplastic cell population of medulloblastoma by electron microscopy can aid in the prevention of diagnostic errors, and may potentially identify subtypes susceptible to alternative therapies.

Introduction

Medulloblastomas are the most common malignant central nervous system tumors in childhood. The estimated annual incidence is 0.5 per 100,000 children. Seventy percent of medulloblastomas occur in patients younger than 16 years of age. The peak age at presentation is 7 years. Both sexes are affected with a slight predilection for male patients.

Histogenetically, medulloblastomas show both a neuroectodermal as well as a mesenchymal origin.

M.A. Hayat (ed.), *Pediatric Cancer, Volume 3: Diagnosis, Therapy, and Prognosis*, Pediatric Cancer 3,
DOI 10.1007/978-94-007-4528-5_16,

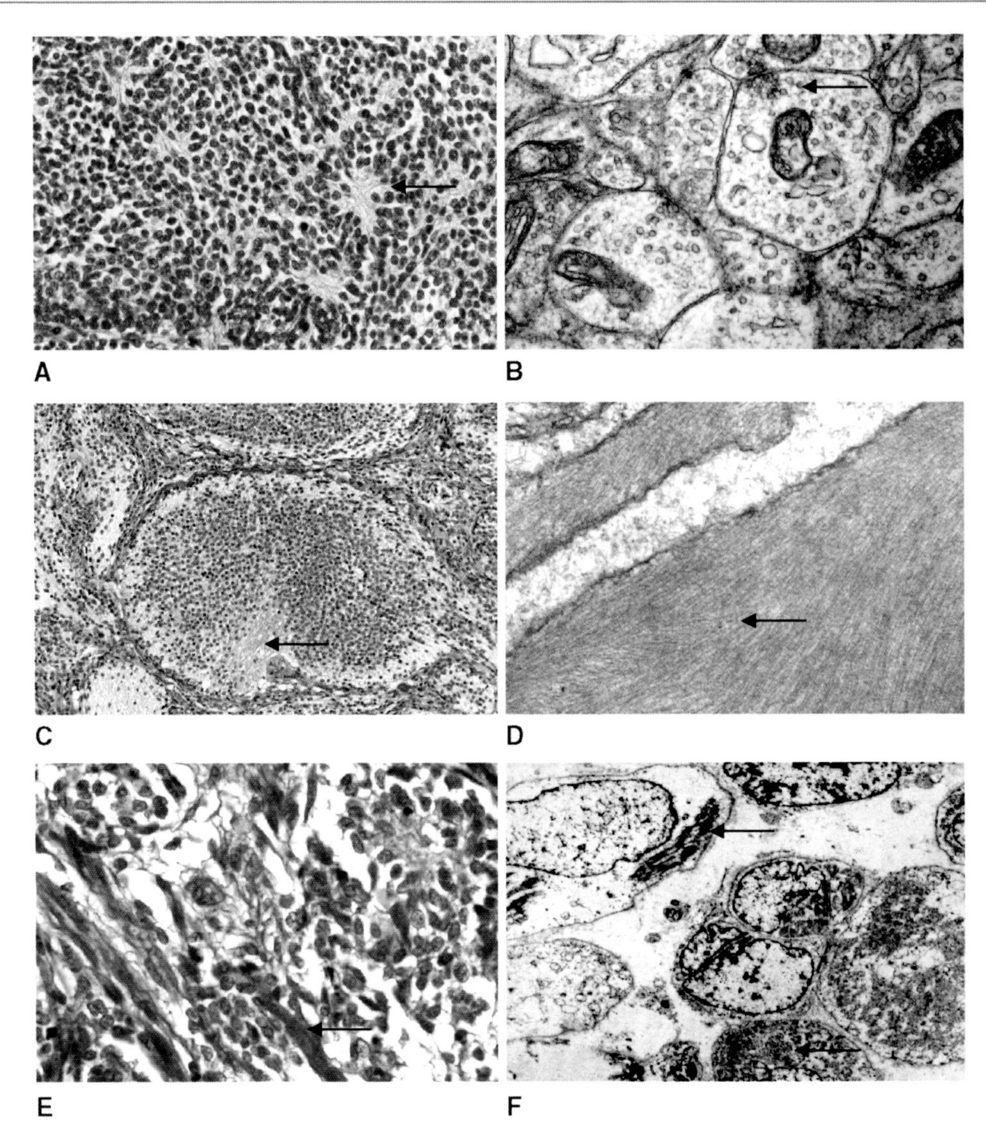

Fig. 16.1 (**a**) Classical medulloblastoma with neuronal differentiation. Densely packed tumor cells with hyperchromatic round-to-oval nuclei and neuroblastic Homer Wright rosettes (*arrow*). GFAP. (**b**) Neuronal cell processes with synaptic vesicles, synaptic densities (*arrow*) and mitochondria. (**c**) Medulloblastoma with extensive nodularity. Densely packed tumor cells with neuronal differentiation next to fibrillary almost cell-free areas with glial differentiation (*arrow*) are surrounded by an internodular tumor component of fibroblasts (*light blue*) and capillaries with mesenchymal differentiation. Masson trichrome. (**d**) Glial cell processes filled with randomly oriented intermediate filaments (*arrow*). (**e**) Medulloblastoma with myogenic differentiation. Round tumor cells with neuronal differentiation are admixed with striated muscle fibers (*arrow*) and few collagenous fibers (*light blue*) with mesenchymal differentiation. Masson trichrome. (**f**) Note the longitudinally or transversally cut striated muscle fibers within the myogenic tumor component (*arrows*) next to smaller medulloblastoma cells with indented and lobulated nuclei surrounded by scanty perinuclear cytoplasm (*center*) within the neuronal tumor component

The neuroectodermal component is characterized by a predominantly neuronal differentiation but also areas with glial (astrocytic) differentiation may occur. The mesenchymal component can be seen in desmoplastic areas with fibroblasts and collagenous fibers as well as in form of striated muscle fibers (Fig. 16.1).

The neuroectodermal histogenesis of a brain tumor such as medulloblastoma is self-explaining. The histogenesis of muscle fibers or fibroblasts as part of this tumor entity is controversial. In the very first publication of medullomyoblastoma, the striated muscle fibers were thought to have originated through a process termed "dysembryogenesis" or from the metaplastic transformation of vascular smooth muscle cells (Marinesco and Goldstein 1933). Another concept was that medullomyoblastoma might represent a variant of a "teratoid" tumor (Ingraham and Bailey 1946). Further, it was suggested that the muscle fibers derive from "unstable" pluripotential mesenchymal cells (Walter and Brucher 1979). Within the CNS, the source of these putative pluripotential cells has been considered to be the embryonic ectomesenchyme, which is derived from the neural crest (Weston 1970). The leptomeninges are considered to be an ectomesenchymal derivative, rarely containing non-neoplastic striated muscle. Intracerebral tumors with a mesenchymal component, such as medullomyoblastoma, gliosarcoma, or intracerebral rhabdomyosarcoma, may originate from the leptomeninges that accompany blood vessels as they penetrate the brain parenchyma. Melanin-containing cells lends further support to a neural crest origin of tumor components within medulloblastoma. However, experimental studies in cell cultures derived from experimental brain tumors in rats or mice suggest that primitive neuroepithelial cells are potentially capable of differentiating along both rhabdomyoblastic and melanocytic lines (Lennon and Peterson 1979; VandenBerg et al. 1981), thus, without necessarily postulating an origin from neural-crest-derived cells. Medulloblastomas have a tendency to metastasize via the CSF pathways, and rarely outside the neuraxis. All variants correspond histologically to WHO grade IV.

The World Health Organization Classification (Louis et al. 2007) describes

- the classical medulloblastoma as clinicopathological entity with distinctive morphology, location, age distribution and biological behavior;
- four variants being reliably identified histologically and having some relevance for clinical outcome but still being part of the overarching entity, namely desmoplastic/nodular medulloblastoma, medulloblastoma with extensive nodularity, anaplastic medulloblastoma, and large cell medulloblastoma;
- and two histological patterns of differentiation with identifiable histological appearances but without distinct clinical or pathological significance, namely medulloblastoma with myogenic differentiation (former medullomyoblastoma), and medulloblastoma with melanotic differentiation.

The investigations reviewed in this chapter have been done using classical methods of transmission electron microscopy (TEM). There is only one publication on medulloblastoma using the wet SEM method (Barshack et al. 2004). Focal rosette formation and poorly developed cell processes were observed. Wet SEM is a technology for imaging fully hydrated tissue samples at atmospheric pressure in a scanning electron microscope (SEM). This method was proposed for rapid intraoperative diagnosis complementing the frozen section diagnosis, but remains restricted to surface imaging. In order to visualize intracellular structures more specialized preparatory techniques such as fracturing and etching would be needed which limits the intraoperative use.

Ultrastructure

Some early reports have not observed any clear differentiating tendency and mention even the lack of differentiation as characteristic for medulloblastomas (Matakas et al. 1970). However, many authors report quite characteristic patterns of neuronal, glial and mesenchymal differentiation (Fig. 16.1), though these differentiation patterns must not be present in every case (Hang and We 1989; Weeks et al. 2003). It is the more differentiated medulloblastomas that can cause the most diagnostic difficulty, as they can simulate other tumor entities such as astrocytoma or ependymoma. Therefore, an electron microscopic investigation may be even more useful with these entities.

Neuronal Differentiation

Neuronal cells are ultrastructurally characterized by several elements:

- First, a cytoskeletal element in the form of elongated, straight, parallel microtubules (neurotubules) with a diameter of 20–25 nm and microfilaments (neurofilaments) with a diameter of 8–11 nm, both occurring in the cell body, dendrites, and axons. Neurotubules together with neurofilaments form neurofibrils.
- A second element is synaptic clear or dense core vesicles (neurotransmitter vesicles) which occur in neuronal terminals and store various neurotransmitters that are released at the synapse. They have a diameter of 35–50 nm and are electron lucent, in which acetylcholine, glutamate, GABA or glycine is the transmitter, or small dense core vesicles, in which norepinephrine, dopamine or serotonin is the transmitter. Large dense core vesicles with a diameter of 70–200 nm contain neuroactive peptides, amines, hormones, or growth factors.
- A third element is synapses composed by presynaptic and postsynaptic cell membrane densities appearing as desmosome-like intercellular junctions.

The classical medulloblastoma cell type consists of densely arranged, poorly differentiated, round to polyhedral cells without a basal lamina. The nuclei are frequently indented and lobulated with a locally condensed chromatin pattern and prominent nucleoli. The scanty perinuclear cytoplasm contains abundant free ribosomes and scarce mitochondria. The Golgi and endoplasmic reticulum complex is poorly developed. Homer Wright rosettes are regarded as expression of neuronal differentiation. In poorly formed cell rosettes, elongated neurite-like cytoplasmic processes joined by specialized adhesion plaques are laden with longitudinally aligned microtubules in parallel array, but little significance has been attached to that appearance alone (Roy 1977). The presence of microtubules and microfilaments, however, is not specific for neuronal cell types since they may play also a role in the extending cytoplasmic processes of medulloblastoma glial progenitors (Maria et al. 1992). Intercellular junctions are often not present, but locally abundant desmosome-like cell junctions, synapses and clear or dense core vesicles may be visible (Hassoun et al. 1975; Moss 1983; Katsetos et al. 1988; Mrak 2002). The exact analysis of the ultrastructural features permits to define an ultrastructural classification of neuronal differentiation (Weeks et al. 2003) into minimal, intermediate or prominent grades (Table 16.1; Fig. 16.2). In one case, the presence of aberrant myelinated neurites has been observed (Kadota et al. 1995). In another case, a neuronal differentiation with microtubules, dense core vesicles, and abortive synaptic densities of metastatases of medullomyoblastoma to an extracranial lymph node is reported (Alwasiak et al. 1991).

Table 16.1 Classification of neuronal differentiation based upon ultrastructural criteria (Weeks et al. 2003)

Prominent	+++ neuritic processes *or* +++ neurosecretory granules
	++ neuritic processes *and* ++ neurosecretory granules
	any synaptic structures
Intermediate	++ neuritic processes *or* ++ neurosecretory granules
Minimal	+ neuritic processes *and/or* + neurosecretory granules

Glial Differentiation

Ultrastructurally typical for glial (astrocytic) differentiation are cytoskeletal elements in form of intermediate filaments with a diameter of 7–10 nm which in immunohistochemistry appear positive for glial fibrillary acidic protein (GFAP). It has to paid attention to the fact that medulloblastomas contain varying numbers of reactive astrocytes, although some cases have a component of neoplastic astrocytes as well. In medulloblastomas, areas of interlacing glial cell processes more or less filled with intermediate filaments 7–10 nm in diameter are visible, in some cases abundantly filled with filaments and strongly resembling astrocytic differentiation (Camins et al. 1980). They are especially located in histologically reticulin-free "pale islands", the latter more often appearing in the desmoplastic/nodular

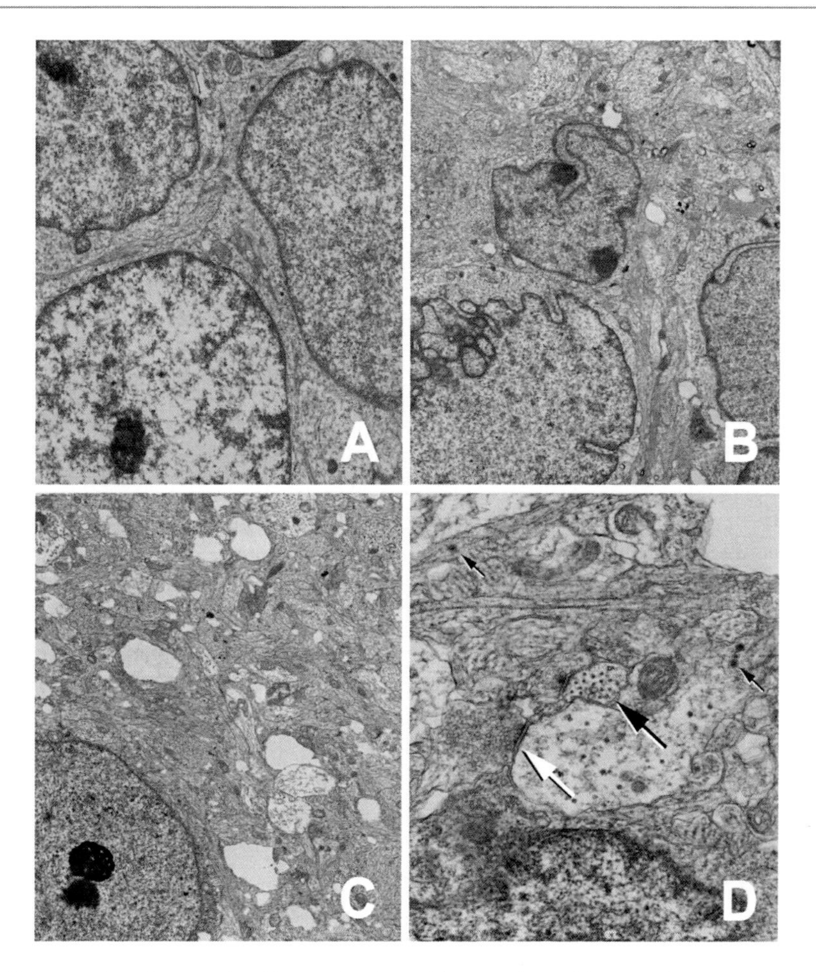

Fig. 16.2 Different grades of neuronal differentiation in medulloblastoma. (**a**) Minimal differentiation with only few (+) neuritic processes and neurosecretory granules. (**b**) Intermediate differentiation with some (++) neuritic processes and neurosecretory granules. (**c**) Prominent differentiation with many (+++) neuritic processes and neurosecretory granules. (**d**) Detail within prominent differentiation illustrating a synapse (*white arrow*), an array of microtubules in cross sectional profile (*large black arrow*), and neurosecretory granules (*small black arrows*)

variant. By some investigators pale islands are regarded as bi-directional glial and neuronal differentiation (Burger et al. 1987).

Myogenic Differentiation

Ultrastructurally typical for myogenic differentiation are contractile myofilaments, a term used for both, actin with a diameter of 7–9 nm and myosin filaments with a diameter of 15 nm together. Actin filaments are fixed in Z-bands which mark the both ends of a sarcomere and are the principal elements for the striated appearance of striated muscle. In medullomyoblastomas, the "medulloblastoma" component is highly cellular in comparison to the less cellular "myoblastic" component. Tumor cells with myogenic differentiation possess a distinct, although often incomplete, basement membrane. They contain nuclei with coarsely clumped nuclear chromatin, abundant cytoplasm with glycogen granules, in places forming huge pools of glycogen, moderate amounts of organelles and bundles of myofilaments with a tendency to form striated myofibers (Walter and Brucher 1979; Dickson et al. 1983; Smith and Davidson 1984; Patt et al. 1989; Labrousse et al. 1990; Dastur and Manghani 1999;

Sakata et al. 2008). The primitive sarcomere units are generally in disarray, and only rudimentary Z-band-like densities in the sense of "early myofibril organization" (Prince 1981) can be observed. But also well-differentiated muscle fibers with thick myosin and thin actin filaments arranged in well-defined sarcomeres may occur, with distinct Z-lines, and A, I, H, and M bands.

Melanotic Differentiation

Ultrastructurally typical for melanotic differentiation are melanosomes which are organelles containing melanin pigment granules. Stage I melanosomes are defined as membrane-bound filaments with definite periodicity. Stage II melanosomes are elongated and have occasional fine zig-zag lines with a periodicity of 8–9 nm. Stage III melanosomes are characterized by melanin granules in parallel lines or spirals following the patterns formed by the zig-zag lines of the stage II melanosomes. Stage IV melanosomes are electron-dense with no discernible internal structure (Fitzpatrick et al. 1971). Medulloblastoma cells with melanotic differentiation are larger and more pleomorphic than the classical medulloblastoma cells. They contain premelanosomes and melanosomes consistent with stage II through stage IV melanosomes. No stage I melanosomes have been found (Boesel et al. 1978; Dolman 1988; Garcia-Bragado et al. 1990).

Medulloblastoma in Tissue Culture

First investigations of tissue cultures from medulloblastoma failed to demonstrate a neuronal or glial differentiation by electron microscopy (Gullotta and Kersting 1972; McAllister et al. 1977). Later studies succeeded in demonstrating differentiation. In the early phase of outgrowth, tumor cells contain prominent nuclei with regularly dispersed or peripheral clumps of chromatin, often with small nucleoli. They have thin cytoplasmic rims with few mitochondria, free ribosomes, polyribosomes (polysomes), occasional dense bodies and scanty microtubules. In later phases, thin neuritic processes containing mitochondria and numerous parallel microtubules 20–25 nm in diameter occur (Markesbery et al. 1980).

In conclusion, electron microscopy is not mandatory for a reliable pathomorphological diagnosis of medulloblastoma, its variants, or its histological patterns of differentiation, because there are no differential decisions to be taken with regard to therapeutic approaches. In future, however, ultrastructural differentiation and its possible basis on genetic differences may open a new window for individualized tumor therapy of ultrastructurally distinguishable medulloblastoma variants.

References

Alwasiak J, Mirecka B, Wozniak L, Liberski PP (1991) Neuroblastic differentiation of metastases of medulloblastoma to extracranial lymph node: an ultrastructural study. Ultrastruct Pathol 15:647–654

Barshack I, Polak-Charcon S, Behar V, Vainshtein A, Zik O, Ofek E, Hadani M, Kopolovic J, Nass D (2004) Wet SEM: a novel method for rapid diagnosis of brain tumors. Ultrastruct Pathol 28:255–260

Boesel CP, Suhan JP, Sayers MP (1978) Melanotic medulloblastoma: report of a case with ultrastructural findings. J Neuropathol Exp Neurol 37:531–543

Burger PC, Grahmann FC, Bliestle A, Kleihues P (1987) Differentiation in the medulloblastoma. A histological and immunohistochemical study. Acta Neuropathol 73:115–123

Camins MB, Cravioto HM, Epstein F, Ransohoff J (1980) Medulloblastoma: an ultrastructural study – evidence for astrocytic and neuronal differentiation. Neurosurgery 6:398–411

Dastur DK, Manghani DK (1999) Ultrastructural changes in medullomyoblastoma. Similarities with foetal rhabdomyoma. Neurol India 47:178–181

Dickson DW, Hart MN, Menezes A, Cancilla PA (1983) Medulloblastoma with glial and rhabdomyoblastic differentiation. A myoglobin and glial fibrillary acidic protein immunohistochemical and ultrastructural study. J Neuropathol Exp Neurol 42:639–647

Dolman CL (1988) Melanotic medulloblastoma. A case report with immunohistochemical and ultrastructural examination. Acta Neuropathol 76:528–531

Fitzpatrick TB, Quevedo WC Jr, Szaba G, Seiji M (1971) Melanocyte system. In: Fitzpatrick TB, Arndt KA, Clark WH, Eisen AL, van Scott EJ, Vaughan JH (eds) Dermatology in general medicine. McGraw-Hill, New York, pp 117–146

García-Bragado F, Cabello A, Guarch R, Ruiz de Azúa Y, Ezpeleta I (1990) Medulloblastoma melanotico.

Estudio ultraestructural e immunohistoquimico de un caso. Arch Neurobiol (Madr) 53:8–12

Gullotta F, Kersting G (1972) The ultrastructure of medulloblastoma in tissue culture. Virchows Arch A (Pathol Anat) 356:111–118

Hang ZB, We YQ (1989) Ultrastructural study of cerebellar medulloblastoma. Zhonghua Bing Li Xue Za Zhi 18:214–216

Hassoun J, Hirano A, Zimmerman HM (1975) Fine structure of intercellular junctions and blood vessels in medulloblastoma. Acta Neuropathol 33:67–78

Ingraham FD, Bailey OT (1946) Cystic teratomas and teratoid tumors of the central nervous system in infancy and childhood. J Neurosurg 3:511–532

Kadota Y, Arai H, Sato K (1995) Neural differentiation and maturation in metastatic medulloblastoma. Case report. Neurol Med Chir (Tokyo) 35:32–35

Katsetos CD, Liu HM, Zacks SI (1988) Immunohistochemical and ultrastructural observations on Homer Wright (neuroblastic) rosettes and the "pale islands" of human cerebellar medulloblastomas. Hum Pathol 19:1219–1227

Labrousse F, Lhermine A, Maunoury R, Daumas-Duport C, Vedrenne C (1990) Médullomyoblastome: étude immunohistochimique et ultrastructurale. Arch Anat Cytol Pathol 38:198–202

Lennon VA, Peterson S (1979) Neuroectoderm markers retained in phenotypical skeletal muscle cells arising from a glial cell line. Nature 281:586–588

Louis DN, Ohgaki H, Wiestler OD, Cavenee WK (eds) (2007) WHO classification of tumours of the central nervous system. IARC, Lyon

Maria BL, Cumming R, Sukhu L (1992) Crown of microfilaments in the extending cytoplasmic processes of medulloblastoma glial progenitors. Can J Neurol Sci 19:23–33

Marinesco G, Goldstein M (1933) Sur une forme anatomique, non encore décrite, de médulloblastome: médullo-myoblastome. Ann Anat Pathol (Paris) 10:513–525

Markesbery WR, Walsh JW, Frye MD (1980) Ultrastructural study of the medulloblastomas in tissue culture. J Neuropathol Exp Neurol 39:30–41

Matakas F, Cervòs-Navarro J, Gullotta F (1970) The ultrastructure of medulloblastomas. Atca. Neuropathol 16:271–284

McAllister RM, Isaacs H, Rongey R, Peer M, Au W, Soukup SW, Gardner MB (1977) Establishment of a human medulloblastoma cell line. Int J Cancer 20: 206–212

Moss TH (1983) Evidence for differentiation in medulloblastomas appearing primitive on light microscopy: an ultrastructural study. Histopathology 7:919–930

Mrak RE (2002) The big eye in the 21st century: the role of electron microscopy in modern diagnostic neuropathology. J Neuropathol Exp Neurol 61:1027–1039

Patt S, Oppel F, Cervós-Navarro J (1989) Zur Frage des Medullomyoblastoms. Zentralbl Allg Pathol Anat 135:445–455

Prince FP (1981) Ultrasturctural aspects of myogenesis found in neoplasms. Acta. Neuropathol 54:315–320

Roy S (1977) An ultrastructural study of medulloblastoma. Neurol India 25:226–229

Sakata H, Kanamori M, Watanabe M, Kumabe T, Tominaga T (2008) Medulloblastoma demonstrating multipotent differentiation: case report. Brain Tumor Pathol 25:39–43

Smith TW, Davidson RI (1984) Medullomyoblastoma. A histologic, immunohistochemical, and ultrastructural study. Cancer 54:323–332

VandenBerg SR, Hess JR, Herman MM, DeArmond S, Halks-Miller M, Rubinstein LJ (1981) Neural differentiation in the OTT-6050 mouse teratoma. Production of a tumor fraction showing melanogenesis in neuroepithelial cells after centrifugal elutriation. Virchows Arch A Pathol Anat Histol 392:295–308

Walter GF, Brucher JM (1979) Ultrastructural study of medullomyoblastoma. Acta Neuropathol 48:211–214

Weeks DA, Malott RL, Goin L, Mierau GW (2003) Ultrastructural spectrum of medulloblastoma with immunocytochemical correlations. Ultrastruct Pathol 27:101–107

Weston TA (1970) The migration and differentiation of neural crest cells. In: Abercrombie M, Brachet J, King TJ (eds) Advances in morphogenesis. Academic Press, New York, pp 41–114

Pediatric Medullomyoblastoma: Immunohistochemical Analyses

17

Masaki Ueno, Masayuki Onodera, Takashi Kusaka, Reiji Haba, Takashi Tamiya, and Haruhiko Sakamoto

Contents

M. Ueno (✉) • M. Onodera • H. Sakamoto
Department of Pathology and Host Defense, Faculty of Medicine, Kagawa University, 1750-1 Ikenobe, Miki-cho, Kita-gun, Kagawa 761-0793, Japan
e-mail: masaueno@med.kagawa-u.ac.jp

T. Kusaka
Maternal Perinatal Center, Faculty of Medicine, Kagawa University, 1750-1 Ikenobe, Miki-cho, Kita-gun, Kagawa 761-0793, Japan

R. Haba
Department of Diagnostic Pathology, Faculty of Medicine, Kagawa University, 1750-1 Ikenobe, Miki-cho, Kita-gun, Kagawa 761-0793, Japan

T. Tamiya
Department of Neurological Surgery, Faculty of Medicine, Kagawa University, 1750-1 Ikenobe, Miki-cho, Kita-gun, Kagawa 761-0793, Japan

Abstract

Medullomyoblastoma is a rare embryonal tumor of the central nervous system and is classified as medulloblastoma with myogenic differentiation according to the most recent WHO classification, 4th edition. The tumor cells have neuroectodermal and myoblastic features. The origin of the myoblastic element of MMB remains to be completely clarified. We reported a case of a 3-year-old girl with medullomyoblastoma in the cerebellar vermis. She underwent total resection of the tumor, followed by chemotherapy and radiotherapy in the brain and spinal cord. The resected specimen mainly consisted of densely packed cells with round-to-oval highly chromatic nuclei surrounded by scanty cytoplasm (indicating neuroectodermal differentiation) and focally of long spindle-shaped cells with elongated nuclei and eosinophilic cytoplasm showing discernible cross-striations (indicating myoblastic differentiation). In addition, the tumor cells showed large nuclei with nucleolus, frequent mitoses, apoptoses, nuclear molding, and cell wrapping, indicating moderate anaplasia. Immunohistochemical staining revealed partial expression of myoglobin and desmin as well as synaptophysin and neurofilament in the tumor cells. Some tumor cells showed double immunopositivity for synaptophysin and myoglobin, suggesting the idea that the neuroectodermal cells may undergo differentiation into rhabdomyoblasts.

M.A. Hayat (ed.), *Pediatric Cancer, Volume 3: Diagnosis, Therapy, and Prognosis*, Pediatric Cancer 3, DOI 10.1007/978-94-007-4528-5_17,

Introduction

Medullomyoblastoma (MMB) is a rare embryonal tumor of the central nervous system (CNS), with only a few dozens of reported cases since its first published description in 1933 (Marinesco and Goldstein 1933). MMB is believed to be a variant of medulloblastoma. Medulloblastomas are the most common malignant CNS tumors of childhood. In the previous World Health Organization (WHO) classification, 3rd edition (Giordana and Wiestler 2000), medulloblastomas were classified into five categories: classic medulloblastoma, desmoplastic medulloblastoma, large cell medulloblastoma, medullomyoblastoma, and melanotic medulloblastoma. Medullomyoblastoma was defined histopathologically as a combination of primitive neuroectodermal and myoblastic elements. According to the most recent WHO classification, 4th edition (Giangaspero et al. 2007; Louis et al. 2007), there are some variants of medulloblastomas: desmoplastic/nodular medulloblastoma, medulloblastoma with extensive nodularity, anaplastic medulloblastoma, and large cell medulloblastoma. In the 4th edition WHO classification, MMB is described as medulloblastoma with myogenic differentiation and considered to be any variant of medulloblastoma because genetic changes in medulloblastoma with myogenic differentiation are similar to those in other medulloblastomas, suggesting that this is not a distinct entity. Prognosis in medulloblastoma with myogenic differentiation is poor according to the descriptions in published papers (Shintaku et al. 1982; Helton et al. 2004), although there have been reports of survival up to 5 or more than 10 years after presentation (Helton et al. 2004; Jaiswal et al. 2005; Lindberg et al. 2007).

Regarding the origin of the myoblastic element of MMB, several theories have been put forward. Some researchers suggested MMB to be a variant of malignant teratoma or teratoid tumor (Ingraham and Bailey 1946; Er et al. 2008), while other groups have proposed that the myoblastic component arises by recruitment of multipotent endothelial (Walter and Brucher 1979) or mesenchymal (Stahlberger and Friede 1977) cells from the tumor microenvironment. In addition, it has been suggested that the primitive neuroectodermal cells may undergo differentiation into rhabdomyoblasts (Smith and Davidson 1984). The last hypothesis is supported by some findings (Helton et al. 2004) showing the same acquired genetic changes in the neuroectodermal as in the myoblastic tumor components.

We reported a case of medulloblastoma with myogenic differentiation, MMB, with aggressive proliferative activity making clinical progression with poor prognosis (Kido et al. 2009). We introduce some immunohistochemical findings of the MMB in this paper.

Clinical and Pathological Findings

Clinical Findings

A 3-year-old girl presented with headache and floating sensation and showed truncal ataxia. Magnetic resonance imaging (MRI) demonstrated a large mass lesion occupying the fourth ventricle in the cerebellum, appearing as hyperintense on T2-weighted MRI and hypointense on T1-weighted MRI. She underwent total resection of the tumor. Postoperative MRI showed no residual lesion. The patient received radiation therapy at a total of 48 Gy to the brain and spine, followed by some cycles of combination chemotherapy. However, she died 1 year after appearance of clinical signs.

Materials and Methods

Pathological samples in this paper were got from an autopsied case of a 3-year-old girl suffered from medullomyoblastoma located in the cerebellar vermis with dissemination of the tumor cells to the subarachnoid space of whole brain and spinal cord. Surgical tissue specimens and autopsied CNS samples were examined by histochemical and immunohistochemical techniques. The primary antibodies used were monoclonal antibodies against synaptophysin (American Research Product (ARP), Belmont, MA, USA), neurofilament (Dako, Glostrup, Denmark), Ki-67 (Dako), desmin (Dako), α-smooth muscle actin (α-SMA) (Dako), HHF-35 (Dako), myoglobin (AbFrontier (AbF), Seoul, Korea), myogenin (Santa Cruz, CA, USA), proliferating cell nuclear antigen (PCNA) (Dako), p-53 (Calbiochem), and rabbit anti-synaptophysin (Zymed (Zym), CA, USA), neurofilament (Millipore, CA, USA), glial fibrillary acidic protein (GFAP) (Dako), and myoglobin (Dako) antibodies. Staining was achieved according to standard immunohistochemical techniques (Kido et al. 2009). For two kinds of double immunofluorescent staining, deparaffinized sections were treated with 2% bovine serum albumin and incubated in mouse anti-myoglobin (AbF) or synaptophysin (ARP) antibody, followed by incubation in Alexa Fluor 488-conjugated anti-mouse IgG antibody (Molecular Probes, OR). After washing in phosphate-buffered saline, the sections were incubated with rabbit anti-synaptophysin (Zym) or myoglobin (Dako) antibody, followed by incubation in Alexa Fluor 594-conjugated anti-rabbit IgG antibody (Molecular Probes), respectively. In addition, the sections were incubated for 15 min in 4′-6-Diamidino-2-Phenylindole (DAPI) (Molecular Probes, Eugene, OR, USA) solution at RT, which was diluted to 400 nM in 1% albumin solution in PBS. The fluorescent signals were viewed under a confocal microscope (Bio-Rad Radiance 2100, Bio-Rad, Osaka, Japan).

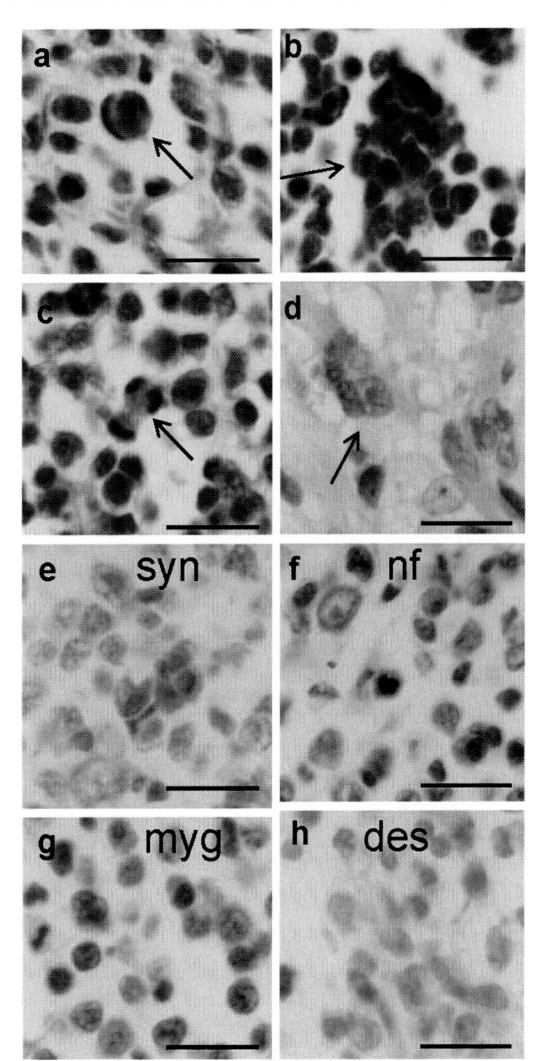

Fig. 17.1 Microscopic images of hematoxylin and eosin (H&E) staining (**a**–**d**) and immunohistochemical staining for synaptophysin (**e**), neurofilament (**f**), myoglobin (**g**), and desmin (**h**). H&E staining shows cell wrapping (**a**: *arrow*), nuclear molding (**b**: *arrow*), and atypical mitosis (**c**: *arrow*) of densely packed tumor cells with round highly chromatic nuclei surrounded by scanty cytoplasm, and moreover long spindle-shaped cells with eosinophilic cytoplasm and large atypical nuclei (**d**: *arrow*). Immunohistochemical staining shows that some tumor cells show partial or focal expression of synaptophysin (**e**: *syn*), neurofilament (**f**: *nf*), myoglobin (**g**: *myg*), and desmin (**h**: *des*). Scale bars indicate 20 μm

Pathological Findings by H&E Staining and Immunohistochemical Techniques

The tumor cells were densely packed cells with round-to-oval highly chromatic large nuclei surrounded by scanty cytoplasm (Fig. 17.1a, b, c). The tumor cells showed cell wrapping (Fig. 17.1a), nuclear molding (Fig. 17.1b), frequent mitoses (Fig. 17.1c), apoptoses, and angulation. Judging from histopathologic grading proposed by Eberhart et al. (2002; Min et al. 2006), the histopathological features in this case represented moderate anaplasia. In addition, long spindle-shaped cells with elongated nuclei and eosinophilic cytoplasm were focally seen in the other area of the tumor (Fig. 17.1d). Immunohistochemical staining revealed partial expression of neuroectodermal markers such as synaptophysin (Fig. 17.1e), neurofilament (Fig. 17.1f), GFAP (not shown), and CD57 (not shown) and focal expression of myoblastic markers such as myoglobin (Fig. 17.1g), desmin (Fig. 17.1h), and HHF-35 (not shown), but not α-smooth muscle actin nor myogenin (Er et al. 2008). A lot of tumor cells showed diffuse expression of Ki-67, whose labeling index was 46%, while the tumor cells showed no clear immunostaining for p-53.

Double Immunostaining for Myoglobin and Synaptophysin

We performed double immunostaining for synaptophysin and myoglobin to examine whether neuroectodermal cells express myoblastic markers such as myoglobin. We used two kinds of combinations of antibodies for myoglobin and synaptophysin. One is a combination of a monoclonal antibody for myoglobin and a polyclonal antibody for synaptophysin (Fig. 17.2a), while the other is a combination of a polyclonal antibody for myoglobin and a monoclonal antibody for synaptophysin (Fig. 17.2b). In any combination, the immunostaining for myoglobin in some tumor cells is seen in contact with the immunostaining for synaptophysin and nuclear staining, suggesting colocalization of myoglobin with synaptophysin in the same cytoplasm of the tumor cell (Fig. 17.2).

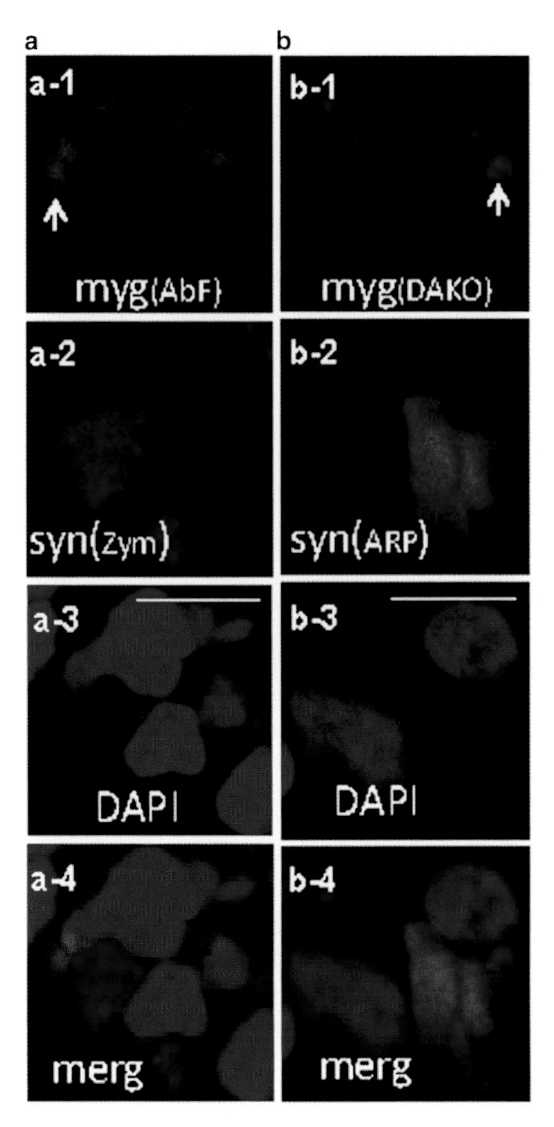

Fig. 17.2 Confocal microscopic images of double immunofluorescent and DAPI staining are shown. Images in (**a**) indicate triple staining using a monoclonal antibody for myoglobin (**a-1**: *myg(AbF)*), a polyclonal antibody for synaptophysin (**a-2**: *syn(Zym)*), DAPI (**a-3**: *DAPI*), and the merged images (**a-4**: *merg*). Images in (**b**) indicate triple staining for a polyclonal antibody for myoglobin (**b-1**: *myg(DAKO)*), a monoclonal antibody for synaptophysin (**b-2**: *syn(ARP)*), DAPI (**b-3**: *DAPI*), and the merged images (**b-4**: *merg*). The immunostaining for myoglobin (**a-1, b-1**: *arrow*) is seen in contact with the immunostaining for synaptophysin and nuclear staining. Scale bars indicate 10 μm

Discussion

Medulloblastoma is the most common pediatric primary malignant intracranial neoplasm. The 5-year survival rates vary from 40% to 70% (Carlotti et al. 2008). In contrast, medulloblastoma with myogenic differentiation, MMB, is a rare disease and the prognosis was originally described as highly unfavorable with few patients surviving for more than 3 years (Mahapatra et al. 1998). Although there have been reports of survival up to more than 10 years after presentation (Helton et al. 2004; Jaiswal et al. 2005), the previous average survival was described as being <2 years, with the caveat that long-term follow-up data often were unavailable (Helton et al. 2004). In our case, the patient died 1 year after the appearance of clinical signs in spite of operation, chemotherapy, and radiotherapy.

Medulloblastoma has more mutations and other genetic changes in developmental genes than in canonical regulators of the cell cycle such as p53 (Giangaspero et al. 2007). Examination of the signaling pathways dysregulated in various medulloblastoma subtypes has also allowed further speculation on the involvement of Wnt activation, Hedgehog activation, and Myc amplification (Giangaspero et al. 2007; Lindberg et al. 2007; Fan and Eberhart 2008; Yokota et al. 2002; Blanc et al. 2005). It is thought in the recent WHO classification that genetic changes in medulloblastoma with myogenic differentiation are similar to those in other medulloblastomas, suggesting that this is not a distinct entity (Giangaspero et al. 2007; Louis et al. 2007). It was described in the previous WHO classification (Giordana and Wiestler 2000) that the growth fraction, as revealed by the fraction of medulloblastoma cells expressing Ki-67, is often >20%. It was reported in a recent paper (Meurer et al. 2008) that the percentage of Ki-67-positive cells was 1.8–54% and 29 patients had over 20% of positive cells while 11 showed less than 20% of positive cells. In contrast, Lindberg et al. (2007) described that the Ki-67 index was 35% in the neuroectodermal component of MMB. Thus, it is likely that the proliferative ability of tumor cells of MMB is high compared with that of tumor cells of medulloblastoma. In this case, the Ki-67 index was high. In addition, the histopathological features in this case represented moderate anaplasia, indicating increasing anaplasia compared with classic medulloblastoma. The high proliferative ability, presumably due to multiple genetic changes, may be related to the poor prognosis. High proliferative ability in the tumor cells and poor prognosis were characteristic in this case. It would be premature to suggest that MMB is not distinct from medulloblastoma regarding prognosis, genetic changes, or treatment.

The double immunopositivity for synaptophysin and myoglobin in the tumor cells of MMB supports the hypothesis that the primitive neuroectodermal cells may undergo differentiation into rhabdomyoblasts (Smith and Davidson 1984) and also suggests that tumor cells of medulloblastoma derive from cerebellar stem cells with multipotent differentiation (Fan and Eberhart 2008).

References

Blanc E, Goldschneider D, Douc-Rasy S, Benard J, Raguenez G (2005) Wnt-5a gene expression in malignant human neuroblasts. Cancer Lett 228: 117–123

Carlotti CG Jr, Smith C, Rutka JT (2008) The molecular genetics of medulloblastoma: an assessment of new therapeutic targets. Neurosurg Rev 31:359–368

Eberhart CG, Kepner JL, Goldtheaite PT, Kun LE, Duffner PK, Friedman HS, Strother DR, Burger PC (2002) Histopathologic grading of medulloblastomas: a pediatric oncology group study. Cancer 94:552–560

Er U, Yigitkanli K, Kazanci B, Ozturk E, Sorar M, Bavbek M (2008) Medullomyoblastoma: teratoid nature of a quite rare neoplasm. Surg Neurol 69:403–406

Fan X, Eberhart CG (2008) Medulloblastoma stem cells. J Clin Oncol 26:2821–2827

Giangaspero F, Eberhart CG, Haapasalo H, Pietsch T, Wiestler OD, Ellison DW (2007) Medulloblastoma. In: Louis DN, Ohgaki H, Wiestler OD, Cavenee WK (eds) World Health Organization classification of tumours of the central nervous system. IARC Press, Lyon, pp 132–140

Giordana M, Wiestler OD (2000) Medullomyoblastoma. In: Kleihues P, Cavenee WK (eds) World Health Organization classification of tumours, pathology and genetics of tumours of the nervous system. IARC Press, Lyon, pp 138–139

Helton KJ, Fouladi M, Boop FA, Perry A, Dalton J, Kun L, Fuller C (2004) Medullomyoblastoma: a radiographic and clinicopathologic analysis of six cases and review of the literature. Cancer 101: 1445–1454

Ingraham F, Bailey O (1946) Cystic teratomas and teratoid tumors of the central nervous system in infancy and childhood. J Neurosurg 3:511–532

Jaiswal AK, Jaiswal S, Mahapatra AK, Sharma MC (2005) Unusually long survival in a case of medullomyoblastoma. J Clin Neurosci 12:961–963

Kido M, Ueno M, Onodera M, Matsumoto K, Imai T, Haba R, Tamiya T, Huang C, Sakamoto H (2009) Medulloblastoma with myogenic differentiation showing double immunopositivity for synaptophysin and myoglobin. Pathol Int 59:255–260

Lindberg E, Persson A, Ora I, Mertens F, Englund E, Gisselsson D (2007) Concurrent gain of 17q and the MYC oncogene in a medullomyoblastoma. Neuropathology 27:556–560

Louis DN, Ohgaki H, Wiestler OD, Cavenee WK, Burger PC, Jouvet A, Scheithauer BW, Kleihues P (2007) The 2007 WHO classification of tumors of the central nervous system. Acta Neuropathol 114:97–109

Mahapatra AK, Sinha AK, Sharma MC (1998) Medullomyoblastoma. A rare cerebellar tumour in children. Childs Nerv Syst 14:312–316

Marinesco G, Goldstein M (1933) On an anatomical form of medulloblastoma not yet described, medullomyoblastoma. Ann Anat Pathol (Paris) 10:513–525

Meurer RT, Martins DT, Hilbig A, Ribeiro MC, Roehe AV, Narbosa-Coutinho LM, Fernandes MC (2008) Immunohistochemical expression of markers Ki-67, NeuN, synaptophysin, p53 and HER2 in medulloblastoma and its correlation with clinicopathological parameters. Arq Neuropsiquiatr 66:385–390

Min HS, Lee YJ, Park K, Cho B-K, Park S-H (2006) Medulloblastoma: histopathologic and molecular markers of anaplasia and biologic behavior. Acta Neuropathol 112:13–20

Shintaku M, Ogura M, Maeda R, Nishiyama T (1982) An autopsy case of medulloblastoma. Brain Nerve 34:105–114

Smith TW, Davidson RI (1984) Medulloblastoma. A histologic, immunohistochemical, and ultrastructural study. Cancer 54:323–332

Stahlberger R, Friede RL (1977) Fine structure of myomedulloblastoma. Acta Neuropathol 37:43–48

Walter GF, Brucher JM (1979) Ultrastructural study of medullomyoblastoma. Acta Neuropathol 48:211–214

Yokota N, Daniels F, Crosson J, Rabb H (2002) Role of Wnt pathway in medulloblastoma oncogenesis. Int J Cancer 101:198–201

Boost Gamma Knife Radiosurgery During Multimodality Management of Medulloblastoma/PNET Tumors

18

Thomas Flannery, Douglas Kondziolka, and L. Dade Lunsford

Contents

Abstract

Medulloblastoma/primitive neuroectodermal tumors (PNETs) are the most common malignant tumors of the central nervous system in children accounting for at least 20% of all childhood brain tumors (Kleihues and Cavenee (eds) Pathology and genetics of tumours of the nervous system. International Agency for Research on Cancer, Lyon, 2000). Multimodal treatment, including maximal feasible resection, fractionated neuraxis radiation therapy, and systemic chemotherapy is considered the standard initial strategy against these tumors. In spite of this, local and metastatic recurrences occur in 30–40% of patients, and

T. Flannery (✉)
Departments of Neurological Surgery and Radiation Oncology, University of Pittsburgh Medical Center, Pittsburgh, PA, USA

Department of Neurosurgery, Royal Hospitals Trust, Belfast, and Leeds Gamma Knife Center, St. James's Institute of Oncology, Leeds, UK
e-mail: t.flannery@qub.ac.uk

D. Kondziolka • L.D. Lunsford
Departments of Neurological Surgery and Radiation Oncology, University of Pittsburgh Medical Center, Pittsburgh, PA, USA

M.A. Hayat (ed.), *Pediatric Cancer, Volume 3: Diagnosis, Therapy, and Prognosis*, Pediatric Cancer 3,
DOI 10.1007/978-94-007-4528-5_18,

such recurrences portend a poor prognosis for survival (Kleihues and Cavenee (eds) Pathology and genetics of tumours of the nervous system. International Agency for Research on Cancer, Lyon, 2000).

Stereotactic radiosurgery has been proposed as a potentially effective adjunctive therapy in the management of recurrent or residual medulloblastoma (as reported by Patrice, Tarbell, Goumnerova, Shrieve, Black, and Loeffler, Pediatr Neurosurg 22:197–203, 2005). At the University of Pittsburgh, Gamma Knife stereotactic radiosurgery (GKRS) was used in the treatment of 7 pediatric and 12 adult patients who underwent a total of 36 procedures for residual, locally recurrent and metastatic medulloblastoma/PNET tumors. GKRS was administered to pediatric patients who failed initial multimodal treatment. The procedure was well tolerated and none of the patients experienced adverse radiation effects. Local tumor control was more likely in patients with smaller irradiated tumor volumes. Ultima-tely, delayed local progression, distant relapse, or leptomeningeal seeding led to the death of all pediatric patients in our series. Further efforts to develop more effective strategies are needed for this patient population.

Introduction

Primitive Neuroectodermal Tumors (PNET) are malignant, invasive tumors of embryonal cell origin with a propensity to spread through the cerebrospinal fluid (CSF) pathways (Kleihues and Cavenee 2000). They account for approximately 20% of childhood CNS malignancies, of which medulloblastoma is the most common subtype. Supratentorial PNET tumors, although similar to medulloblastoma, originate in other parts of the brain (Kleihues and Cavenee 2000). Medulloblastomas are more prevalent in younger children; the peak age at diagnosis is 7 years with over 70% of tumors observed in children less than 16 years of age. In adults, medulloblastoma is rare, comprising less than 2% of CNS malignancies (Selected Childhood Primary Brain and CNS Tumor Age-Specific Incidence rates. Central Brain Tumor Registry of the United States, 1998–2002).

Pathology of Medulloblastomas

Four different subtypes of medulloblastoma are recognized by the WHO: desmoplastic medulloblastoma, large cell medulloblastoma, medullomyoblastoma, and melanocytic medulloblastoma (Kleihues and Cavenee 2000). Significant attention has focused on medulloblastomas that display anaplastic features, including increased nuclear size, marked cytological pleomorphism, numerous mitoses, and apoptotic bodies (Kleihues and Cavenee 2000). Molecular genetic profiles are also being incorporated into evaluation and may radically alter classification in the future (Pomeroy et al. 2002).

Staging of Medulloblastoma

Evidence suggests that medulloblastomas originate in the granular cells of the cerebellum near the roof of the fourth ventricle. The tumors may spread contiguously to the cerebellar peduncle, along the floor of the fourth ventricle, into the cervical spine, or above the tentorium (Kleihues and Cavenee 2000). At the time of diagnosis there is spread via the cerebrospinal fluid (CSF) in up to one-third of patients. Every patient with newly diagnosed medulloblastoma should undergo disease staging with diagnostic imaging of the entire neuroaxis and, when possible, lumbar CSF analysis for free-floating tumor cells. Magnetic resonance imaging (MRI) is the method of choice to evaluate for intracranial or spinal cord subarachnoid metastases.

Prognostic Factors

Medulloblastoma patients are currently stratified into two groups: standard-risk and high-risk. High-risk patients are those <3 years of age, have residual tumor mass after surgery of >1.5 cm^2, or metastatic disease at diagnosis. The use of multiagent chemotherapy has allowed for the use of reduced-dose craniospinal radiotherapy (CSRT) to 24 Gy with improved cure rates, reflected by a >80% 5-year event-free survival in standard-risk patients (Rossi et al. 2008). For other than standard-risk medulloblastoma, the dose of CSRT is 36 Gy with a boost dose to the primary tumor to 54 Gy followed by adjuvant chemotherapy. The 5-year event free survival rates for high-risk disease is 50–60% (Rossi et al. 2008).

A host of biologic (including chromosomal 17p loss and B-catenin immunostaining) and histopathologic features (including large cell variant, anaplasia, and desmoplasia) have been shown to correlate with outcome (Kleihues and Cavenee 2000; Gaijjar et al. 2004). These biologic findings may be utilized in the future in combination with extent of dissemination at time of diagnosis, patient age, and amount of residual disease after surgery to better categorize patients with medulloblastoma into risk subgroups.

Treatment Options

Surgery is usually the initial treatment for children with medulloblastoma, both to confirm diagnosis and to remove as much tumor as is safely possible. Evidence suggests that more extensive surgical resections are related to an improved rate of survival, primarily in children with nondisseminated disease at the time of diagnosis (Albright et al. 1996; Taylor et al. 2004).

Fractionated radiation therapy (RT) is usually initiated after surgery with or without concomitant chemotherapy (Taylor et al. 2004). Clinical trials suggest that adjuvant chemotherapy given during and after RT improves overall survival for children with both average-risk and high-risk disease (Kortmann et al. 2000; Taylor et al. 2004).

Children of all ages are susceptible to the adverse effects of radiation on brain development. Debilitating effects on growth and neurologic/cognitive development have been frequently observed, especially in younger children (Ris et al. 2001). For this reason, the role of chemotherapy in allowing a delay in the administration of RT has been extensively studied. High-dose chemotherapy however may also contribute to longterm endocrine dysfunction (Laughton et al. 2008).

Surveillance testing is a part of all ongoing medulloblastoma studies (Saunders et al. 2003). Although most treatment failures in patients newly diagnosed with medulloblastoma will occur within the first 18 months post-diagnosis, relapses many years after diagnosis have been noted (Jenkin 1996). In addition, secondary tumors have been increasingly diagnosed in long-term survivors (Stavrou et al. 2001). As with initial management, long-term management is complex and requires a multidisciplinary approach.

Treatment of Recurrent Medulloblastoma

Disease may recur at the primary site or may be disseminated at the time of relapse. Sites of noncontiguous relapse may include the spinal leptomeninges, intracranial sites, and cerebrospinal fluid, in isolation or in any combination, and is variably associated with primary tumor relapse (Taylor et al. 2004).

At the time of relapse, a complete evaluation for extent of recurrence is recommended for all PNET tumors. Biopsy or surgical resection may be necessary for confirmation of relapse because other entities such as secondary tumors and treatment-related brain necrosis may be clinically indistinguishable from tumor recurrence. The need for surgical intervention must be individualized on the basis of the initial tumor type, the length of time between initial treatment and the reappearance of the lesion, and clinical symptomatology. Extraneural disease relapse may occur but is rare and is seen primarily in patients treated with RT alone.

Patients with recurrent tumors who have already received radiation therapy and chemotherapy may be candidates for salvage chemotherapy and/or stereotactic irradiation (Abe et al. 2006). These tumors can be responsive to chemotherapeutic agents used singularly or in combination. Approximately 30–50% of these patients will have objective responses to conventional chemotherapy, but long-term disease control is rare.

For selected patients with recurrent medulloblastoma, primarily infants and young children who were treated at the time of diagnosis with chemotherapy alone and developed local recurrence, long-term disease control may be obtained after further treatment with chemotherapy plus local RT (Ridola et al. 2007). For patients who have previously received radiation therapy, higher-dose chemotherapeutic regimens, supported with autologous bone marrow rescue or peripheral stem-cell support, have been used (Butturini et al. 2009). With such regimens, objective response is frequent, occurring in 50–75% of patients; however, long-term disease control is obtained in fewer than 30% of patients and is primarily seen in patients in first relapse and in those with only localized disease at relapse (Bowers et al. 2007). Long-term disease control for patients with disseminated disease is infrequent and drug toxicity can be a limiting factor (Rosenfeld et al. 2010).

Rational for Stereotactic Radiosurgery

Although PNETs are associated with a high propensity for diffuse seeding, the predominant pattern of failure after standard treatment is local disease recurrence. However, diffuse leptomeningeal disease progression may develop in spite of local disease control and widespread dissemination in the CNS may be present when MR imaging appears to show only local recurrence. The failure of conventional treatment to control local and distant disease and the poorer outcome seen in high-risk patients indicates the need for additional therapeutic modalities.

Stereotactic radiosurgery (SRS) was first proposed as an effective and safe treatment option in the management of medulloblastoma by Patrice et al. (1995). Using a modified linear accelerator, SRS was used as a technique for boosting sites of post-treatment residual disease and as salvage therapy in patients with recurrent tumors. After SRS, in no patient did the treatment fail locally within the radiosurgical target volume, whereas six of the patients (43%) had failure outside the posterior fossa. The authors' experience suggested that SRS was capable of controlling small, locally recurrent disease and was an effective adjunct to craniospinal irradiation for patients with newly diagnosed medulloblastoma. While other forms of SRS are available, our experience at the University of Pittsburgh has been with Gamma Knife stereotactic radiosurgery.

Gamma Knife Stereotactic Radiosurgery

The principle of Gamma Knife stereotactic radiosurgery (GKRS) is based on the mechanical focusing of up to 201 radiation sources, resulting in an extremely limited irradiated volume. By the addition of several focuses (isocentres), virtually any geometrical structure can be matched, thereby allowing the exclusive irradiation of the target within the brain. Significantly, the Gamma Knife provides a steep radiation dose fall-off ensuring that the surrounding tissue is exposed to only limited radiation and consequently is 'protected' against undesired radiation effects. The necessary precision of GKRS requires stereotactic frame fixation followed by a magnetic resonance imaging (MRI) study prior to planning and irradiation.

The 3D precision of the radiation focus and dose gradient features of stereotactic radiosurgery allow for treatment in a single session. Unlike fractionated radiotherapy, which may involve lengthy hospitalisation plus potential side effects affecting the patient's quality of life, single-session Gamma Knife can be carried out without interrupting the patient's systemic treatment. The consequent minimal disruption is important to patients and their families where quality of life is extremely important.

GKRS also appears to provide good local control rates for tumors that are otherwise resistant to conventional fractionated external-beam radiation therapy – a potentially important factor for "radiation-resistant" embryonal tumors.

The Gamma Knife Procedure

Although GKRS treatment is usually performed under local anesthesia, for younger children a general anaesthetic is administered. The Leksell Model G stereotactic head frame (Elekta AB) is placed on the patient's head after induction of general anesthesia and endotracheal intubation and stereotactic MR images are obtained for computer dose planning. We obtain a 3D contrast-enhanced volume acquisition by using fast spoiled gradient–recalled acquisition in steady state sequences (matrix 512×256, 2 excitations), covering the entire tumor volume and surrounding critical structures. Additional MR imaging sequences, including long repetition time images, may be obtained as required. Dose planning is performed using Leksell GammaPlan software. A conformal radiosurgery plan in which multiple isocenters are used is created. The margin dose is usually prescribed to the 50% isodose line and the maximal dose jointly selected by a team of radiation oncologists, neurosurgeons, and medical physicists. The final plan is exported to the Gamma Knife unit, and the radiation delivered by robotically positioning the head of the patient at the planned target coordinates.

Follow-Up Imaging

In the host institute (University of Pittsburgh), patients are typically evaluated based on MR imaging studies at 3-month intervals, or earlier if there is clinical evidence of disease progression. The follow-up images are compared with the GKRS treatment images, and tumor dimensions measured in the axial, coronal, and sagittal planes. A complete response is defined as complete disappearance of enhancing or nonenhancing tumor; partial response defined as >25% shrinkage of the tumor volume; stable disease defined as between ≤25% shrinkage of the tumor volume and up to ≤25% growth in tumor volume; and progressive disease defined as >25% increase in the size of the enhancing or nonenhancing tumor.

GKRS for Pediatric Medulloblastoma/PNET Tumors

Patient Cohort

Our experience with pediatric medulloblastoma and PNET tumors comprises seven patients (age <13 years) treated with GKRS between 1989 and 2006 (Fig. 18.1; Table 18.1) (Flannery et al. 2009). These seven patients underwent nine treatments for local recurrences and six for distant intracranial metastases (15 GKRS sessions in total). Five patients had tumors located solely in the posterior fossa, and two had primary tumors located in the region of the pineal gland and in the temporoparietal lobe.

All patients underwent ≥1 sessions of boost GKRS after failing initial standard therapies (maximal feasible resection, adjuvant chemotherapy, and fractionated radiation therapy). The mean interval from diagnosis to first stereotactic radiosurgery was 25.8 months (range 11–35 months). Chemotherapeutic trials included CCG-99701 in three patients, CCG-9921 in two patients, and "8 in 1" and "Baby POG" for the remaining two patients. The series consisted of three male and four female patients whose ages at the time of diagnosis ranged from 1 to 12.3 years (mean 4.9 years; see Table 18.1). No patient had evidence of spinal disseminated disease on MR imaging studies, and all had negative results on cytological analysis of CSF obtained prior to GKRS.

Results of GKRS

At the conclusion of multimodality therapy and ≥1 GKRS procedures, the patient population could be separated into two outcome groups: one group had early progressive local or distant disease (two patients); the other group had late progressive disease after an initial response to GKRS (five patients). The late progressive group included three patients who had a complete tumor response. One patient who exhibited a partial response later developed local relapse as well as distant metastatic disease (which required additional GKRS). The average age of these patients was 6.2 years at diagnosis; their median survival from time of diagnosis was 59 months, and median survival following initial GKRS treatment was 30 months.

Two patients had early disease progression, one of whom developed disseminated leptomeningeal disease in spite of complete tumor response

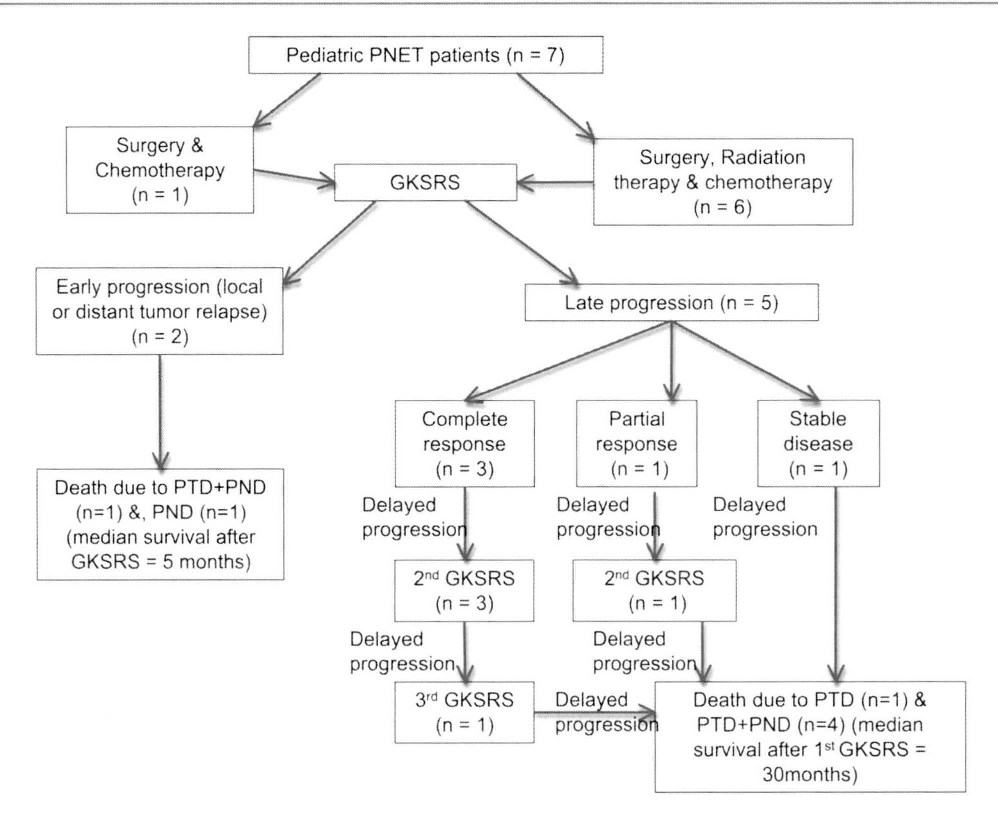

Fig. 18.1 Outcome diagram of seven patients who underwent boost *GKRS* procedures during multimodality management of PNETs. *PND* progressive new disease (including disseminated leptomeningeal disease), *PTD* progressive *GKRS*-treated disease (Figure reproduced with permission by Journal of Neurosurgery Pediatrics 2009;3:205–210)

to GKRS. Their mean age at time of diagnosis was 1.9 years. These patients' median survival from time of diagnosis was 27 months, and the median survival after GKRS was 5 months. The two patients who had early disease progression tended to have larger tumors (mean 10.8 cm^3) than those with late progressive disease (mean 2.83 cm^3, range 1.1–11 cm^3) ($p<0.005$, unpaired t-test). The mean tumor dose for the group who had early disease progression (14.5 Gy) did not differ significantly from that for the late progression group (14.6 Gy). No adverse radiation effects secondary to GKRS were observed in any patient.

Although local disease control was initially observed for five patients with late progression, in total they underwent 13 GKS procedures for either local recurrence or distant relapse (Fig. 18.2; Table 18.1). Four of these patients were retreated with GKRS for disease relapse because of their initial response and in the apparent absence of alternative effective therapies. These patients had end-stage recurrent disease after failure of maximal initial treatment. Additional chemotherapy in two of the four patients who received repeat GKRS also had no apparent effect (Table 18.1).

All patients eventually died (median survival from time of diagnosis, 37 months; median survival from the time of initial GKRS, 15 months). The cause of death was progressive new disease and/or progressive GKRS-treated disease. Progressive new disease included death from distant disease and/or disseminated leptomeningeal disease. One patient died of progressive treated disease, one patient of progressive new disease, and five of progressive new and progressive treated disease (Table 18.1).

Table 18.1 Characteristics in seven patients with GKRS-treated pediatric PNET tumors

				1st SRS			2nd SRS			3rd SRS					
Case No.	Age (years), sex	Initial tumor site	RT dose; WB/B/SC (Gy)	Int. (mos)/ Indic.	TV (cm³)/ dose (Gy)	Resp. (mos)	Int (mos)/ indic.	TV (cm³)/ Dose (Gy)	Resp. (mos)	Int. (mos)/ Indic.	TV (cm³)/ dose (Gy)	Resp. (mos)	Chemo during/ after GKS	Survival from Dx (mos from 1st SRS)	Cause of death
1	2.4, M	Temporo-parietal	24/24/23	25/LR	11/13	PR (4)	30/MR	3.0/9	PR (2)				Yes	33(8)	PND + PTD
		Third ventricle					30/DR	1.1/12	CR (2)						
		Lateral ventricle					30/DR	1.1/13	CR (2)						
		Basal ganglia					30/DR	3.0/12	CR (2)						
2	2.7, F	Posterior Fossa	23/28/23	33/LR	8.4/16	CR (2)							Yes	37(4)	PND
3	1.0, M	Posterior Fossa	0/0/0	11/DR	13.1/13	PD (2)							Yes	17(6)	PND + PTD
4	3.3, F	Posterior Fossa	24/24/23	35/LR	2.7/15	CR(36)	79/MR	1.3/16	CR(36)				No	126 (91)	PND + PTD
5	2.2, F	Posterior Fossa	0/51/0	18/DR	4.6/16	CR(10)	30/DR	1.1/14	NA				Yes	33(15)	PND + PTD
6	12.3, M	Posterior Fossa	23/32/23	29/LR	1.2/20	SD(12)							Yes	59(30)	PND + PTD
7	10.7, M	Pineal	36/18/23	30/LR	3.3/16	CR(17)	47/MR	1.6/16	CR (6)	53/MR	1.7/16	CR (2)	No	67(37)	PTD

Values in parentheses denote duration of response to GKS or earliest evidence of progressive GKS-treated disease.
BG basal ganglia, *Chemo* chemotherapy, *CR* complete response, *DR* distant recurrence, *Ind.* indication, *Int.* interval, *LR* local recurrence, *mos* Month, *MR* marginal recurrence adjacent to site of previous GKS, *NA* data not available, *PD* progressive disease, *PF* posterior fossa, *PND* progressive new disease (including disseminated leptomeningeal disease), *PR* partial response, *PTD* progressive GKS-treated disease, *Resp.* response, *RT* fractionated radiation therapy to craniospinal axis, *SD* stable disease, *TP* temporoparietal, *TV* tumor volume, *vent* ventricle, *WB/B/SC* whole brain/boost to initial tumor site/spinal cord

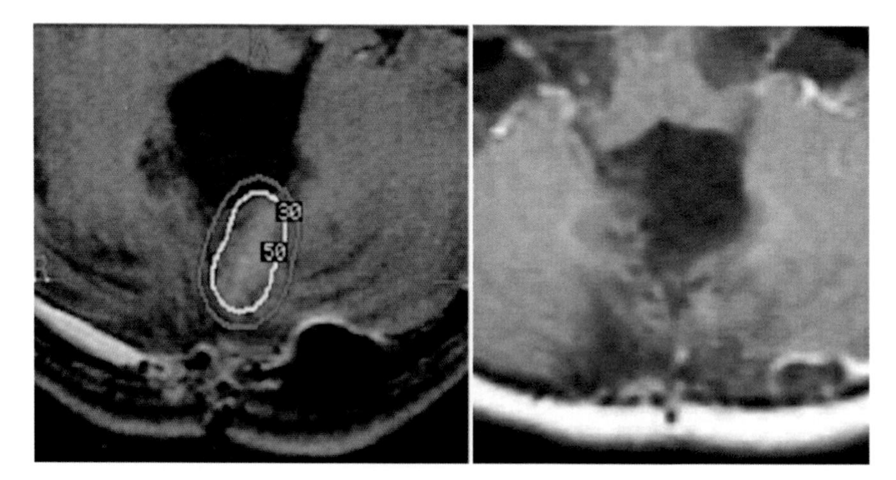

Fig. 18.2 Case 4, second *GKRS* treatment. *Left*: Axial contrast-enhanced MR image of the posterior fossa depicting a conformal *GKRS* plan. A steep dose falloff is observed, with the inner contour representing 50% isodose and the outer contour representing 30% isodose. *Right*: Axial contrast-enhanced MR image showing tumor volume reduction 6 months after GKRS (Figure reproduced with permission by Journal of Neurosurgery Pediatrics 2009;3:205–210)

GKRS for Adult Medulloblastoma

The outcomes of adult medulloblastoma patients treated with GKRS in University of Pittsburgh was also reviewed recently (Germanwala et al. 2008). Some similarities may exist between children and adult medulloblastoma in terms of overall survival and response to XRT and chemotherapy (Curran et al. 2009). However, the same study found that infants fared significantly worse compared to children and adult groups. Twelve adult patients (mean age of 33.8 years, range; 19–52 years) with histologically proven medulloblastoma or supratentorial PNET tumor underwent ≥1 sessions of GKRS for post-treatment residual or recurrent tumors (six tumors in each group). Before GKRS, all patients had undergone a maximal feasible resection followed by craniospinal irradiation. Nine patients also received systemic chemotherapy. Stereotactic radiosurgery was applied to residual and recurrent posterior fossa tumor as well as to foci of intracranial medulloblastoma metastases. The median time interval from initial diagnosis to the first GKRS treatment was 24 months (range 2–37 months). The mean GKRS-treated tumor volume was 9.4 cm^3 (range 0.5–39 cm^3).

Following adjunctive radiosurgery, five patients had no evidence of tumor on magnetic resonance (MR) imaging, three had stable tumor burden and four had evidence of tumor progression locally with or without intracranial metastases. All patients with tumor progression died. Eight patients survived with a mean cumulative follow-up of 72.4 months (range 21–152 months). No acute radiation toxicity or delayed radiation necrosis was observed among any of the 12 patients. The majority of patients who achieved tumor eradication (80%) and tumor stabilization (67%) after GKRS had residual tumor as the reason for their referral for GKRS. The best outcomes were attained in patients with residual disease who were younger, had smaller tumor volumes, had no evidence of metastatic disease, and had received higher cumulative GKRS doses.

Observations on Our Experience with GKRS for Medulloblastoma/PNET Tumors

GKRS Is Well Tolerated

GKRS is well tolerated by children (and adults) who have previously undergone craniospinal irradiation and chemotherapy. Although the impact of radiosurgery on the quality of overall survival was not examined in either study, the outpatient nature of the procedure and the minimal additional risks were well received by the parents and the patients.

Treated Tumor Volume Influences Response

Although the number of cases in both studies is small, our findings confirm the observation that tumor size influences response to treatment. Mean marginal dose delivered to the tumor was on average 14–15 Gy.

Response to GKRS May Be Influenced by Histology

Our cohort of multiply recurrent pediatric tumors includes two with supratentorial PNET. The recent fourth edition of the World Health Organization (Louis et al. 2007) classification of tumors of the central nervous system (CNS) made substantial revisions to the category of embryonal tumors recognizing the heterogeneity of different subgroups. Despite shared histopathologic features with medulloblastomas, PNETs are considerably more aggressive and have different genetic characteristics (Russo et al. 1999). In addition, medulloblastomas and PNET tumors harboring anaplastic/large cell features appear to be associated with a worse outcome (Behdad and Perry 2010). Desmoplastic/nodular sub-type of medulloblastoma has a better prognosis than classic histology despite traditional adverse clinical features of metastatic disease and incomplete surgical resection (Kleihues and Cavenee 2000). This spectrum of histologic subtypes among PNET tumors may partially explain the varying response to treatment (including GKRS) and overall survival.

Younger Patients Harbor More Aggressive Disease

Children who had late progression following GKRS were generally older than those who had early progression. Their mean age at time of diagnosis was 6.2 years versus 1.9 years for the early progression group.

This confirms the observation that younger children harbor more biologically aggressive or radiation-resistant tumors. In a Canadian review of 96 medulloblastoma cases under the age of 3 years (median age at diagnosis of 19.5 months), there was a significant increase in survival time in patients who received RT compared to those who were not treated with this modality, as well as for those who were over 18 months at diagnosis compared to those under 18 months (Johnston et al. 2009).

Given the time course of our case series, which extends back to 1989, some of the younger cases may in fact be atypical teratoid rhabdoid tumor (AT/RT) – a tumor which behaves more aggressively than standard medulloblastoma and is most common in younger children. Diagnosis of AT/RT is often confirmed by the lack of nuclear expression of INI1. Two series have encountered subgroups of PNET cases that on review were more consistent with AT/RT histology and these cases were also associated with a worse outcome (Haberler et al. 2006; Behdad and Perry 2010).

Adjuvant GKS Following Resection

In our series, children who had the longest survival times had maximal repeat resection of their local recurrence, followed by GKRS to the tumor bed. Children who underwent GKRS alone survived for 15 months, whereas those who underwent repeat resection followed by GKRS enjoyed a median survival of 33.5 months. Microscopic tumor deposits have been confirmed in arachnoid and CSF spaces adjacent to the site of surgery (Souweidane et al. 2009). Radiosurgery to the resection bed may improve local control by targeting these microscopic deposits. Indeed there is evidence that adjuvant radiation may reduce medulloblastoma cell invasiveness, a factor which may promote local tumor recurrence (Ranger et al. 2009).

Difficulties with Data Interpretation Using Multimodal Therapies

Given that all of these children were treated with other salvage therapies in addition to SRS, one cannot reliably comment on how GKRS impacted survival time. Because of the multiply recurrent nature of the disease and failure of initial treatment, various second and third-line treatments had been implemented by the time GKRS was administered. Through future international collaboration of pediatric CNS tumor databases and the standardization of treatment options for recurrent pediatric CNS tumors, future analyses should become easier.

Future Therapeutic Strategies

The Need for Better Disease Surveillance

Although patients were selected for SRS based on the best available medical evidence and after failure of standard management, unrecognized micrometastatic disease may have been the source of delayed distant progression. In addition, local disease may progress if tumors are relatively resistant to radiation doses compatible with satisfactory risk to adjacent critical brain structures. Better surveillance tools are required to select patients appropriately, based on who is more likely to benefit from radiosurgery. However, based on our experience of more than 9,300 patients undergoing GKRS, there is no better modality than high-resolution MR imaging performed at the time of referral of the patient.

The Importance of Tumor Control Versus Risk of Longterm Treatment-Related Sequelae

Fractionated radiotherapy is an established modality in the treatment of PNET tumors. However, with the improvement in disease control, there is an increasing recognition of the delayed effects of RT in terms of development of new CNS neoplasms and cognitive/endocrine sequelae. In addition, delayed disease relapse is a common occurrence. In a recent study by Armstrong et al. (2009), cumulative late mortality at 30 years was 25.8% due primarily to recurrence and/or progression of primary disease. Patients who received cranial RT of 50 Gy or more had a cumulative incidence of a subsequent neoplasm within the CNS of 7.1% at 25 years from diagnosis compared with 1.0% for patients who had no RT. Survivors had higher risk than siblings of developing new endocrine, neurological, or sensory complications 5 or more years after diagnosis. Neurocognitive impairment was high and proportional to radiation dose for specific tumor types. There was a dose-dependent association between RT to the frontal and/or temporal lobes and lower rates of employment, and marriage.

In another longterm follow-up study by Frange et al. (2009), only patients whose primary treatment included craniospinal radiation were considered. At a median follow-up from diagnosis of 14.4 years (in 45 surviving patients), late sequelae were frequent, particularly neurological deficits (71%) and endocrine complications (52%). Impairments of psychosocial functioning, including employment, driving capacity, independent living, and marital status, were identified in most patients. Most long-term medulloblastoma survivors suffer persistent deficits in several domains, with a significant impact on their psychosocial functioning (Frange et al. 2009).

The need to minimize longterm cognitive/endocrine sequelae yet maximize tumor control has been recognized by the drive to deliver the least radiation dose that can be considered effective for the areas of brain with highest risk of recurrence. In addition, patients with delayed focal disease relapse may not be candidates for further fractionated radiotherapy mandating a role for repeat surgery, SRS and other focal therapies. These studies highlight the differing therapeutic challenges presented by the malignant brain tumours of early childhood, the importance of surgical approaches and the need to explore individualised brain sparing approaches.

Role of SRS in Children Under 3 Years of Age

One of the potential benefits of GKRS is its application in children who are unsuitable for initial or additional fractionated radiation therapy because of the increased risk of neurotoxicity and poor long-term neurocognitive outcomes. These children also fall within the high-risk category, necessitating alternative therapeutic modalities for local disease control. GKRS administered to primary and metastatic tumor sites may allow for disease control until the child is old enough to receive fractionated radiation therapy.

The Role of New Chemotherapeutic Regimens

One of the key findings of our study is that recurrent PNET after prior multimodality therapy is a systemic illness, not a localized disease. Even though all of our available tests might suggest that the recurrence is local, six of seven children ultimately died of disseminated disease Therefore, using a focal therapy such as SRS may offer some degree of palliation, but only systemic therapy will afford the chance of a cure.

In light of our increasing understanding of the molecular biology of medulloblastomas, future progress will depend on developing optimised surgical strategies, and designing chemotherapy/drug strategies tailored to different biological categories. In light of these new chemotherapeutic agents, the role of intrathecal drug delivery may also be revisited.

As highlighted by the eventual disseminated disease in most of our pediatric cohort, systemic therapy will be needed to achieve disease control. Combined international efforts and continued investment is needed to develop systemic therapies that may provide even more benefit for these difficult tumors. It is our hope that until better treatment strategies are developed, GKRS will be considered as an important but palliative additional tool in the fight against treatment-resistant medulloblastomas.

Conclusions

GKRS is a management option for patients who fail initial treatment for medulloblastoma/PNET tumors. Ultimately, delayed local progression, distant relapse, or leptomeningeal seeding led to the death of all pediatric patients in our series. Further efforts to develop more effective strategies are needed.

Acknowledgements/Disclosures Drs. Lunsford, Kondziolka, and Niranjan are consultants with AB Elekta. Dr. Lunsford is a stockholder in AB Elekta. The work described in this report was funded by a grant to Dr. Flannery from the Irish Institute of Clinical Neuroscience, the Ethicon Foundation Fund R.C.S. (Edinburgh), Friends of the Royal Travel Fund, Northern Ireland Medical & Dental Training Agency, and the Congress of Neurological Surgeons. The authors report no other potential conflicts of interest.

References

Abe M, Tokumaru S, Tabuchi K, Kida Y, Takagi M, Imamura J (2006) Stereotactic radiation therapy with chemotherapy in the management of recurrent medulloblastomas. Pediatr Neurosurg 42:81–88

Albright AL, Wishoff JH, Zelter PM, Boyett JM, Rorke LB, Stanley P (1996) Effects of medulloblastoma resections on outcome in children: a report from the Children's Cancer Group. Neurosurgery 38:265–271

Armstrong GT, Liu Q, Yasui Y, Huang S, Ness KK, Leisenring W, Hudson MM, Donaldson SS, King AA, Stovall M, Krull KR, Robison LL, Packer RJ (2009) Long-term outcomes among adult survivors of childhood central nervous system malignancies in the childhood cancer survivor study. J Natl Cancer Inst 101(13):946–958

Behdad A, Perry A (2010) Central nervous system primitive neuroectodermal tumors: a clinicopathologic and genetic study of 33 cases. Brain Pathol 20(2):441–450

Bowers DC, Gargan L, Weprin BE, Mulne AF, Elterman RD, Munoz L, Giller CA, Winick NJ (2007) Impact of site of tumor recurrence upon survival for children with recurrent or progressive medulloblastoma. J Neurosurg 107(1 Suppl):5–10

Butturini AM, Jacob M, Aguajo J, Vander-Walde NA, Villablanca J, Jubran R, Erdreich-Epstein A, Marachelian A, Dhall G, Finlay JL (2009) High-dose chemotherapy and autologous hematopoietic progenitor cell rescue in children with recurrent medulloblastoma and supratentorial primitive neuroectodermal tumors: the impact of prior radiotherapy on outcome. Cancer 115(13):2956–2963

Curran EK, Le GM, Sainani KL, Propp JM, Fisher PG (2009) Do children and adults differ in survival from medulloblastoma? A study from the SEER registry. J Neurooncol 95(1):81–85

Flannery T, Kano H, Martin JJ, Niranjan A, Flickinger JC, Lunsford LD, Kondziolka D (2009) Boost radiosurgery as a strategy after failure of initial management of pediatric primitive neuroectodermal tumors. J Neurosurg Pediatr 3:205–210

Frange P, Alapetite C, Gaboriaud G, Bours D, Zucker JM, Zerah M, Brisse H, Chevignard M, Mosseri V, Bouffet E, Doz F (2009) From childhood to adulthood: long-term outcome of medulloblastoma patients. The Institut Curie experience (1980–2000). J Neurooncol 95(2):271–279

Gaijjar A,Hernan R, Kocak M, Fuller C,Lee Y, McKinnon PJ, Wallace D, Lau C, Chintagumpala M, Ashley DM, Kellie SJ, Kun L, Gilbertson RJ (2004) Clinical, histopathologic, and molecular markers of prognosis: toward a new disease risk stratification system for medulloblastoma. J Clin Oncol 22(6): 984–993

Germanwala AV, Mai JC, Tomycz ND, Niranjan A, Flickinger JC, Kondziolka D, Lunsford LD (2008) Boost Gamma Knife surgery during multimodality management of adult medulloblastoma. J Neurosurg 108:204–209

Haberler C, Laggner U, Slavic I, Czech T, Ambros IM, Ambros PF, Budka H, Hainfellner JA (2006) Immunohistochemical analysis of INI1 protein in malignant pediatric CNS tumors: lack of INI1 in atypical teratoid/rhabdoid tumors and in a fraction of primitive neuroectodermal tumors without rhabdoid phenotype. Am J Surg Pathol 30:1462–1468

Jenkin D (1996) Long-term survival of children with brain tumors. Oncology (Williston Park) 10(5):715–719

Johnston DL, Keene D, Bartels U, Carret AS, Crooks B, Eisenstat DD, Fryer C, Lafay-Cousin L, Larouche V, Moghrabi A, Wilson B, Zelcer S, Silva M, Brossard J, Bouffet E (2009) Medulloblastoma in children under the age of three years: a retrospective Canadian review. J Neurooncol 94(1):51–56

Kleihues P, Cavenee WK (eds) (2000) Pathology and genetics of tumours of the nervous system. International Agency for Research on Cancer, Lyon

Kortmann RD, Kühl J, Timmermann B, Mittler U, Urban C, Budach V, Richter E, Willich N, Flentje M, Berthold F, Slavic I, Wolff J, Meisner C, Wiestler O, Sorensen N, Warmuth-Metz M, Bamberg M (2000) Postoperative neoadjuvant chemotherapy before radiotherapy as compared to immediate radiotherapy followed by maintenance chemotherapy in the treatment of medulloblastoma in childhood: results of the German prospective randomized trial HIT '91. Int J Radiat Oncol Biol Phys 46(2):269–279

Laughton SJ, Merchant TE, Sklar CA, Kun LE, Fouladi M, Broniscer A, Morris EB, Sanders RP, Krasin MJ, Shelso J, Xiong Z, Wallace D, Gajjar A (2008) Endocrine outcomes for children with embryonal brain tumors after risk-adapted craniospinal and conformal primary-site irradiation and high-dose chemotherapy with stem-cell rescue on the SJMB-96 trial. J Clin Oncol 26(7):1112–1118

Louis DN, Ohgaki H, Wiestler OD, Cavenee WK (eds) (2007) WHO classification of tumours of the central nervous system. IARC Press, Lyon

Patrice SJ, Tarbell NJ, Goumnerova LC, Shrieve DC, Black PM, Loeffler JS (1995) Results of radiosurgery in the management of recurrent and residual medulloblastoma. Pediatr Neurosurg 22:197–203

Pomeroy SL, Tamayo P, Gaasenbeek M, Sturla LM, Angelo M, McLaughlin ME, Kim JY, Goumnerova LC, Black PM, Lau C, Allen JC, Zagzag D, Olson JM, Curran T, Wetmore C, Biegel JA, Poggio T, Mukherjee S, Rifkin R, Califano A, Stolovitzky G, Louis DN, Mesirov JP, Lander ES, Golub TR (2002) Prediction of central nervous system embryonal tumour outcome based on gene expression. Nature 415(6870):436–442

Ranger A, McDonald W, Bauman GS, Del Maestro R (2009) Effects of surgical excision and radiation on medulloblastoma cell invasiveness. Can J Neurol Sci 36(5):631–637

Ridola V, Grill J, Doz F, Gentet JC, Frappaz D, Raquin MA, Habrand JL, Sainte-Rose C, Valteau-Couanet D, Kalifa C (2007) High-dose chemotherapy with autologous stem cell rescue followed by posterior fossa irradiation for local medulloblastoma recurrence or progression after conventional chemotherapy. Cancer 110(1):156–163

Ris MD, Packer R, Goldwein J, Jones-Wallace D, Boyett JM (2001) Intellectual outcome after reduced-dose radiation therapy plus adjuvant chemotherapy for medulloblastoma: a Children's Cancer Group study. J Clin Oncol 19(15):3470–3476

Rosenfeld A, Kletzel M, Duerst R, Jacobsohn D, Haut P, Weinstein J, Rademaker A, Schaefer C, Evans L, Fouts M, Goldman S (2010) A phase II prospective study of sequential myeloablative chemotherapy with hematopoietic stem cell rescue for the treatment of selected high risk and recurrent central nervous system tumors. J Neurooncol 97(2):247–255

Rossi A, Caracciolo V, Russo G, Reiss K, Giordano A (2008) Medulloblastoma: from molecular pathology to therapy. Clin Cancer Res 14:971–976

Russo C, Pellarin M, Tingby O, Bollen AW, Lamborn KR, Mohapatra G, Collins VP, Feuerstein BG (1999) Comparative genomic hybridization in patients with supratentorial and infratentorial primitive neuroectodermal tumors. Cancer 86:331–339

Saunders DE, Hayward RD, Phipps KP, Chong WK, Wade AM (2003) Surveillance neuroimaging of intracranial medulloblastoma in children: how effective, how often, and for how long? J Neurosurg 99(2):280–286

Souweidane MM, Morgenstern PF, Christos PJ, Edgar MA, Khakoo Y, Rutka JT, Dunkel IJ (2009) Intraoperative arachnoid and cerebrospinal fluid sampling in children with posterior fossa brain tumors. Neurosurgery 65(1): 72–78

Stavrou T, Bromley CM, Nicholson HS, Byrne J, Packer RJ, Goldstein AM, Reaman GH (2001) Prognostic factors and secondary malignancies in childhood medulloblastoma. J Pediatr Hematol Oncol 23(7):431–436

Taylor RE, Bailey CC, Robinson KJ, Weston CL, Ellison DW, Ironside J, Lucraft H, Gilbertson R, Tait DM, Walker DA, Pizer BL, Lashford LS (2004) Impact of radiotherapy parameters on outcome in the International Society of Paediatric Oncology/United Kingdom Children's Cancer Study Group PNET-3 study of preradiotherapy chemotherapy for M0-M1 medulloblastoma. Int J Radiat Oncol Biol Phys 58(4):1184–1193

Early Childhood Medulloblastoma: Prognostic Factors

19

André O.von Bueren and Stefan Rutkowski

Contents

A.O. von Bueren, MD • S. Rutkowski, MD, PhD (✉)
Department of Pediatric Hematology and Oncology, University Medical Center Hamburg-Eppendorf, Martinistr 52, D-20246 Hamburg, Germany
e-mail: s.rutkowski@uke.de

Abstract

Clinical management of medulloblastoma, the most common malignant childhood central nervous system tumor, is particularly challenging in young children due to the vulnerability of the developing central nervous system. Most recent studies have aimed to utilize chemotherapy in order to avoid, delay or reduce radiotherapy. Identification of prognostic markers for young children with medulloblastoma which may help to stratify patients is of enormous interest. The nodular desmoplastic histological variants of medulloblastoma, with medulloblastoma with extensive nodularity at the end of the spectrum, has been shown in several studies to be a strong independent positive prognostic marker in young children, and is therefore a candidate to improve risk-adapted treatment stratification – in addition to clinical risk factors such as presence or absence of metastases and postoperative residual disease status. Consequently, stratification according to histologic variants has been implemented in current multicenter studies of cooperative groups in Europe and North America. In contrast, management of young children with classic, anaplastic or large-cell medulloblastoma remains challenging, as sustained tumor control after intensified treatment strategies including high-dose chemotherapy and local conformal or craniospinal radiotherapy has only be achieved in a minority of children so far. The histological variants reflect at least in part the insights into medulloblastoma

M.A. Hayat (ed.), *Pediatric Cancer, Volume 3: Diagnosis, Therapy, and Prognosis*, Pediatric Cancer 3,
DOI 10.1007/978-94-007-4528-5_19, © Springer Science+Business Media Dordrecht 2012

biology, with at least four distinct entities being recently identified by different gene expression profiling. Future treatment recommendations may be based on robust histopathological and biological prognostic parameters to decrease or intensify the risk of tumor relapse and treatment-related late effects.

Introduction

Medulloblastoma, the most frequent primary malignant brain tumor of childhood, occurs in ~33% of cases in the first 3 years and ~50% of cases in the first 5 years of life (Kaatsch et al. 2001). Unfavorable prognosis of early childhood medulloblastoma, survival rates of young children with medulloblastoma ranged from 20% to 50% until the last decade, might be explicable be several reasons. First, it is generally assumed that early childhood medulloblastoma share a more aggressive clinical/biological behavior and presence of metastases is frequent (Zeltzer et al. 1999; Packer et al. 2003; Rutkowski 2006). Second, misclassifications of atypical teratoid/rhabdoid tumor (AT/RT) – a clinically aggressive tumor, primarily occurring in children aged <3 years, which has been recognized only since the last decade – might have contributed also to the poor survival of young children with medulloblastoma. Third, there is a treatment limitation as the immature brain is particularly susceptible to radiotherapy-induced neurocognitive deficits (Kiltie et al. 1997) resulting in reluctance to use radiotherapy in young children with medulloblastoma (Warren and Packer 2004; Kalifa and Grill 2005; Rutkowski 2006). Finally, some young children with medulloblastoma may not have been treated with a curative approach in times when subgroups with favorable prognoses were not yet identified. In general, all treatment strategies used in young children with medulloblastoma may cause neuroendocrine, behavioral, and deficits of neurocognitive function. Current treatment strategies for young children with medulloblastoma aim to increase survival while improving quality of life and decreasing treatment induced sequelae. Many studies designed to delay or avoid radiotherapy by several approaches using conventional systemic chemotherapy and radiotherapy, high-dose chemotherapy with autologous stem cell rescue given either in primary treatment or at relapse, or by substituting radiotherapy by the use of intraventricular methotrexate (Rutkowski 2006). The establishment of solid prognostic markers, which may help to stratify young children with medulloblastoma to different risk adapted treatments, is of particular value. Thus far, histological subtype, stage of disease, and amount of postoperative residual disease appear to be most helpful to use in the future for risk adapted treatment decisions in young children with medulloblastoma. However, assignment of medulloblastoma patients to the respective subgroups based on distinct molecular expression profiles may become standard for risk-adapted stratification of treatment in future (Kool et al. 2008; Northcott et al. 2011; Cho et al. 2011).

Histology and Biology

Five histological variants of medulloblastoma have been recognized in the latest World Health Organization (WHO) classification of central nervous system tumors (Louis et al. 2007): classic medulloblastoma, desmoplastic/nodular medulloblastoma, medulloblastoma with extensive nodularity, large cell medulloblastoma, and anaplastic medulloblastoma. Classic histopathological variant are described to be composed of sheets of generally small round to oval or carrot-like hyperchromatic nuclei and scant cytoplasms. The desmoplastic/nodular variant is characterized by nodular reticulin-free tumor islands surrounded by areas with densely packed, proliferative tumor cells which produce a dense intercellular reticulin fiber network. The variant medulloblastoma with extensive nodularity shows a similar biphasic pattern as the desmoplastic/nodular medulloblastoma but is differing from desmoplastic/nodular variant by expanded lobular architecture and reduced internodular reticulin-rich components. Typically, the MBEN variant has a characteristic grape-like growth pattern which may be

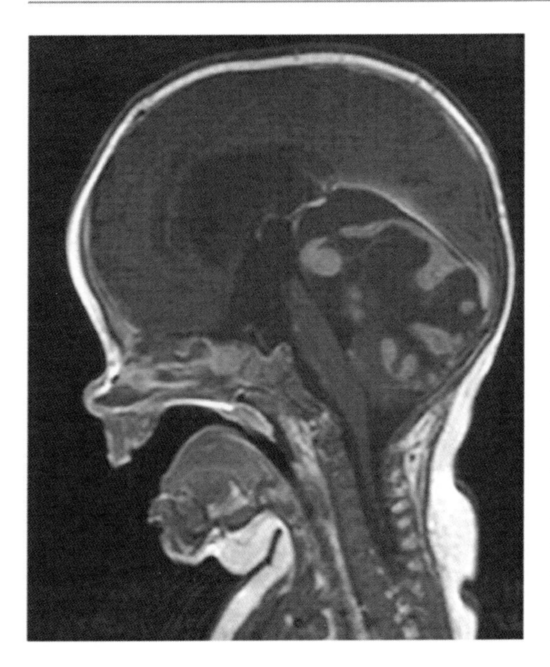

Fig. 19.1 Sagittal T1-weighted MRI with gadolinium. Medulloblastoma with extensive nodularity (MBEN) with characteristic grape-like growth pattern. Frontal bossing and macrocephalia may indicate Gorlin's syndrome

identifiable on preoperative magnetic resonance imaging (MRI) scanning (Fig. 19.1).

Anaplastic medulloblastoma shows marked cytological pleomorphism and high mitotic and apoptotic counts. Large cell medulloblastoma is characterized by its groups of uniform large round cells with a single nucleolus, and frequently in association with groups of anaplastic cells. Frequency of the histological subtypes varies at different ages. It has been shown in several studies that desmoplastic/nodular medulloblastoma and medulloblastoma with extensive nodularity account together for >40% of early childhood medulloblastoma cases (Rutkowski et al. 2005, 2010; von Bueren et al. 2011). In the same age group, more than 50% of the cases are described as having the classic histopathological variant, whereas large cell and anaplastic medulloblastoma are less frequent. Of note, frequency of histological subtypes differs in older children. Desmoplasia is infrequent in patients aged >3 years (~5–15%) and the classic variant accounts for >80% of cases. The HIT-SKK'92 trial of the Society of Pediatric Oncology and Hematology in Germany, Austria and Switzerland (GPOH) for children aged <3 years demonstrated that 20 patients with desmoplastic/nodular medulloblastoma or medulloblastoma with extensive nodularity, respectively, had a better outcome than 23 patients with classic medulloblastoma, independent of presence or absence of metastases or postoperative residual tumor (Rutkowski et al. 2005). The consecutive trial HIT-SKK'2000BIS4 confirmed the prognostic impact of histology in young children (von Bueren et al. 2011). Nineteen patients with desmoplastic/nodular medulloblastoma or medulloblastoma with extensive nodularity, respectively, had better event-free survival and overall survival (5-year rates: 95% ± 5% and 100% ± 0%) than 23 patients with classic medulloblastoma (5-year rates: 30% ± 11% and 68% ± 10%, $p < 0.001$ for event-free survival, $p = 0.008$ for overall survival) (von Bueren et al. 2011). The multivariable Cox regression analysis identified histology as an independent prognostic factor in both studies (Rutkowski et al. 2005; von Bueren et al. 2011). A similar finding was obtained in a retrospective analysis of the HIT-SKK 87 GPOH pilot study for young children with malignant brain tumors (Rutkowski et al. 2009). Finally, an international meta-analysis from more than 250 children younger than 5 years treated within prospective trials of five national study groups confirmed histopathological subtypes as strong independent prognostic factor (Rutkowski et al. 2010). Interestingly, differences of survival rates between histological subtypes remained significant in the subgroups of children with nonmetastatic medulloblastoma without postoperative residual disease (M0, R0), in the subgroup of children with nonmetastatic medulloblastoma and incomplete resection (M0, R+), and in the subgroup of children with metastatic medulloblastoma (M+) (Rutkowski et al. 2010). Patients with desmoplastic/nodular medulloblastoma and medulloblastoma with extensive nodularity had more favorable survival rates (8-year event-free survival, 55% ± 5%, 8-year overall survival, 76% ± 4%), followed by patients with classic medulloblastoma (8-year event-free survival, 27% ± 4%, 8-year overall survival, 42% ± 4%), and children with large-cell/anaplastic medulloblastoma (7.5-year event-free survival, 14%±13%, 7.5-year overall survival, 14%±13%). Of note, patients who had a diagnosis of medulloblastoma with extensive nodularity had the most favorable survival rates (8-year event-free survival, 86%±8%, 8-year overall survival, 95%±5%). Survival rates of patients with medulloblastoma with extensive nodularity in the trials HIT-SKK'92 and HIT-SKK'2000BIS4 were excellent (5-year event-free survival and overall survival rates for seven children in the HIT-SKK'92 trial (Rutkowski et al. 2005), and for six children in the HIT-SKK'2000BIS4 trial (von Bueren et al. 2011) were 100%±0%). Important results have been reported with regards to age-dependent occurrence of Gorlin syndrome in medulloblastoma variants (Garre et al. 2009). Five of 82 patients (6%) were diagnosed with Gorlin syndrome, all these cases had a medulloblastoma with extensive nodularity variant. When medulloblastoma is associated with Gorlin syndrome, nevoid basal cell carcinoma and irradiation-induced meningioma may occur after radiotherapy. On the basis that Gorlin syndrome is in particular frequent in children with medulloblastoma with extensive nodularity (5 out of 12 patients) (Garre et al. 2009), they should be examined very carefully at time of diagnosis (family history, clinical and dermatological examinations), and during follow-up. Genetic counseling, and investigation of *PTCH* mutations should be considered to exclude or confirm the diagnosis of Gorlin syndrome.

Gene expression studies are suggesting 4–6 molecular subtypes of medulloblastoma (Kool et al. 2008; Northcott et al. 2011; Cho et al. 2011). All studies have demonstrated a subgroup of medulloblastoma showing wingless (WNT) activation, a second group with sonic hedgehog (SHH) signaling activation, and 2–4 non-WNT/non-SHH groups. Children and adolescents with WNT tumors are typically aged 6–20 years (median, 10.4 years) (Kool et al. 2008). WNT tumors are 2–3 times more commonly identified in females than males (Northcott et al. 2011). In addition, this group is characterized to have classic histology, absence of metastases, and excellent prognosis. Genetics hallmarks of these tumors are monosomy 6, and mutations in *CTNNB1*, the gene encoding ß-catenin, a downstream effector of the WNT pathway. Gene expression analysis identified overexpression of many genes of the WNT pathway (Kool et al. 2008).

Patients with SHH tumors are typically either very young children (aged ≤3 years) or adults (aged ≥16 years), and tumors are often nonmetastatic (Kool et al. 2008). Desmoplastic medulloblastoma constitutes more than 50% of the SHH tumors; classic, large cell, and anaplastic phenotypes are less frequent. Young children with desmoplastic histology (SHH tumors) appear to have an excellent outcome even without application of radiotherapy (Rutkowski et al. 2005, 2010; von Bueren et al. 2011). Adults with desmoplastic histology (SHH tumors) have an intermediate outcome (Kool et al. 2008). On the basis of genetics, 9q loss and *MYCN* amplification are characteristic for these tumors. Mechanisms of activation of the SHH pathway include mutations in *PTCH1* (patched1) and others genes. These tumors are characterized by overexpression of genes involved in the SHH signaling. In the article of Northcott et al. non-WNT/non-SHH tumors are subdivided in Group C and Group D tumors. Patients with Group C tumors (corresponding to Kool et al. cluster E tumors) are young children (median, 3.8 years; range, 2–15 years), classic medulloblastoma is the most common histological phenotype, up to 70% of those children do have metastases (Kool et al. 2008), and children of this molecular subgroup share an unfavorable prognosis (Kool et al. 2008; Northcott et al. 2011; Cho et al. 2011). Gene amplification of *c-MYC* has been reported to be specific for group C tumors (Northcott et al. 2011; Cho et al. 2011). Gain of chromosome 18, loss of X chromosome, and isochromosome 17q (usually having one copy of 17p and three copies of 17q) are common in group C and group D tumors. High expression of c-MYC mRNA is frequent in the WNT tumors and the group C tumors. Patients with group D tumors (corresponding to Kool et al. cluster C and cluster D) are generally older children with a median age at diagnosis of 9 years (Northcott et al. 2011), around one third of the patients do have metastases (Kool et al. 2008), classic medulloblastoma is the most frequent histology, and prognosis of these patients is intermediate. As described above, genetic characteristics are similar compared to group C tumors.

In summary, molecular subgroups may provide additional explanations for the less favorable prognoses of young children with medulloblastoma. Patients with WNT tumors show an excellent prognosis and have been reported only to be evident in older children and adolescents. Young children with desmoplastic histopathological phenotype (SHH tumors) are doing extremely well and precise explanation for that is still elusive. Non-WNT/non-SHH tumors are characterized by a poor prognosis, and young children clustering in those medulloblastoma profiles may have a very poor prognosis because of age-related limitations of treatment options.

Table 19.1 illustrates the different molecular subgroups defined by several research groups (Kool et al. 2008; Northcott et al. 2011; Cho et al. 2011).

Extent of Tumor Resection and Disseminated Disease

The Chang classification (T/M) system is based on the extent of the primary tumor, on macroscopic metastases, diagnosed by craniospinal magnetic resonance imaging, and on dissemination of tumor cells within the cerebrospinal fluid. The Chang classification (T/M) system was introduced in the year 1969 (Chang et al. 1969), and the staging system is currently used in a modified form. Preoperative tumor (T) stage was determined based on tumor size, extent, and invasion. T stage is rarely assigned. Metastasis (M) stage is now defined with craniospinal magnetic resonance imaging (MRI) scanning of the entire neuraxis as well as a lumbar puncture for cerebrospinal fluid cytology. The extent of disease has been demonstrated to be a prognostic marker in several studies (Albright et al. 1996; Zeltzer et al. 1999). Difference in prognosis was mainly seen in older children with nonmetastatic medulloblastoma. Most of the international trials excluded patients with residual tumors larger than 1.5 cm^2 from "standard-risk" trials, and therefore this factor was not studied extensively lately. However, for young children with medulloblastoma, the data on postoperative residual tumor are still limited. Previous studies have provided evidence that the ability to achieve a gross-total resection of the tumor may represent a positive prognostic indicator for survival (Rutkowski et al. 2005; Duffner et al. 1993; Kalifa and Grill 2005; Grill et al. 2005; Rutkowski 2006). On the other hand, several large studies found that incomplete resection did not affect survival (Walter et al. 1999; Johnston et al. 2009; Rutkowski et al. 2009; Geyer et al. 2005). In the previous study HIT-SKK'2000BIS4, 39 patients without postoperative residual tumor >1.5 cm^2 appeared to have a better event-free survival and overall survival than six patients with postoperative residual tumor >1.5 cm^2 (von Bueren et al. 2011). However, in the multivariable Cox regression analysis, histology but not extent of resection was identified as an independent prognostic factor (von Bueren et al. 2011).

According to the Chang staging system, the following M-stages are defined: M0: No evidence of metastasis; M1: Presence of tumor cells in the cerebrospinal fluid; M2: Gross nodular seeding demonstrated in cerebellar, cerebral subarachnoid space, or in the third or lateral ventricles; M3: Gross nodular seeding in spinal subarachnoid space; M4: Tumor spread to areas outside the central nervous system. Metastatic status in young children with medulloblastoma has not consistently demonstrated to be of significant prognostic value (Halperin et al. 2001; Rutkowski et al. 2005, 2010; Walter et al. 1999; Zeltzer et al. 1999).

The largest analysis performed so far in young children with medulloblastoma has evaluated the prognostic value of histology, extent of tumor resection, and M-stages (Rutkowski et al. 2010). Interestingly, children with desmoplastic/nodular medulloblastoma as well as children with medulloblastoma with extensive nodularity had lower M-stages and gross-total resection was achieved more frequently than in children with classic medulloblastoma. Multivariable analysis identified in addition to the histopathological medulloblastoma variant the combination of extent of

Table 19.1 Summary of principal clinical and biological characteristics of different medulloblastoma subgroups as defined by several research groups

Kool	Cluster A	Cluster B	Cluster E	Cluster C/D
Northcott	WNT	SHH	Group C	Group D
Cho	C_6	C_3	C_1/C_5	C_2/C_4
Age and sex characteristics	Older children (>6 years); females > males	Young children and adults (<3 years; >16 years)	Young children (median age, ~3.5 years)	Children (median age, ~9 years)
Predominant M-stage	Nonmetastatic	Nonmetastatic	Metastatic	Metastatic
Predominant histology	Classic	Desmoplastic Classic, LC/A	Classic LC/A	Classic LC/A
Prognosis	Favorable	Favorable (young children), intermediate (adults)	Unfavorable	Intermediate
Genetic characteristics	−6, CTNNB1 mutations	−9q, MYCN amplification, PTCH/SMO/SUFU mutations	i(17q), +18, −X, c-MYC amplification	i(17q), +18, −X, MYCN amplification
Expression characteristics	WNT signaling, c-MYC↑	SHH signaling	Photoreceptor markers, c-MYC↑	Neuronal and photoreceptor markers

resection and metastases (M+ versus M0R+ versus M0R0) as independent factors for event-free survival and overall survival. Confirmation of the prognostic relevance of tumor resection in combination with M-stage on event-free survival and overall survival supports the effort to achieve a maximal safe surgery at diagnosis without increasing the risk of the patient unnecessarily for postoperative neurologic deficits.

Late Effects

Treatment strategies currently used in young children with medulloblastoma may all potentially induce neurocognitive and neuroendocrine deficits, among others. Many long-term survivors have limitations of social and daily life. Of note, to analyze the impact of the different treatment modalities (surgery, radiotherapy, systemic chemotherapy, and intraventricular chemotherapy) appears to be challenging. Moreover, the disease by itself and the surgery may cause a decrease of the neuroendocrine and neurocognitive functions. Large and comprehensive reports investigating the quality of life, the endocrine and neurocognitive functions are still elusive. Many studies are differing from each other with regards of inclusion criteria (e.g., age), with regards of the treatment applied, and finally with regards of the tests used to examine the neurocognitive functions. Intelligence quotient (IQ) scores have been used over many years to measure changes in cognitive function after treatment. However, the studies performed thus far are limited by low numbers of patients, and intelligence quotient (IQ) scores need to be sensitive, reproducible, and comparable between different cohorts of patients. Effect of craniospinal radiotherapy on neurocognitive functions, neurocognitive skills, and growth impairments of bone and soft-tissue has been investigated (Duffner et al. 1985; Rutkowski 2006; Silber et al. 1992). Mean loss of 2–4 Intelligence quotient (IQ) points per year have been reported after craniospinal radiotherapy (Mulhern et al. 2004; Rutkowski 2006). Omission of radiotherapy appears to be of highest importance in children with Gorlin's syndrome, which appears to be especially frequent among children with medulloblastoma with extensive nodularity.

Future Directions

In future studies, improved criteria for risk-adapted treatment stratification will lead to further decreasing numbers of patients in the different treatment arms. Consequently, the Society of Pediatric Oncology and Hematology in Germany, Austria and Switzerland (GPOH), the French Society of Pediatric Oncology (SFOP), and the United Kingdom Children's Cancer Study Group (UKCCSG) are planning to implement a clinical trial for young children with medulloblastoma: Children aged less than 3–5 years with a centrally confirmed desmoplastic/nodular medulloblastoma as well as children with medulloblastoma with extensive nodularity will be eligible to be treated with HIT-SKK chemotherapy (Rutkowski et al. 2005; von Bueren et al. 2011), as it has been shown that patients with desmoplastic histopathological phenotype do have an excellent prognosis when treated with postoperative HIT-SKK chemotherapy (Rutkowski et al. 2005; von Bueren et al. 2011). Of note, before start of chemotherapy, 2 years, and 5 years after diagnosis neuropsychological assessments will be performed. Efficacy and toxicity of systemic chemotherapy (cyclophosphamide, vincristine, methotrexate, carboplatin and etoposide) will be evaluated versus the same systemic chemotherapy combined with intraventricular methotrexate (36 single doses of 2 mg). Improved strategies are needed for non-desmoplastic/non-nodular medulloblastoma. Based on the fact that they share poorer survival, intensification of primary treatment through the use of high-dose chemotherapy with stem cell rescue, with or without radiotherapy, will be evaluated until targeted therapies become available. For better comparability of results, it is planned that inclusion criteria as well as late effect measures will be harmonized between upcoming studies both in North America (Children's Oncology Group (COG)) and Europe. Finally, the next protocols for young children with medulloblastoma should also focus on biology to provide prospective, and age-dependent validation of already known factors and to investigate currently unknown markers of the disease that may be targeted in the future with novel treatment approaches.

References

Albright AL, Wisoff JH, Zeltzer PM, Boyett JM, Rorke LB, Stanley P (1996) Effects of medulloblastoma resections on outcome in children: a report from the Children's Cancer Group. Neurosurgery 38:265–271

Chang CH, Housepian EM, Herbert C (1969) An operative staging system and a megavoltage radiotherapeutic technic for cerebellar medulloblastomas. Radiology 93:1351–1359

Cho YJ, Tsherniak A, Tamayo P, Santagata S, Ligon A, Greulich H, Berhoukim R, Amani V, Goumnerova L, Eberhart CG, Lau CC, Olson JM, Gilbertson RJ, Gajjar A, Delattre O, Kool M, Ligon K, Meyerson M, Mesirov JP, Pomeroy SL (2011) Integrative genomic analysis of medulloblastoma identifies a molecular subgroup that drives poor clinical outcome. J Clin Oncol 29:1424–1430. doi:JCO.2010.28.5148 [pii] 10.1200/JCO.2010.28.5148

Duffner PK, Cohen ME, Thomas PR, Lansky SB (1985) The long-term effects of cranial irradiation on the central nervous system. Cancer 56:1841–1846

Duffner PK, Horowitz ME, Krischer JP, Friedman HS, Burger PC, Cohen ME, Sanford RA, Mulhern RK, James HE, Freeman CR et al (1993) Postoperative chemotherapy and delayed radiation in children less than three years of age with malignant brain tumors. N Engl J Med 328:1725–1731

Garre ML, Cama A, Bagnasco F, Morana G, Giangaspero F, Brisigotti M, Gambini C, Forni M, Rossi A, Haupt R, Nozza P, Barra S, Piatelli G, Viglizzo G, Capra V, Bruno W, Pastorino L, Massimino M, Tumolo M, Fidani P, Dallorso S, Schumacher RF, Milanaccio C, Pietsch T (2009) Medulloblastoma variants: age-dependent occurrence and relation to Gorlin syndrome – a new clinical perspective. Clin Cancer Res 15:2463–2471

Geyer JR, Sposto R, Jennings M, Boyett JM, Axtell RA, Breiger D, Broxson E, Donahue B, Finlay JL, Goldwein JW, Heier LA, Johnson D, Mazewski C, Miller DC, Packer R, Puccetti D, Radcliffe J, Tao ML, Shiminski-Maher T (2005) Multiagent chemotherapy and deferred radiotherapy in infants with malignant brain tumors: a report from the Children's Cancer Group. J Clin Oncol 23:7621–7631

Grill J, Sainte-Rose C, Jouvet A, Gentet JC, Lejars O, Frappaz D, Doz F, Rialland X, Pichon F, Bertozzi AI, Chastagner P, Couanet D, Habrand JL, Raquin MA, Le Deley MC, Kalifa C (2005) Treatment of medulloblastoma with postoperative chemotherapy alone: an SFOP prospective trial in young children. Lancet Oncol 6:573–580

Halperin EC, Watson DM, George SL (2001) Duration of symptoms prior to diagnosis is related inversely to presenting disease stage in children with medulloblastoma. Cancer 91:1444–1450

Johnston DL, Keene D, Bartels U, Carret AS, Crooks B, Eisenstat DD, Fryer C, Lafay-Cousin L, Larouche V, Moghrabi A, Wilson B, Zelcer S, Silva M, Brossard J, Bouffet E (2009) Medulloblastoma in children under the age of three years: a retrospective Canadian review. J Neurooncol 94:51–56

Kaatsch P, Rickert CH, Kuhl J, Schuz J, Michaelis J (2001) Population-based epidemiologic data on brain tumors in German children. Cancer 92:3155–3164

Kalifa C, Grill J (2005) The therapy of infantile malignant brain tumors: current status? J Neurooncol 75:279–285

Kiltie AE, Lashford LS, Gattamaneni HR (1997) Survival and late effects in medulloblastoma patients treated with craniospinal irradiation under three years old. Med Pediatr Oncol 28:348–354

Kool M, Koster J, Bunt J, Hasselt NE, Lakeman A, van Sluis P, Troost D, Meeteren NS, Caron HN, Cloos J, Mrsic A, Ylstra B, Grajkowska W, Hartmann W, Pietsch T, Ellison D, Clifford SC, Versteeg R (2008) Integrated genomics identifies five medulloblastoma subtypes with distinct genetic profiles, pathway signatures and clinicopathological features. PLoS One 3:e3088

Louis DN, Ohgaki H, Wiestler OD, Cavenee WK (2007) WHO classification of tumours of the central nervous system. IARC Press, Lyon

Mulhern RK, Merchant TE, Gajjar A, Reddick WE, Kun LE (2004) Late neurocognitive sequelae in survivors of brain tumours in childhood. Lancet Oncol 5:399–408

Northcott PA, Korshunov A, Witt H, Hielscher T, Eberhart CG, Mack S, Bouffet E, Clifford SC, Hawkins CE, French P, Rutka JT, Pfister S, Taylor MD (2011) Medulloblastoma comprises four distinct molecular variants. J Clin Oncol 29:1408–1414. doi: JCO.2009.27.4324 [pii] 10.1200/JCO.2009.27.4324

Packer RJ, Rood BR, MacDonald TJ (2003) Medulloblastoma: present concepts of stratification into risk groups. Pediatr Neurosurg 39:60–67

Rutkowski S (2006) Current treatment approaches to early childhood medulloblastoma. Expert Rev Neurother 6:1211–1221

Rutkowski S, Bode U, Deinlein F, Ottensmeier H, Warmuth-Metz M, Soerensen N, Graf N, Emser A, Pietsch T, Wolff JE, Kortmann RD, Kuehl J (2005) Treatment of early childhood medulloblastoma by postoperative chemotherapy alone. N Engl J Med 352:978–986

Rutkowski S, Gerber NU, von Hoff K, Gnekow A, Bode U, Graf N, Berthold F, Henze G, Wolff JE, Warmuth-Metz M, Soerensen N, Emser A, Ottensmeier H, Deinlein F, Schlegel PG, Kortmann RD, Pietsch T, Kuehl J (2009) Treatment of early childhood medulloblastoma by postoperative chemotherapy and deferred radiotherapy. Neuro Oncol 11:201–210

Rutkowski S, von Hoff K, Emser A, Zwiener I, Pietsch T, Figarella-Branger D, Giangaspero F, Ellison DW, Garre ML, Biassoni V, Grundy RG, Finlay JL, Dhall G, Raquin MA, Grill J (2010) Survival and prognostic factors of early childhood medulloblastoma: an international meta-analysis. J Clin Oncol 28:4961–4968. doi: JCO.2010.30.2299 [pii] 10.1200/JCO.2010.30.2299

Silber JH, Radcliffe J, Peckham V, Perilongo G, Kishnani P, Fridman M, Goldwein JW, Meadows AT (1992) Whole-brain irradiation and decline in intelligence: the influence of dose and age on IQ score. J Clin Oncol 10:1390–1396

von Bueren AO, von Hoff K, Pietsch T, Gerber NU, Warmuth-Metz M, Deinlein F, Zwiener I, Faldum A, Fleischhack G, Benesch M, Krauss J, Kuehl J, Kortmann RD, Rutkowski S (2011) Treatment of young children with localized medulloblastoma by chemotherapy alone: results of the prospective, multicenter trial HIT 2000 confirming the prognostic impact of histology. Neuro Oncol 13:669–679. doi:nor025 [pii] 10.1093/neuonc/nor025

Walter AW, Mulhern RK, Gajjar A, Heideman RL, Reardon D, Sanford RA, Xiong X, Kun LE (1999) Survival and neurodevelopmental outcome of young children with medulloblastoma at St Jude Children's Research Hospital. J Clin Oncol 17:3720–3728

Warren KE, Packer RJ (2004) Current approaches to CNS tumors in infants and very young children. Expert Rev Neurother 4:681–690

Zeltzer PM, Boyett JM, Finlay JL, Albright AL, Rorke LB, Milstein JM, Allen JC, Stevens KR, Stanley P, Li H, Wisoff JH, Geyer JR, McGuire-Cullen P, Stehbens JA, Shurin SB, Packer RJ (1999) Metastasis stage, adjuvant treatment, and residual tumor are prognostic factors for medulloblastoma in children: conclusions from the Children's Cancer Group 921 randomized phase III study. J Clin Oncol 17:832–845

Part III

Retinoblastoma

Trilateral Retinoblastoma: Diagnosis Using Magnetic Resonance Imaging

20

Elżbieta Jurkiewicz, Olga Rutynowska, and Danuta Perek

Contents

E. Jurkiewicz (✉) • O. Rutynowska • D. Perek
Department of Radiology, MR Unit, The Children's Memorial Hospital Health Institute, Warsaw, Poland
e-mail: e-jurkiewicz@o2.pl

Abstract

Retinoblastoma is the most common pediatric intraocular neoplasm and accounts for ~3% of pediatric malignant tumors, affecting approximately 1 in 18,000 children under 5 years of age in the U.S. It is a highly malignant tumor of the primitive neural retina. Histologically, retinoblastoma develops from immature retinal cells and replaces the retina and other intraocular tissues. Neoplastic cell proliferation is caused by the inactivation of both copies of a tumor suppressor gene (Rb1) that participates in the control of cell cycling. Occasionally patients with ocular hereditary retinoblastoma have an associated independent primary midline intracranial neuroblastic tumor. This syndrome is called trilateral retinoblastoma. Midline intracranial tumors are typically located in the pineal region, but occurrences in the sellar and suprasellar regions are also found. The prognosis for trilateral retinoblastoma is markedly worse, with a high rate of subarachnoid tumor spread. The mean survival in this group of patients after treatment is about 9 months. An association between pineal cysts and hereditary retinoblastoma has been described in the recent literature, found that the prevalence of pineal cysts in children with bilateral, hereditary retinoblastoma was statistically significant compared with that in patients with unilateral retinoblastoma. Pineal cysts are supposed to be a benign variant of trilateral retinoblastoma. MR imaging has become a very useful diagnostic tool in

M.A. Hayat (ed.), *Pediatric Cancer, Volume 3: Diagnosis, Therapy, and Prognosis*, Pediatric Cancer 3,
DOI 10.1007/978-94-007-4528-5_20,

evaluation of patients with retinoblastoma. MR is the imaging modality of choice in detection of leptomeningeal spread of the tumor and evaluation of primary intracranial tumors that can be associated with retinoblastoma. On the basis of some cases in which intracranial midline tumors were diagnosed earlier than intraocular lesions, we strongly recommend very careful ophthalmologic and imaging examinations of orbits in all children below 4 years of age with a intracranial midline primary tumor.

A screening schedule for patients with the hereditary form of retinoblastoma should be established, especially for those children with a pineal cyst.

Introduction

Retinoblastoma is the most common pediatric intraocular neoplasm and accounts for about 3% of pediatric malignant tumors, affecting approximately 1 in 18,000 children under 5 years of age in the U.S. (Devesa 1975). According to the population-based registry data compiled and published by the International Agency for Research in Cancer (IARC), incidence rates are generally similar in North America, Europe, and Australia (Parkin et al. 1998), and higher in developing countries. In some countries in Central and South America, retinoblastoma is one of the most common solid tumor malignancies in children (Leal-Leal et al. 2004). The reason for this higher incidence is not clear. Lower socioeconomic status and the presence of human papilloma virus sequences in retinoblastoma tissue have been implicated (Orjuela et al. 2000). Retinoblastoma occurs primarily in children under the age of 5 years, with a median age at diagnosis of 24 months in children with unilateral disease and 9–12 months in children with bilateral disease (Goddard et al. 1999; Butros et al. 2002). According to the literature, about 35% of these tumors are bilateral (Provenzale et al. 2004).

Retinoblastoma is a highly malignant tumor of the primitive neural retina. Histologically, retinoblastoma develops from immature retinal cells and replaces the retina and other intraocular tissues. It displays a high mitotic and apoptotic rate, and because of this elevated turnover of tumor cells, there are many areas of necrosis and dystrophic calcification.

Neoplastic cell proliferation is caused by the inactivation of both copies of a tumor suppressor gene (Rb1) that participates in the control of cell cycling (Friend et al. 1986). In 1971, Alfred Knudson was the first to present the two-hit hypothesis of retinoblastoma oncogenesis and showed that retinoblastoma is a tumor that occurs in germline (40%) and sporadic (60%) forms (Knudson 1971). Germline disease includes patients with a positive family history (hereditary disease) and those who have inherited a germline mutation from an unaffected parent – de novo mutation. This hereditary predisposition to retinoblastoma is caused by a mutant allele occurring at the q14 band of chromosome 13 (13q14.2) (Friend et al. 1986; Cho et al. 2002). Hereditary retinoblastoma is characterized by the presence of a germline mutation, earlier clinical manifestation of disease with disease detectable in utero in children with known familial disease, and very elevated risk of developing secondary malignancies. All children with bilateral tumors, and roughly 15% of children with unilateral tumors, have this form of disease. Some authors suppose that increased paternal age is associated with a greater risk for hereditary retinoblastoma (Moll et al. 1996; Yip et al. 2006). This could be due to an increased risk of new germ cell mutations by way of increased opportunity for mutations arising in dividing spermatocytes (Moll et al. 1996). But other authors have found that advanced maternal age is significantly predictive of increased risk of having a child with retinoblastoma (Yip et al. 2006).

Data published by Yip et al. (2006) showed that maternal risk factors can contribute to the likelihood of developing hereditary (bilateral) retinoblastoma despite new mutations being expected to occur on the paternal allele given prior findings.

Although much is understood about the effects of the *RB1* mutations underlying the formation of retinoblastoma, little is known about the etiology of these mutations in germinal or retinal cells. New germline mutations are known to occur preferentially on the paternal allele, implicating paternal preconception risk factors (Zhu et al. 1989; Kato et al. 1994; Dryja et al. 1989). There is no knowledge, however, about the etiology of retinal cell mutations or their time of occurrence, and little is known about the causes of unilateral disease. The crucial period for mutation development in retinoblastoma may be during retinal formation in early embryonal development between the 4th and 8th week of gestation, or during infancy, as retinal cells continue to divide until about the age of 2 years.

Occasionally patients with ocular hereditary retinoblastoma have an associated independent primary midline intracranial neuroblastic tumor. This syndrome is called trilateral retinoblastoma. The combination of bilateral intraocular retinoblastoma and a midline primary intracranial neoplasm was described by Jakobiec in 1977 (Jakobiec et al. 1977). Later, the term trilateral retinoblastoma was used to indicate bilateral intraocular tumors associated with an intracranial tumor of similar histopathologic features (Bader et al. 1980). Midline intracranial tumors are typically located in the pineal region, but occurrences in the sellar and suprasellar regions are also found. Localization in the third or fourth ventricle has also been described (Bagley et al. 1996; Katayama et al. 1991; Bejjani et al. 1996; Finelli et al. 1995). The survival rate for intraocular retinoblastoma is generally good because of early diagnosis. Survival rates of 92–93% at 5 years have been reported. The prognosis for trilateral retinoblastoma is markedly worse, with a high rate of subarachnoid tumor spread. The mean survival in this group of patients after treatment is about 9 months (Provenzale et al. 1995).

Methodology

We retrospectively reviewed the medical data of 202 patients with unilateral and bilateral retinoblastoma treated at our Institute between 1996 and 2009. The median age at the time of diagnosis was 12 months for bilateral and 22 months for unilateral tumor. In this group of patients there were only three cases of trilateral retinoblastoma (TRB). This rare syndrome constitutes ~1.5% in our group of patients.

We present MR examinations of one boy and two girls with this syndrome, aged 16, 5, and 10 months at the time of diagnosis, respectively.

All MR brain examinations were performed with a 1.5 T scanner using a phased-array 8-channel head coil. Conventional MR images were obtained using a standard protocol consisting of: axial T1-weighted (467/10[TR/TE]), T2-weighted (3870/100), FLAIR(2500/9000/111[IR/TR/TE]), fatsat (531/12[TR/TE]), slice thickness 5 mm; sagittal T1-weighted (470/11), T2-weighted (4160/111), thickness 3 mm; coronal T1-weighted (467/10), T2-weighted (4130/112), thickness 3 mm. Field of view: 16×20 mm. T1-weighted images in three planes, after contrast administration, were performed in each patient (gadolinium was administered intravenously at a standard dose of 0.1 mmol/L per kilogram).

Spinal canal examinations were obtained with sagittal T2-weighted (4000/104) and T1-weighted (486/10) images before and after gadolinium injection; slice thickness 3 mm, field of view: 340×340 mm.

MR images of the brain were reviewed for detection of a primary neoplasm (pineal and suprasellar region) or metastatic lesions (evidence of leptomeningeal spread as curvilinear or nodular areas of contrast enhancement).

Case Reports

In case 1 (a 16-month-old boy) and in case 2 (a 5-month-old girl), ocular symptoms led to ophthalmologic examination and diagnosis of bilateral retinoblastoma (Fig. 20.1). After that, in both patients MRI examinations were performed as a standard diagnostic procedure to evaluate the structures of the brain. Intracranial midline lesions were found in both cases and the diagnosis of trilateral retinoblastoma was made eventually.

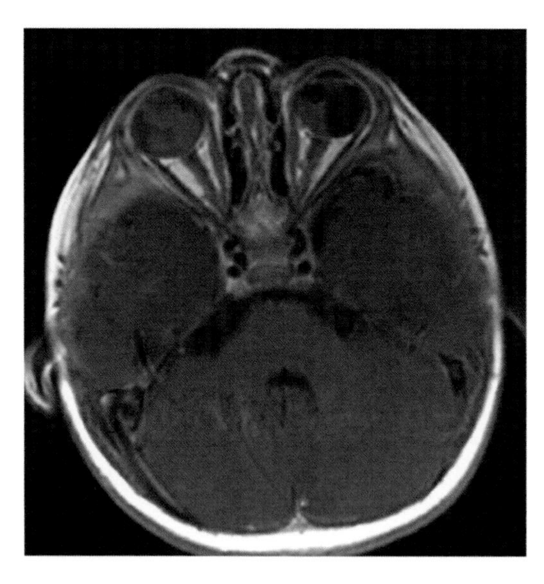

Fig. 20.1 Axial T1-weighted image at the level of the orbits reveals the enhancing bilateral, intrabulbar lesions

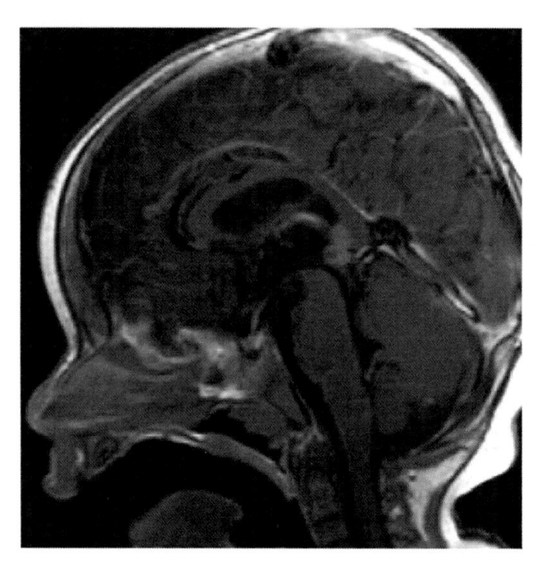

Fig. 20.2 Contrast-enhanced T1-weighted sagittal image shows slightly enhanced mass in the pineal region

Case 1
The intracranial mass was detected in the pineal region. No neurological signs were observed. The size of the pineal tumor was relatively small in the first MR examination. A homogenous, slightly enhanced lesion measured 11 mm × 14 mm and disappeared in the next MR follow-up after chemotherapy (Fig. 20.2). Due to disease progression 3 months from completion of treatment, the patient underwent right eye globe enucleation and conformal pineal tumor irradiation. Cryosurgical therapy and brachytherapy were applied to the left eye because of progression of bulbar lesions. The patient is in good clinical condition 30 months after diagnosis with no signs of intracranial tumor progression, but with progression of intraocular lesions. He is still under systemic treatment – second line chemotherapy was implemented.

Case 2
In this patient the intracranial mass was found in the sellar and suprasellar regions. No neurological or endocrine signs were observed. The tumor was non-homogenous and densely enhanced after contrast administration. It measured 19 mm × 13 mm. After two courses of chemotherapy the brain lesion diminished to 7 mm × 6 mm and remains stable. Lesions in both eyes completely regressed after five courses of chemotherapy. The patient underwent the full chemotherapy protocol for primary CNS malignant tumors for children under 3 years of age. The girl is in complete remission 31 months after diagnosis and 13 months after completing treatment.

Case 3
The third patient, a 10-month-old girl, presented severe neurological symptoms of increased intracranial pressure, failure to thrive, vomiting, cachexia and a tumor of the sellar and suprasellar regions at diagnosis. Biopsy revealed neuroblastic tumor (PNET). The treatment started with the CNS tumor chemotherapy protocol. The intrabulbar tumor of the right eye was evaluated in control CT examination 1 month after diagnosis of the intracranial mass. Strabismus developed in the further course of the disease. The patient underwent ophthalmologic examination in which diagnosis of intrabulbar lesions in both eyes was confirmed. In this case we observed a spectacular decrease of the tumor mass, which was about 100 mm in the first examination and diminished to 25 mm after 17 courses of chemotherapy (Fig. 20.3). The brain lesion remains stable to date. The patient underwent right eye bulb enucleation due to severe retinal detachment with

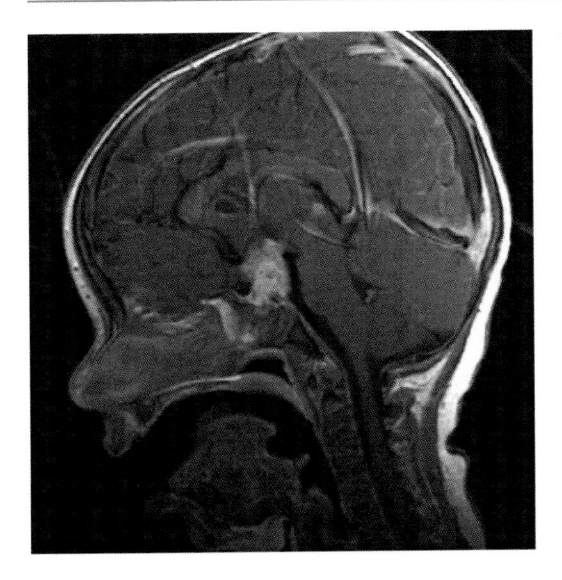

Fig. 20.3 Post-gadolinium sagittal T1-weighted scan shows densely enhanced tumor in the sellar and suprasellar localizations

ophthalmologic signs of a still active retinoblastoma focus. The intracranial mass is unresectable due to invasion of the hypothalamus. She underwent radiation therapy on the region of the brain tumor and left eye globe. The child is in good clinical condition 30 months after diagnosis.

To date in our all cases there was no evidence of leptomeningeal spread. None of the patients have a positive family history.

Discussion

The median age of our patients at diagnosis of TRB was 10 months, earlier than that reported in the literature, 26 months, because there was no latent period between detection of the retinoblastoma and appearance of the brain tumor (Provenzale et al. 2004; Mouratova 2005; Kivelä 1999). In other reports, bilateral RB and intracranial tumor were found at the same time in 13 of 93 children (Kivelä 1999) and in 2 of 8 children (Provenzale et al. 2004). The median age of those patients was also 10 months. According to several studies, however, a latent period between the diagnosis of the ocular disease and the intracranial lesion is usually observed. Ocular lesions are usually detected earlier than the intracranial lesion. The mean time from diagnosis of retinoblastoma to detection of the associated primary intracranial tumor is about 23–24 months (Provenzale et al. 2004). To date, in our retinoblastoma patient group we have not observed a metachronic intracranial tumor after RB treatment.

In two of our patients with TRB (cases 1 and 2), intrabulbar and intracranial lesions were found simultaneously in the first MR examinations. In one patient (case 3) a huge sellar and suprasellar tumor (PNET) was detected earlier than the intrabulbar lesions and trilateral retinoblastoma was diagnosed after detection of the midline tumor. A similar case was reported by Amoaku et al. 1996. The authors described a 4-month-old infant also with PNET in the suprasellar region treated as the primary intracranial tumor. In this case, calcified RB was found in both eyes 13 months after diagnosis of the intracranial lesion. In our case, as in that mentioned above, the intracranial tumor was situated in the suprasellar region. This also confirms previous reports of other authors that the diagnosis of a primary midline intracranial tumor may predate detection of intraocular retinoblastoma and that the brain tumor is usually located in the suprasellar region in these cases (Amoaku et al. 1996). No explanation is currently available for this phenomenon. We strongly recommend that a very careful ophthalmologic examination be performed in all children below 4 years of age with a intracranial midline primary tumor.

All our patients had bilateral RB associated with an intracranial mass. In previous published reports, 86–89% children with TRB had bilateral RB and 11–12% children with TRB had unilateral RB (Mouratova 2005; Kivelä 1999; Ibarra and O'Brien 2000).

Intracranial tumors associated with intraocular retinoblastoma usually occur in the pineal and sellar-suprasellar regions. The pineal region is the more common localization (Provenzale et al. 2004; Cho et al. 2002). Other localizations, e.g. a primitive neuroectodermal tumor in the fourth ventricle, are very rare, but also possible (Finelli et al. 1995). In our cases we found the brain lesion in the pineal region in one case and in the sellar and suprasellar regions in two cases.

In all of our cases, the size of the intracranial masses markedly diminished after chemotherapy and, in all of the patients, the tumor size correlates well with clinical outcome thus far. In case 1, the size of the pineal tumor was relatively small in the first examination. The mass measured 11 mm×14 mm and disappeared in the next follow-up after chemotherapy. In case 2, the sellar and suprasellar tumor diminished from 19 to 7 mm after chemotherapy. In case 3, we observed a spectacular decrease of the huge sellar and suprasellar mass from 100 mm×90 mm to 15 mm×16 mm after chemotherapy.

All lesions have remained stable so far and there is no evidence of metastases. This correlates well with the good clinical status of the patients. In one report, the size of the intracranial masses also diminished to variable degrees after chemotherapy or radiation therapy, yet correlated poorly with clinical outcome because, although the tumor size decreased markedly in three patients, they had fatal outcomes with leptomeningeal dissemination (Provenzale et al. 2004). In other reports the tumor size at the time of diagnosis was similar. The largest size was from 30 (Mouratova 2005) to 90 mm (Kivelä 1999), but no information was provided in these reports about changes in tumor size over time.

In our patients we observed different patterns of the tumor signal. In case 1, the midline lesion was relatively isointense compared with gray matter on T2-weighted images and homogenously enhanced after contrast administration. In case 2 and 3, the brain tumors showed heterogenous signal intensity on T2-weighted images and variable contrast enhancement. Similar reports of tumor images were found in the literature (Cho et al. 2002; Provenzale et al. 1995). MR imaging has become a very useful diagnostic tool in evaluation of patients with retinoblastoma and, because it reduces exposure to radiation, MR has progressively replaced computed tomography. The high radiosensitivity of patients with the hereditary form of retinoblastoma is well known.

Although ophthalmoscopy and US are of great value in the diagnosis of intraocular lesions, MRI is the method of choice in evaluation of primary intracranial tumors that can be associated with retinoblastoma and for detection of leptomeningeal spread.

Not all tumor findings, in particular, extraocular extension, choroidal infiltration, and optic nerve infiltration, can be assessed during ophthalmologic examinations. Magnetic resonance imaging is the method of choice for assessing local extensions to the optic nerve, anterior chamber and orbital fat. The intraocular mass has a signal equivalent to or slightly more intense than that of the vitreous on T1-weighted sequences, with a relatively low-intensity signal on T2-weighted sequences. After contrast injection, enhancement of the retinoblastoma is less visible than the uvea. MRI may be useful for distinguishing retinoblastoma from pseudotumoral conditions such as Coats disease or eye malformations (Brisse et al. 2001). There are, however, some problems with precise visualization of ocular lesions. Artifacts connected with eye motion and no possibility of detecting calcifications are known.

According to other studies, the mean survival of patients with TRB is about 9–13 months from diagnosis (Provenzale et al. Cho et al. 2004; Kivelä 1999). The short survival is caused mainly by cerebrospinal metastases, especially in patients with pineal tumors (Provenzale et al. 1995). All of our patients are alive from 18 (case 3) to 19 months (case 2 and 3) from diagnosis and no leptomeningeal metastases have developed thus far. This is longer than the mean survival time in literature, even in case 3 with the PNET in the suprasellar region, for which the median survival is 6 months (Mouratova 2005; Paulino 1999).

It is well known that children with a positive family history are particularly predisposed to TRB syndrome and should be examined very carefully. In many studies authors recommend neuroimaging screening in patients with familial bilateral RB until the age of 4 years to detect early asymptomatic pineal and suprasellar tumors, because the prognosis for such patients is much better than that for symptomatic patients (Mouratova 2005; Amoaku et al. 1996; De Potter et al. 1994). In our patients, however, no evidence of familial retinoblastoma was found, so, as in several other reports, we suggest that patients with sporadic bilateral RB should also undergo MRI follow-up, because they may have a germline mutation (Amoaku et al. 1996).

Screening by neuroimaging may improve the cure rate if cases of trilateral retinoblastoma are detected during the first year after diagnosis of RB. It has been recommended that children with germline retinoblastoma should be screened using magnetic resonance neuroimaging every 3 months for the first year after diagnosis and at least 2 times a year for the next 3 years (Kivelä 1999).

TRB was not described until 1977. This may be explained by misdiagnosis, especially before the advent of CT scans, but some authors report that bilateral sporadic retinoblastomas may represent new germinal mutations in the RB gene (Amoaku et al. 1996). This is in line with our observations, because we found that in the group of 202 patients with RB treated at our Institute from 1996 to 2008, only three patients had TRB and it is noteworthy that all three cases were detected in the last 2 years.

Non-neoplastic lesions such as pineal cysts are relatively common incidental benign lesions whose distinction becomes crucial for the patient for both prognostic and therapeutic reasons. Small (0.5–1 cm) pineal cysts are encountered in 25–40% of autopsy cases. According to the literature, pineal cysts are relatively rare in young children but are most often discovered in women younger than 30 years of age. MRI can distinguish a normal pineal gland and benign pineal cysts from pineal neoplasms. Pinealoblastoma is described as a large, nodular, solid mass that typically shows diffuse enhancement after administration of contrast material. In contrast, pineal cysts normally show a fine rim of cyst wall enhancement, but the cyst itself does not enhance after administration of contrast material. There is no lobularity or nodularity in the margin of cysts and wall thickness is no more than 2 mm. Pineal cysts usually measure more than 5 mm, are hypointense on T1-weighted images, and present a signal like CSF on T2 images. Follow-up MRI on a 2- to 4-month basis confirms lack of progression (Barboriak et al. 2001; Fleege et al. 1994; Sener 1995).

An association between pineal cysts and hereditary retinoblastoma has been described in the recent literature (Beck Popovic et al. 2006; Popovic et al. 2007; Karatza et al. 2006). Popovic et al. in 2007, found that the prevalence of pineal cysts in children with bilateral, hereditary retinoblastoma was statistically significant compared with that in patients with unilateral retinoblastoma. Pineal cysts are supposed to be a benign variant of trilateral retinoblastoma. The authors presented the hypothesis that trilateral retinoblastoma with hereditary retinoblastoma coexists with benign cystic pineal tumors. This is possible because both the pineal gland and retinoblastoma originate from the neuroectoderm and the pineal gland is considered a photoreceptor organ in lower vertebrates (the 3rd eye). Another hypothesis considers the cysts to be spontaneous or treatment-induced cystic regression of a solid pineal tumor. The mechanism is the same as in retinoma, which is considered to be spontaneous regression of retinoblastoma (Aaby et al. 1983). Popovic et al. in 2007, mentioned that development of pineal cysts may be related to CT performed for intraocular diagnosis, type of Tx, and radiation therapy. The small number of patients does not allow this suggestion to be confirmed. Because of lack of information on the behavior of pineal cysts in retinoblastoma patients, a suggestion has been made to conduct 6-month clinical and MR follow-up for 5 years from the diagnosis of bilateral retinoblastoma (Beck Popovic et al. 2006).

Further studies are needed to establish how often and how long screening for intracranial tumor development of patients with the hereditary form of retinoblastoma should be conducted. The modern treatment approach to retinoblastoma patients consists of neoadjuvant chemotherapy (chemoreduction). Some authors believe that this treatment modality may prevent or delay neuroblastic tumor development (Shields et al. 2001). Nonetheless, longer and more frequent MRI screening is very expensive and its clinical usefulness needs to established (Kivelä 1999).

Conclusions

MR imaging has become a very useful diagnostic tool in evaluation of patients with retinoblastoma. MR is the imaging modality of choice in detection of leptomeningeal spread of the tumor and evaluation of primary intracranial tumors that can be associated with retinoblastoma. On the basis of some cases in which intracranial midline tumors were diagnosed earlier than intraocular lesions, we strongly recommend very careful ophthalmologic and imaging examinations of orbits in all children below 4 years of age with a intracranial midline primary tumor.

A screening schedule for patients with the hereditary form of retinoblastoma should be established, especially for those children with a pineal cyst.

References

Aaby AA, Price RL, Zakov ZN (1983) Spontaneously regressing retinoblastomas, retinoma, or retinoblastoma group O. Am J Ophthalmol 96:315–320

Amoaku WMK, Willshaw HE, Parkes SE, Shah KJ, Mann JR (1996) Trilateral retinoblastoma: a report of five patients. Cancer 78:858–863

Bader JL, Miller RW, Meadows AT, Zimmerman LE, Champion LA, Voute PA (1980) Trilateral retinoblastoma. Lancet 2:582–583

Bagley LJ, Hurst RW, Zimmerman RA, Shields JA, Shields CL, De Potter P (1996) Imaging in the trilateral retinoblastoma syndrome. Neuroradiology 38:166–170

Barboriak DP, Lee L, Provenzale JM (2001) Serial MR imaging of pineal cysts: Implication for natural history and follow-up. AJR Am J Roentgenol 176:737–743

Beck Popovic M, Balmer A, Maeder P, Braganca T, Munier FL (2006) Benign pineal cysts in children with bilateral retinoblastoma: a new variant of trilateral retinoblastoma? Pediatr Blood Cancer 46:755–761

Bejjani GK, Donahue DJ, Selby D, Cohen PH, Packer R (1996) Association of a suprasellar mass and intraocular retinoblastoma: a variant of pineal trilateral retinoblastoma? Pediatr Neurosurg 25:269–275

Brisse HJ, Lumbroso L, Fréneaux PC, Validire P, Doz FP, Quintana EJ, Berges O, Desjardins LC, Neuenschwander SC (2001) Sonographic, CT, and MR imaging findings in diffuse infiltrative retinoblastoma: report of two cases with histologic comparison. AJNR Am J Neuroradiol 22:499–504

Butros LJ, Abramson DH, Dunkel IJ (2002) Delayed diagnosis of the retinoblastoma: analysis of degree, cause, and potential consequences. Pediatrics 109(3):E45

Cho EY, Suh Y-L, Shin H-J (2002) Trilateral retinoblastoma: a case report. J Korean Med Sci 17:137–140

De Potter P, Shields CL, Shields JA (1994) Clinical variations of trilateral retinoblastoma: a report of 13 cases. J Pediatr Ophthalmol Strabismus 31:26–31

Devesa SS (1975) The incidence of retinoblastoma. Am J Ophthalmol 80:263–265

Dryja TP, Mukai S, Rapaport JM, Yandell DW (1989) Parental origin of mutations of the retinoblastoma gene. Nature 339:556–558

Finelli DA, Shurin SB, Bardenstein DS (1995) Trilateral retinoblastoma: two variations. AJNR Am J Neuroradiol 16:166–170

Fleege MA, Miller GM, Fletcher GP, Fain JS, Scheithauer BW (1994) Benign glial cysts of the pineal gland: unusual imaging characteristics with histologic correlation. AJNR Am J Neuroradiol 15:161–166

Friend SH, Bernards R, Rogelj S, Weinberg RA, Rapaport JM, Albert DM, Dryja TP (1986) A human DNA segment with properties of the gene that predisposes to retinoblastoma and osteosarcoma. Nature 323:643–646

Goddard AG, Kingston JE, Hungerford JL (1999) Delay in diagnosis of retinoblastoma: risk factors and treatment outcome. Br J Ophthalmol 83:1320–1323

Ibarra MS, O'Brien JM (2000) Is screening for primitive neuroectodermal tumours in patients with unilateral retinoblastoma necessary? J AAPOS 4:54–56

Jakobiec FA, Tso MO, Zimmerman LE, Danis P (1977) Retinoblastoma and intracranial malignancy. Cancer 39(5):2048–2058

Karatza EC, Shield EJ, Flader EA, Gonzalez M, Shields JA (2006) Pineal cyst simulating pinealoblastoma in 11 children with retinoblastoma. Arch Ophthalmol 124:595–597

Katayama Y, Tsubokawa T, Yamamoto T, Nemoto N (1991) Ectopic retinoblastoma within the 3rd ventricle: case report. Neurosurgery 28:158–161

Kato MV, Ishizaki K, Shimizu T, Ejima Y, Tanooka H, Takayama J, Kaneko A, Toguchida J, Sasaki MS (1994) Parental origin of germ-line and somatic mutations in the retinoblastoma gene. Hum Genet 94:31–38

Kivelä T (1999) Trilateral retinoblastoma: a meta-analysis of hereditary retinoblastoma associated with primary ectopic intracranial retinoblastoma. J Clin Oncol 17(6):1829–1837

Knudson AG (1971) Mutation and cancer: statistical study of retinoblastoma. Proc Natl Acad Sci U S A 68:820–823

Leal-Leal C, Flores-Rojo M, Medina-Sanson A, Cerecedo-Díaz F, Sánchez-Félix S, González-Ramella O, Pérez-Pérez F, Gómez-Martínez R, Quero-Hernández A, Altamirano-Álvarez E, Alejo-González F, Figueroa-Carbajal J, Ellis-Irigoyen A, Tejocote-Romero I, Cervantes-Paz R, Pantoja-Guillén F, Vega-Vega L, Carrete-Ramírez F (2004) A multicentre report from the Mexican Retinoblastoma Group. Br J Ophthalmol 88:1074–1077

Moll AC, Imhof SM, Kuik DJ, Bouter LM, Den Otter W, Bezemer PD, Koten JW, Tan KE (1996) High parental age is associated with sporadic hereditary retinoblastoma: the Dutch Retinoblastoma Register 1862–1994. Hum Genet 98:109–112

Mouratova T (2005) Trilateral retinoblastoma: a literature review, 1971–2004. Bull Soc Belge Ophtalmol 297:25–35

Orjuela M, Castaneda VP, Ridaura C, Lecona E, Leal C, Abramson DH, Orlow I, Gerald W, Cordon-Cardo C (2000) Presence of human papilloma virus in tumor tissue from children with retinoblastoma: an alternative mechanism for tumor development. Clin Cancer Res 6:4010–4016

Parkin DM, Kramarowa E, Draper GJ, Masuyer E, Michaelis J, Neglia JP, Quereshi S, Stiller CA (1998) International incidence of childhood cancer. International Agency for Research on Cancer, Lyon

Paulino AC (1999) Trilateral retinoblastoma: is the location of the intracranial tumour important? Cancer 86:135–141

Popovic MB, Diezi M, Kuchler H, Abouzeid H, Maeder P, Balmer A, Munier FL (2007) Trilateral retinoblastoma with suprasellar tumor and associated pineal cyst. J Pediatr Hematol Oncol 29:53–56

Provenzale JM, Weber A, Klintworth GK, McLendon RE (1995) Radiologic-pathologic correlation. Bilateral retinoblastoma with coexistent pinealoblastoma (trilateral retinoblastoma). AJNR Am J Neuroradiol 16:157–165

Provenzale JM, Gururangan S, Klintworth G (2004) Trilateral retinoblastoma: clinical and radiologic progression. Am J Roentgenol 183(2):505–511

Sener RN (1995) The pineal gland: a comparative MR imaging study in children and adults with respect to normal anatomical variations and pineal cysts. Pediatr Radiol 25:245–248

Shields CL, Meadows AT, Shields JA, Carvalho C, Smith AF (2001) Chemoreduction for retinoblastoma may prevent intracranial neuroblastic malignancy (Trilateral retinoblastoma). Arch Ophtalmol 119:1269–1272

Yip BH, Pawitan Y, Czene K (2006) Parental age and risk of childhood cancers: a population-based cohort study from Sweden. Int J Epidemiol 35:1495–1503

Zhu X, Dunn J, Philips R, Goddard A, Paton K, Becker A, Gallie B (1989) Preferential germ line mutation of the paternal allele in retinoblastoma. Nature 340:312–313

21 Pediatric Intraocular Retinoblastoma: Treatment

Parag K. Shah, Saurabh Aurora, V. Narendran, and N. Kalpana

Contents

P.K. Shah (✉) • S. Aurora • V. Narendran • N. Kalpana
Department of Pediatric Retina and Ocular Oncology, Aravind Eye Hospital, Avinashi Road, Coimbatore 641 014, Tamil Nadu, India
e-mail: drshahpk2002@yahoo.com

Abstract

The management of retinoblastoma has evolved remarkably for the past century, and lately there is a drift towards focal conservative treatments. The challenge remains, however, in maintaining the eye and vision. Tumor reduction by diverse first-line chemotherapy protocols followed by local treatments like cryotherapy, laser photocoagulation, thermotherapy, and plaque radiotherapy is now accepted as treatment strategy for intraocular retinoblastoma with the goal of avoiding external beam radiotherapy (EBRT) or enucleation. However in most eyes with large tumors with diffuse vitreous and subretinal seeds, the EBRT or enucleation is eventually required. Chemoprophylaxis is necessary for preventing metastases in tumors with high-risk pathology features (tumor extending beyond lamina cribrosa of the optic nerve, tumor extending till the surgical margin of the optic nerve, massive choroidal invasion, scleral involvement or anterior segment involvement). Intensified chemotherapy with autologous stem cell rescue appears effective for patients with metastatic retinoblastoma. Recently, ophthalmic intra-arterial infusion with melphalan is proved as an excellent globe conserving treatment option in advanced retinoblastoma cases with minimal systemic side effects. Progress in the clinical recognition and management of retinoblastoma has led to high survival rates.

M.A. Hayat (ed.), *Pediatric Cancer, Volume 3: Diagnosis, Therapy, and Prognosis*, Pediatric Cancer 3,
DOI 10.1007/978-94-007-4528-5_21,

Introduction

Retinoblastoma is the most common intraocular malignancy of childhood (Shields and Shields 1999). It is now known as a curable cancer (Shields and Shields 2008). It is caused by a mutation on band 14 on the long arm of chromosome 13 (13q14). RB1 gene is a tumor suppressor gene and both the genes have to be mutated to cause this disease. When both the mutations involve only the retinal cells (somatic cells) then the child develops a non-germinal type of disease, which is non-heritable. However when one mutation involves the germinal cell then the child develops germinal type of disease, which is transmittable to next generation. Among the most important objectives in the management of a child with retinoblastoma is survival of the child, and preservation of the globe. The focus on visual acuity comes last, after safety of the child and globe is established. Therapy is customized to each individual case and based on the overall anatomical situation, including threat of metastatic disease, laterality of the disease, the number, size and location of the tumor(s), evidence of subretinal fluid, localized or diffuse vitreous seeding, risks for secondary tumors, systemic status, and estimated visual prognosis.

International Classification of Retinoblastoma

The classification currently used for staging and grouping retinoblastoma is "The International Classification of Retinoblastoma." It has replaced the older Reese Ellsworth classification, as it could not be applied to current treatment modalities. This classification consists of two parts:

1. Staging for the patient.
2. Grouping for each eye.

Staging

There are five stages (Chantada et al. 2006).

1. Stage 0: When the child presents with intra ocular retinoblastoma with no regional or systemic metastasis and no enucleation has been performed.
2. Stage 1: When enucleation has been done in one eye. High-risk pathology features may be present in the enucleated specimen. It may be present in the other eye.
3. Stage 2: When residual orbital tumor is seen at the cut end of optic nerve during enucleation.
4. Stage 3: When there is an overt orbital extension with involvement of pre-auricular or cervical lymph nodes.
5. Stage 4: Distant metastasis. It is subdivided into:
   (a) Stage 4a: Non central nervous system (CNS) spread
   (b) Stage 4b: CNS spread.

Grouping for Each Eye

This also has five groups (Murphree 2005).

1. Group A: Small tumors which are<3 mm in size and should be located at least 3 mm from the foveola and 1.5 mm from optic disc (Fig. 21.1a).
2. Group B: Any tumor>3 mm in size (except smaller tumors which are very close to fovea and optic disc as specified in group A). Cuff of exudative retinal detachment<5 mm from tumor base or<1 quadrant is allowed (Fig. 21.1b).
3. Group C: Any tumor with localized tumor dissemination i.e. vitreous seeds or sub retinal seeds, which are<3 mm from tumor surface (Fig. 21.1c).
4. Group D: Any tumor with diffuse vitreous or sub retinal seeds (Fig. 21.1d).
5. Group E: End stage disease (Fig. 21.2). For Example:
   (a) Neovascular glaucoma.
   (b) Tumor or retinal detachment touching the lens.
   (c) Anterior segment involvement.
   (d) Aseptic orbital cellulitis, etc.

In addition, a proposal for a sub staging (according to the histopathological features of enucleated specimens) may further help to differentiate patients with intraocular disease. The intraorbital staging is based on magnetic resonance imaging (MRI), which must be performed in almost all patients. Radiological visible extension to the retro laminar optic nerve must be investigated, especially in case of optic disc involvement, as it determines the

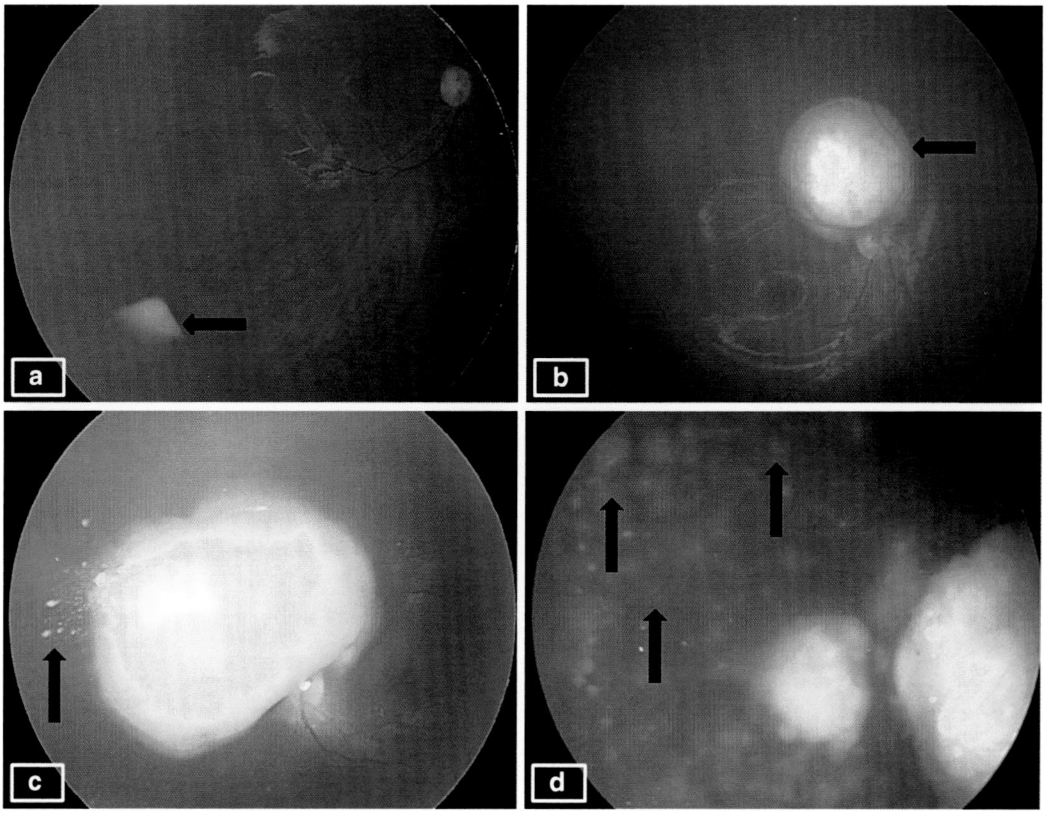

Fig. 21.1 (**a**) Fundus photo of right eye showing small tumor (<3 mm) in infero temporal quadrant (*arrow*). This is group A retinoblastoma. (**b**) Large tumor (>3 mm) seen superior to disc (*arrow*), suggestive of group B disease. (**c**) Left eye showing large tumor with localized vitreous seeds (*arrow*) suggestive of group C retinoblastoma. (**d**) Large tumors with multiple, diffuse sub-retinal seeds (*arrows*) suggestive of group D retinoblastoma

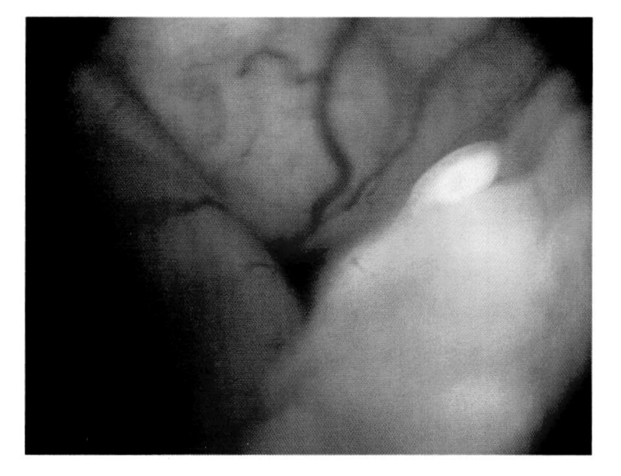

Fig. 21.2 Fundus photo showing total exudative retinal detachment with large sub-retinal mass (not seen in the photo), suggestive of group E retinoblastoma

surgical approach for enucleation. Lumbar puncture and bone marrow aspiration for distant staging is done only when there are features of extra ocular spread (Moscinski et al. 1996). There are several options for treatment of retinoblastoma, and the ocular oncologist should be thoroughly familiar with the indications, technique and expected results of all treatment methods as well as the expected systemic and visual problems.

Treatment of Intraocular Retinoblastoma

The currently available treatment methods for retinoblastoma include.

Group A

Only local treatment in the form of cryotherapy, laser photocoagulation or thermotherapy.

1. Cryotherapy involves freezing the tumor till its apex with a cryo probe and thawing it for 1 min. This is done thrice and is called triple freeze thaw cryotherapy. This treatment is preferred for anterior tumors (Shields et al. 1989). The disadvantage is that the scar formed is much bigger than the tumor size.
2. Laser photocoagulation involves surrounding the tumor with two to three rows of green laser (532 nm). This cuts off the blood supply and leads to regression of the tumor. This is preferred for posterior tumors (Shields 1994). However, here also the scar formed is much bigger than the initial tumor and high power if used on tumor surface can cause iatrogenic vitreous seeding (Shields et al. 1995).
3. Transpupillary Thermotherapy (TTT) is a method of applying localized heat to tissue that is below the coagulative threshold and thus sparing the retinal vessels from photocoagulation (Shields et al. 1999). The goal is to deliver a temperature of 42–60°C using a diode infrared (810 nm) laser system and induce tumor necrosis. The advantage of TTT is that the scar formed is not bigger than the tumor size.

Group B

Here in addition to local therapy, the tumor needs to be reduced in size with the help of chemotherapy. Here at least three cycles of chemotherapy (carboplatin, vincristine with or without etoposide) are needed along with local therapy before every cycle. Primary epi-scleral brachytherapy using either Ru 106 or I 125 seeds is also an option here.

Group C

Most retinoblastoma centers now adopt a protocol of three-agent chemotherapy using Vincristine (0.05 mg/kg), Etoposide (5 mg/kg) and Carboplatin (18.6 mg/kg) (VEC) delivered 3 weekly over 6 cycles to allow for adequate tumor reduction along with local therapy before each cycle. In addition to this 2 ml of sub-tenon carboplatin (STC) can be given to tackle the avascular vitreous or sub-retinal seeds on the day of chemo cycle 2, 3 and 4. However it causes lot of periocular inflammation and might cause a frozen orbit. STC should be avoided along with cryotherapy as this combination can lead to rhegmatogenous retinal detachment (Tawansy et al. 2006). A strikingly fewer numbers of trilateral retinoblastoma were noted in children who were treated with chemotherapy and so Shields concluded that chemotherapy might be protecting against the highly fatal intracranial neuroblastic tumors (Shields et al. 2001a). This observation is particularly important in children with bilateral or familial retinoblastoma who are at greatest risk for this brain tumor.

Group D

In addition to the treatment above for group C, a reduced dose of 36 Gy of whole globe EBRT (standard dose is 46 Gy) would be required if reactivation of tumor is seen. EBRT may induce a second cancer among the patients with familial disease. Babies who are younger than 12 months of age have a greater risk for second cancers than patients over 12 months of age (Abramson and Frank 1998) in the field of irradiation. The 30-year cumulative incidence for second cancers in bilateral retinoblastoma (germinal mutation) has been reported at 35% for patients who received radiation therapy compared with 6% for those who did not receive radiation (Roarty et al. 1988). This was found to be dependent on patient age at the time of irradiation as well as other factors. Primary enucleation is still an option in unilateral group D cases.

Group E

The ideal treatment option for this group is Enucleation. The idea is to gently remove the intact eye without seeding the malignancy into the orbit (Shields et al. 1993). Orbital implants are routinely placed in children at the time of initial surgery and give excellent cosmetic results with improved prosthesis motility (Christmas et al. 2000). After enucleation, on histo-pathology if high-risk pathology features are present then the child will require six cycles of prophylactic chemotherapy to prevent distant metastasis. In rare cases of bilateral group E, treatment as specified in group D can be attempted. Brachytherapy can also be used as a secondary treatment to salvage a globe that fail to respond to laser therapy, thermotherapy, cryotherapy or chemoreduction, and it is less successful for those that fail to respond to EBRT (Shields et al. 2001b). On the basis of the International Classification of Retinoblastoma, treatment success was found in 100% of group A eyes, 93% of group B eyes, and 90% of group C eyes (Shields et al. 2006). Group D eyes showed 48% success but, more recently, these eyes have been managed with additional sub-tenon's carboplatin to improve control.

Tumour Regression Patterns

The interpretation of tumor regression can be challenging as retinoblastoma can regress in one of several patterns including type 0 (no remnant visible), type 1 (calcified remnant), type 2 (non-calcified or fish flesh remnant), type 3 (partially calcified with fish flesh remnant), and type 4 (flat scar) (Shields et al. 2009). These regression patterns are defined post EBRT. However post chemotherapy, types 2 and 3 patterns should be closely watched as they have a high chance of reactivation.

Intra Arterial Chemotherapy

The strategy of direct infusion of chemotherapy into the ophthalmic artery allows the delivery of high concentrations of the drug to the *eye* (and to the cancer), with far lower concentrations when given systemically. Intra-arterial chemotherapy for retinoblastoma was first described as "instillation under direct observation into the internal carotid artery on the side of the involved eye" (Reese et al. 1954). Later, a group in Japan revisited this delivery technique, and they pioneered the use of selective administration of chemotherapy to the ophthalmic vasculature to deliver localized treatment to retinoblastoma tumors (Mohri 1993).

This recent treatment modality was successful in sparing enucleation in seven of nine children with advanced retinoblastoma, with acceptable ocular toxicity and minimal systemic toxicity (Abramson et al. 2008), and that many treated eyes could retain or even improve retinal function (Brodie et al. 2009). In a 3-year experience with this technique on advanced retinoblastoma, only 1 of 28 eyes required enucleation and none required adjuvant systemic chemotherapy or radiation (Abramson et al. 2010). Cannulization was successful in 100%, with patients requiring a mean of 3.2 infusions of melphalan only or melphalan combined with topotecan or carboplatin. Estimates of globe-salvage were shown to be 100% at 1 year and 89% at 2 years.

They also reported on the use of tandem therapy, or bilateral infusions, during the same session for cases with bilateral retinoblastomas. Subsequently indications for this modality expanded to be used as a primary treatment (Abramson et al. 2010).

Several benefits of Intra-arterial chemotherapy should be realized, including the localized chemotherapy injection, few necessary sessions (approximately 2 doses), 1-day delivery, and systemic tolerance (Shields et al. 2011).

This procedure is performed under general anesthesia with endotracheal intubation. Alternate single femoral artery is punctured, and a standard dose of heparin (70 IU/kg) is administered. A straight microcatheter, such as the Marathon microcatheter (ev3, Irvine, California) or the Magic 1.5 microcatheter (Balt, Montmorency, France), is passed till the internal carotid artery. The tip of the catheter is placed at the ostium of the ophthalmic artery followed by selective angiography. In cases of unsuitable anatomy alternative techniques used are ipsilateral middle meningeal artery anastomosis to the orbit or the

"Japanese technique," with placement of a temporary balloon to occlude the internal carotid artery above the origin of the ophthalmic artery and infusion into the internal carotid artery below the balloon (Yamane et al. 2004).

The drugs that can be used are melphalan (most common) with or without topotecan hydrochloride or carboplatin. Drug dosage is 5 mg for melphalan, 0.3 mg for topotecan and 30 mg for carboplatin. The decision to use 1 or 2 drugs is based on clinical judgment with eyes that were more extensively involved (especially widespread seeding) receiving two agents at once (Abramson et al. 2010). Melphalan is diluted with saline to obtain a volume of 30 ml of solution, which is injected manually by repeated small bolus (pulsatile injection) at a rate of 1 ml/min. After drug delivery, the catheter is removed and hemostasis of the femoral artery is obtained with manual compression. Efficacy and toxicity are judged during the examination under anesthesia performed 3–4 weeks after each treatment. Efficacy is judged on tumor shrinkage and regression, disappearance or calcifications of vitreous and subretinal seeds, and absence of new tumor growth. Toxicity is estimated with electro retino graph study.

The mild short-term effects included eyelid edema, blepharoptosis, and orbital congestion, sometimes with temporary dysmotility (Shields et al. 2011). These findings were common and typically resolved within a few months, leaving minimal or no residual and without need for surgical repair. The more serious ocular adverse events include arterial occlusion, retinal bleeding, and orbital inflammation in the early phase and chorioretinal atrophy and ischemic chorioretinopathy in the late phase (Suzuki et al. 2011). Another drawback of this therapy is that even if enucleation is avoided in some advanced group E eyes, there is a risk of distant metastasis as that child would have received prophylactic chemotherapy if high-risk pathology features were seen on enuleated specimen (Shields et al. 2011). There could also be a risk of inducing second cancers in patients with germinal mutation if repeated fluoroscopy was done for this procedure (Shields et al. 2011).

In conclusion, retinoblastoma continues to be a challenge both diagnostically and therapeutically. It is important to first clearly establish the correct diagnosis at an early stage before embarking on therapy. With the improvements and advances in the management protocols and various options available, the prognosis for life and for preservation of vision has improved remarkably in recent years.

References

Abramson DH, Frank CM (1998) Second nonocular tumors in survivors of bilateral retinoblastoma: a possible age effect on radiation-related risk. Ophthalmology 105:573–579

Abramson DH, Dunkel IJ, Brodie SE, Kim JW, Gobin YP (2008) A phase I/II study of direct intraarterial (ophthalmic artery) chemotherapy with melphalan for intraocular retinoblastoma initial results. Ophthalmology 115:1398–1404

Abramson DH, Dunkel IJ, Brodie SE, Marr B, Gobin YP (2010) Superselective ophthalmic artery chemotherapy as primary treatment for retinoblastoma (chemosurgery). Ophthalmology 117:1623–1629

Brodie SE, Pierre Gobin Y, Dunkel IJ, Kim JW, Abramson DH (2009) Persistence of retinal function after selective ophthalmic artery chemotherapy infusion for retinoblastoma. Doc Ophthalmol 119:13–22

Chantada G, Doz F, Antoneli CB, Grundy R, Clare Stannard FF, Dunkel IJ, Grabowski E, Leal-Leal C, Rodríguez-Galindo C, Schvartzman E, Popovic MB, Kremens B, Meadows AT, Zucker JM (2006) A proposal for an international retinoblastoma staging system. Pediatr Blood Cancer 47:801–805

Christmas NJ, Van Quil IK, Murray TG, Gordon CD, Garonzik S, Tse D, Johnson T, Schiffman J, O'Brien JM (2000) Evaluation of efficacy and complications: primary pediatric orbital implants after enucleation. Arch Ophthalmol 118:503–506

Mohri M (1993) The development of a new system of selective ophthalmic arterial infusion for the patients of intraocular retinoblastoma (in Japanese). Keio Igaku (J Keio Med Soc) 70:679–687

Moscinski LC, Pendergrass TW, Weiss A, Hvizdala E, Buckley KS, Kalina RE (1996) Recommendations for the use of routine bone marrow aspiration and lumbar punctures in the follow-up of patients with retinoblastoma. J Pediatr Hematol Oncol 18:130–134

Murphree AL (2005) Intraocular retinoblastoma: the case for a new group classification. Ophthalmol Clin North Am 18:41–53

Reese AB, Hyman GA, Merriam GR Jr, Forrest AW, Kligerman MM (1954) Treatment of retinoblastoma by radiation and triethylenemelamine. AMA Arch Ophthalmol 53:505–513

Roarty JD, McLean IW, Zimmerman LE (1988) Incidence of second neoplasms in patients with retinoblastoma. Ophthalmology 95:1583–1587

Shields JA (1994) The expanding role of laser photocoagulation for intraocular tumors. The 1993 H. Christian Zweng Memorial Lecture. Retina 14:310–322

Shields JA, Shields CL (1999) Retinoblastoma. In: Atlas of intraocular tumors. Lippincott Williams & Wilkins, Philadelphia, pp 207–232

Shields JA, Shields CL (2008) Retinoblastoma. In: Atlas of intraocular tumors. Lippincott Williams & Wilkins, Philadelphia, pp 293–365

Shields JA, Parsons H, Shields CL, Giblin ME (1989) The role of cryotherapy in the management of retinoblastoma. Am J Ophthalmol 108:260–264

Shields CL, Shields JA, De Potter P, Singh AD (1993) Lack of complications of the hydroxyapatite orbital implant in 250 consecutive cases. Trans Am Ophthalmol Soc 91:177–189

Shields CL, Shields JA, Kiratli H, De Potter PV (1995) Treatment of retinoblastoma with indirect ophthalmoscope laser photocoagulation. J Pediatr Ophthalmol Strabismus 32:317–322

Shields CL, Santos MC, Diniz W, Gunduz K, Mercado G, Cater JR, Shields JA (1999) Thermotherapy for retinoblastoma. Arch Ophthalmol 117:885–893

Shields CL, Meadows AT, Shields JA, Carvalho C, Smith AF (2001a) Chemoreduction for retinoblastoma may prevent intracranial neuroblastic malignancy (trilateral retinoblastoma). Arch Ophthalmol 119:1269–1272

Shields CL, Shields JA, Cater J, Othmane I, Singh AD, Micaily B (2001b) Plaque radiotherapy for retinoblastoma: long-term tumor control and treatment complications in 208 tumors. Ophthalmology 108:2116–2121

Shields CL, Mashayekhi A, Au AK, Czyz C, Leahey A, Meadows AT, Shields JA (2006) The international classification of retinoblastoma predicts chemoreduction success. Ophthalmology 113:2276–2280

Shields CL, Palamar M, Sharma P, Ramasubramanian A, Leahey A, Meadows AT, Shields JA (2009) Retinoblastoma regression patterns following chemoreduction and adjuvant therapy in 557 tumors. Arch Ophthalmol 127:282–290

Shields CL, Bianciotto CG, Jabbour P, Griffin GC, Ramasubramanian A, Rosenwasser R, Shields JA (2011) Intra-arterial chemotherapy for retinoblastoma: report no. 2, treatment complications. Arch Ophthalmol 129:1407–1415

Suzuki S, Yamane T, Mohri M, Kaneko A (2011) Selective ophthalmic arterial injection therapy for intraocular retinoblastoma: the long-term prognosis. Ophthalmology 118:2081–2087

Tawansy KA, Samuel MA, Shammas M, Murphree AL (2006) Vitreoretinal complications of retinoblastoma treatment. Retina 26(7 Suppl):S47–S52

Yamane T, Kaneko A, Mohri M (2004) The technique of ophthalmic arterial infusion therapy for patients with intraocular retinoblastoma. Int J Clin Oncol 9:69–73

Part IV

Glioma

Pediatric High-Grade Glioma: Role of Microsatellite Instability

22

Marta Viana-Pereira, Chris Jones, and Rui Manuel Reis

Contents

M. Viana-Pereira
Life and Health Sciences Research Institute (ICVS), School of Health Sciences, University of Minho, Braga, Portugal

C. Jones
Section of Paediatric Oncology, Institute of Cancer Research, Sutton, Surrey, UK

R.M. Reis (✉)
Molecular Oncology Research Center, Barretos Cancer Hospital, Rua Antenor Duarte Villela, 1331 CEP 14784 400, Barretos, S. Paulo, Brazil
e-mail: rreis@ecsaude.uminho.pt

Abstract

Microsatellite instability (MSI) frequency in pediatric high-grade glioma remains a controversial research topic, and there is lack of clarity in the literature. Overall, it has been shown that MSI-positivity in adult high-grade glioma is a rare event, whereas in pediatric tumors reported frequencies are highly variable, probably due to the lack of consistency in the screening strategies. Furthermore, in contrast to colorectal MSI-positive tumors that harbor Type B MSI, high-grade gliomas have been reported as presenting Type A MSI, increasing the difficulty of an accurate analysis. In this chapter, we will review the type of MSI mostly found in pediatric high-grade gliomas and the distinct approaches to detect it, the role of the mismatch repair system (MMR) in these tumors, as well as the relation of MSI with other genomic abnormalities and the frequency of MSI target genes mutations.

Introduction

The mismatch repair (MMR) system is the major pathway responsible for repairing insertions, deletions and misincorporation of bases that occur during DNA replication and recombination, avoiding frameshift mutations and base-substitutions (Arana and Kunkel 2010; Nigg 2005). While the fidelity of replicating DNA polymerases is insufficient to generate an error-free copy of genomic DNA, the MMR system

M.A. Hayat (ed.), *Pediatric Cancer, Volume 3: Diagnosis, Therapy, and Prognosis*, Pediatric Cancer 3,
DOI 10.1007/978-94-007-4528-5_22,

ensures that the human genome can be duplicated without mutations (Arana and Kunkel 2010). Effective repair requires the MutS (MSH2, MSH3 and MSH6) and MutL (MLH1 and PMS2) homologues, which function as a complex (Jiricny 2006; Nigg 2005). Microsatellites are repeated-sequence motifs, which are present throughout the genome (International Human Genome Sequencing Consortium 2001). Due to the repetitive nature of the microsatellites, during DNA synthesis the primer and template strands can dissociate and re-anneal incorrectly, requiring the MMR system to correct these errors. In the absence of MMR, these frameshift mutations remain uncorrected, leading to the expansion or retraction of the number of repeats, the microsatellite instability (MSI) phenotype (Ionov et al. 1993).

In 1993, the existence of a causal link between inherited mutations in the MMR genes and the colon cancer predisposition syndrome *hereditary nonpolyposis colorectal cancer* (HNPCC) or Lynch Syndrome was described (Ionov et al. 1993). Subsequently, hundreds of studies about the frequency and characterization of MSI-positivity in cancer of different organs have been published (Jiricny 2006; Nigg 2005). Tumors with defects in *MLH1*, *MSH2* and *PMS2* generally present MSI, whereas defects in *MSH6* are thought to not cause the same high frequency of MSI, probably due to the ability of cells to compensate for MSH6 absence (Boland and Goel 2010). In addition, it was found that also sporadic cancers could be MMR defective, mainly due to promoter hypermethylation of *MLH1* gene (Jiricny 2006; Nigg 2005).

In high-grade gliomas, the presence and frequency of MSI is a controversial and poorly addressed issue. Literature reports have indicated an absence or rare incidence of MSI in adult patients, while in children the results have been contradictory, with reported frequencies in pediatric gliomas varying between 0% and 44% (Alonso et al. 2001; Amariglio et al. 1995; Cheng et al. 1999; Dams et al. 1995; Eckert et al. 2007; Izumoto et al. 1997; Kanamori et al. 2000; Leung et al. 1998; Martinez et al. 2005; Pollack et al. 2010; Sobrido et al. 2000; Vladimirova et al. 2007; Viana-Pereira et al. 2011). This chapter will review the potential role of MSI in pediatric high-grade glioma.

Classification of Microsatellite Instability (MSI)

Due to the particular clinical characteristics and the differential response of MSI-positive colorectal cancer to therapeutic agents, MSI screening of this malignancy is of particular interest, and guidelines for HNPCC and MSI diagnosis have been standardized (Umar et al. 2004). Tumors should be analyzed using standard panels of five microsatellite markers, and the classification of MSI more commonly adopted considers the number of markers presenting frameshift alterations. Considering the number of markers presenting alterations cancers would be classified as MSI-negative or (microsatellite stable (MSS)), or MSI-positive, that are further divided into MSI-High or MSI-Low, according to the number of markers (microsatellites) altered (Buhard et al. 2006; Umar et al. 2004).

One of the key considerations in the assessment of MSI frequency is the choice of the panel of markers used. The guidelines for HNPCC and MSI diagnosis recommend the use of the classic National Cancer Institute panel of markers (two mononucleotide markers: BAT26 and BAT25; and three dinucleotide markers: D2S123, D5S346 and D17S250), for which germline DNA of the patient should be studied in parallel, or of a pentaplex of quasimonomorphic mononucleotide markers (NR27, NR21, NR24, BAT25 and BAT26), which overcomes the need for using matching germline DNA, required for the dinucleotide polymorphic markers (Buhard et al. 2006; Umar et al. 2004; Wong et al. 2006). Regardless, when using the panel of mononucleotide markers, there is still the need for optimization of the quasi-monomorphic variation range (QMVR) for each marker, as the allelic size estimation of the markers can be influenced by the use of specific reagents or by the specifications of the sequencing instrument (Goel et al. 2010).

The MSI frequency of high-grade glioma has been evaluated using different methodologies in recent years, which certainly has contributed for the diversity of frequencies reported. The earlier studies have assessed MSI frequencies in gliomas using polynucleotide markers only, with frequencies ranging from 0% to 37% (Amariglio et al. 1995; Dams et al. 1995; Izumoto et al. 1997; Sobrido et al. 2000). Including both mononucleotide and polynucleotides repeat markers did not improve consistency, with contrasting results varying between 0% and 44% in pediatric gliomas cohorts (Cheng et al. 1999; Kanamori et al. 2000; Leung et al. 1998; Martinez et al. 2005; Pollack et al. 2010). Using mononucleotides alone also provided contradictory results of 0–27% MSI in pediatric gliomas (Alonso et al. 2001; Eckert et al. 2007; Vladimirova et al. 2007). In addition to the heterogeneity of markers used to assess MSI frequency that likely accounts for much of the variability in the data, many of the previous studies did not refer the establishment of the QMVR or a direct comparison between tumor and germline DNA (for other markers), which most likely impaired the classification of MSI in high-grade gliomas.

An alternative classification of MSI relies on the size of the allelic shifts within the markers, rather than the number of markers with alterations. In this classification, samples presenting small length allelic shifts (≤ 6 bp) are considered Type A MSI, while those presenting more drastic alterations (> 6 bp) are described as Type B MSI (Oda et al. 2005).

MSI-positive colorectal cancers mostly present Type B MSI, whereas high-grade gliomas have been consistently shown to harbor Type A MSI (Giunti et al. 2009; Viana-Pereira et al. 2011). This feature of the MSI-positive high-grade glioma can be one of the main responsible for the high variation frequency of MSI in these tumors reported in the literature, since many authors do not consider type A MSI (Alonso et al. 2001; Amariglio et al. 1995; Cheng et al. 1999; Dams et al. 1995; Eckert et al. 2007; Izumoto et al. 1997; Kanamori et al. 2000; Leung et al. 1998; Martinez et al. 2005; Sobrido et al. 2000; Vladimirova et al. 2007).

Taking into account all these important considerations of MSI analysis, we have recently studied a series of 71 pediatric high-grade glioma and described a frequency of about 20% MSI in these tumors (Viana-Pereira et al. 2011). In parallel, we analyzed 73 adult high-grade glioma and confirmed that the frequency of MSI was significantly higher in pediatric than in adult tumors, reflecting the majority of the previous literature reports (Alonso et al. 2001; Cheng et al. 1999; Kanamori et al. 2000; Leung et al. 1998; Martinez et al. 2005).

Role of MMR System in High-Grade Glioma

Mismatch repair deficiencies have been associated with pediatric high-grade glioma particularly in a hereditary context, such as Turcot syndrome and also "mismatch repair-deficiency (MMR-D) syndrome" (Louis et al. 2007).

Turcot syndrome is an autosomal dominant disorder characterized by the occurrence of colorectal and brain tumours, mainly glioblastomas or medulloblastomas (Louis et al. 2007). This syndrome can be further divided in type 1 (glioma-polyposis) and type 2 patients (medulloblastoma-polyposis). Turcot type 1 patients present glioblastoma and colorectal cancer, presenting germline mutations in the DNA MMR genes *MLH1*, *PMS2*, *MSH2* and *MSH6* (Louis et al. 2007). Turcot type 2 patients typically develop medulloblastoma, presenting familial adenomatous polyposis, together with mutations in the *APC* gene (Louis et al. 2007).

Case reports have described biallelic MMR germline mutations combined with NF1-like clinical features, particularly café-au-lait spots, in children presenting high-grade glioma, described as a "mismatch repair-deficiency (MMR-D) syndrome" (Giunti et al. 2009; Roy et al. 2009; Toledano et al. 2009; Viana-Pereira et al. 2011; Wimmer and Etzler 2008). These patients develop childhood malignancies, particularly hematological cancers and brain tumors as well as very early-onset colorectal cancer. The most frequent brain tumors in MMR-D patients are astrocytomas, particularly glioblastomas (Wimmer and Etzler 2008).

The role of MMR deficiencies in sporadic high-grade glioma, even in those described as MSI-positive is less clear. Nevertheless, *MSH6* mutations have been demonstrated to arise in adult gliomas as a consequence of treatment with temozolomide, and have been implicated in drug resistance and the presence of a hypermutated phenotype (The Cancer Genome Atlas Research Network [TCGA] 2008).

Relation of MSI to Other Genomic Abnormalities

In colorectal and gastric cancer, microsatellite and chromosomal instability have been considered to be mutually exclusive, and although recent reports have demonstrated that a minority of tumors can present both MSI-H and chromosomal instability, the frequency and degree of chromosomal alterations in MSS tumors is much higher than in the MSI-H cases (Jones et al. 2005). Interestingly, pediatric high-grade gliomas differ from their adult counterparts by comprising a proportion of tumors with few or no detectable copy number changes (Bax et al. 2010). In our recent publication (Viana-Pereira et al. 2011), together with the presence of MSI in a significant number of childhood high-grade glioma, we have also described a tendency of association between MSI-positive pediatric tumors and a stable genomic profile at the chromosomal level, even if microsatellite and chromosomal instability were not mutually exclusive. As mentioned, the presence of a proportion of tumors with few or absent copy number alterations distinguishes pediatric high-grade gliomas from their adult counterparts and therefore we hypothesize that MSI might represent an alternative form of genetic instability, at least in a proportion of these pediatric tumors with no gross chromosome number alterations.

MSI Target Genes in MSI-positive High-Grade Glioma

The widespread presence of microsatellites in DNA implies that several mutations are expected to accumulate in the genome of tumor cells due to MMR deficiency, and some of these will potentially contribute to tumorigenesis (Woerner et al. 2006). Genes that present frameshift mutations in microsatellites due to MMR deficiency are commonly designated MSI target genes. Several MSI target genes have already been described, particularly in colorectal and gastric cancers, however their relevance in carcinogenesis and cancer development is not always clear-cut (Woerner et al. 2006). In high-grade gliomas, only a small number of the "classical" MSI target genes have been reported: IGFIIR (Leung et al. 1998) and PTEN (Kanamori et al. 2000), each of them in a single case of MSI high-grade gliomas, and TGFβRII, reported in 71% of samples (Izumoto et al. 1997), although this result was never confirmed (Kanamori et al. 2000; Leung et al. 1998). We have performed a screening of 18 MSI target genes, frequently mutated in colorectal and gastric cancers, in our series of high-grade gliomas (Viana-Pereira et al. 2011). Three additional alterations, not previously reported in pediatric high-grade gliomas, were identified in genes involved in different DNA repair pathways: mutations in the DNAPKcs and MSH6 genes. Still, it seems that the "classical" MSI target genes in other tumor types are not frequently mutated in high-grade gliomas. In this perspective, a bioinformatic approach for the identification of glioma-specific MSI target genes would be of major importance to the research area.

In conclusion, lack of specific screening strategies for MSI analysis in high-grade gliomas has confounded an accurate assessment of the frequency of MSI-positivity in these tumors. Nevertheless, the use of the most sensitive and robust techniques has allowed the identification of MSI in a fraction of pediatric high-grade gliomas, a distinguishing feature compared with adult tumors. Further studies are needed to evaluate the biological and clinical impact of this type of genetic instability in pediatric high-grade gliomas.

References

Alonso M, Hamelin R, Kim M, Porwancher K, Sung T, Parhar P, Miller DC, Newcomb EW (2001) Microsatellite instability occurs in distinct subtypes of pediatric but not adult central nervous system tumors. Cancer Res 61:2124–2128

Amariglio N, Friedman E, Mor O, Stiebel H, Phelan C, Collins P, Nordenskjold M, Brok-Simoni F, Rechavi G (1995) Analysis of microsatellite repeats in pediatric brain tumors. Cancer Genet Cytogenet 84:56–59

Arana ME, Kunkel TA (2010) Mutator phenotypes due to DNA replication infidelity. Semin Cancer Biol 20:304–311

Bax DA, Mackay A, Little SE, Carvalho D, Viana-Pereira M, Tamber N, Grigoriadis AE, Ashworth A, Reis RM, Ellison DW, Al-Sarraj S, Hargrave D, Jones C (2010) A distinct spectrum of copy number aberrations in pediatric high grade gliomas. Clin Cancer Res 16:3368–3377

Boland CR, Goel A (2010) Microsatellite instability in colorectal cancer. Gastroenterology 138(6):2073–2087.e3. Review

Buhard O, Cattaneo F, Wong YF, Yim SF, Friedman E, Flejou JF, Duval A, Hamelin R (2006) Multipopulation analysis of polymorphisms in five mononucleotide repeats used to determine the microsatellite instability status of human tumors. J Clin Oncol 24:241–251

Cheng Y, Ng HK, Zhang SF, Ding M, Pang JC, Zheng J, Poon WS (1999) Genetic alterations in pediatric high-grade astrocytomas. Hum Pathol 30:1284–1290

Dams E, Van de Kelft EJ, Martin JJ, Verlooy J, Willems PJ (1995) Instability of microsatellites in human gliomas. Cancer Res 55:1547–1549

Eckert A, Kloor M, Giersch A, Ahmadi R, Herold-Mende C, Hampl JA, Heppner FL, Zoubaa S, Holinski-Feder E, Pietsch T, Wiestler OD, von Knebel Doeberitz M, Roth W, Gebert J (2007) Microsatellite instability in pediatric and adult high-grade gliomas. Brain Pathol 17:146–150

Giunti L, Cetica V, Ricci U, Giglio S, Sardi I, Paglierani M, Andreucci E, Sanzo M, Forni M, Buccoliero AM, Genitori L, Genuardi M (2009) Type A microsatellite instability in pediatric gliomas as an indicator of Turcot syndrome. Eur J Hum Genet 17:919–927

Goel A, Nagasaka T, Hamelin R, Boland CR (2010) An optimized pentaplex PCR for detecting DNA mismatch repair-deficient colorectal cancers. PLoS One 5:e9393

International Human Genome Sequencing Consortium (2001) Initial sequencing and analysis of the human genome. Nature 409:860–921

Ionov Y, Peinado MA, Malkhosyan S, Shibata D, Perucho M (1993) Ubiquitous somatic mutations in simple repeated sequences reveal a new mechanism for colonic carcinogenesis. Nature 363:558–561

Izumoto S, Arita N, Ohnishi T, Hiraga S, Taki T, Tomita N, Ohue M, Hayakawa T (1997) Microsatellite instability and mutated type II transforming growth factor-beta receptor gene in gliomas. Cancer Lett 112:251–256

Jiricny J (2006) The multifaceted mismatch-repair system. Nat Rev Mol Cell Biol 7:335–346

Jones AM, Douglas EJ, Halford SE, Fiegler H, Gorman PA, Roylance RR, Carter NP, Tomlinson IP (2005) Array-CGH analysis of microsatellite-stable, near-diploid bowel cancers and comparison with other types of colorectal carcinoma. Oncogene 24:118–129

Kanamori M, Kon H, Nobukuni T, Nomura S, Sugano K, Mashiyama S, Kumabe T, Yoshimoto T, Meuth M, Sekiya T, Murakami Y (2000) Microsatellite instability and the PTEN1 gene mutation in a subset of early onset gliomas carrying germline mutation or promoter methylation of the hMLH1 gene. Oncogene 19:1564–1571

Leung SY, Chan TL, Chung LP, Chan AS, Fan YW, Hung KN, Kwong WK, Ho JW, Yuen ST (1998) Microsatellite instability and mutation of DNA mismatch repair genes in gliomas. Am J Pathol 153:1181–1188

Louis DN, Ohgaki H, Wiestler OD, Cavenee WK (eds) (2007) WHO classification of tumours of the central nervous system. IARC, Lyon

Martinez R, Schackert HK, Appelt H, Plaschke J, Baretton G, Schackert G (2005) Low-level microsatellite instability phenotype in sporadic glioblastoma multiforme. J Cancer Res Clin Oncol 131:87–93

Nigg EA (2005) Genome instability in cancer development. Springer, New York

Oda S, Maehara Y, Ikeda Y, Oki E, Egashira A, Okamura Y, Takahashi I, Kakeji Y, Sumiyoshi Y, Miyashita K, Yamada Y, Zhao Y, Hattori H, Taguchi K, Ikeuchi T, Tsuzuki T, Sekiguchi M, Karran P, Yoshida MA (2005) Two modes of microsatellite instability in human cancer: differential connection of defective DNA mismatch repair to dinucleotide repeat instability. Nucleic Acids Res 33:1628–1636

Pollack IF, Hamilton RL, Sobol RW, Nikiforova MN, Nikiforov YE, Lyons-Weiler MA, LaFramboise WA, Burger PC, Brat DJ, Rosenblum MK, Gilles FH, Yates AJ, Zhou T, Cohen KJ, Finlay JL, Jakacki RI, Children's Oncology Group (2010) Mismatch repair deficiency is an uncommon mechanism of alkylator resistance in pediatric malignant gliomas: a report from the Children's Oncology Group. Pediatr Blood Cancer 55:1066–1071

Roy S, Raskin L, Raymond VA, Thibodeau SN, Mody RJ, Gruber SB (2009) Pediatric duodenal cancer and biallelic mismatch repair gene mutations. Pediatr Blood Cancer 53:116–120

Sobrido MJ, Pereira CR, Barros F, Forteza J, Carracedo A, Lema M (2000) Low frequency of replication errors in primary nervous system tumours. J Neurol Neurosurg Psychiatry 69:369–375

The Cancer Genome Atlas Research Network [TCGA] (2008) Comprehensive genomic characterization defines human glioblastoma genes and core pathways. Nature 455:1061–1068

Toledano H, Goldberg Y, Kedar-Barnes I, Baris H, Porat RM, Shochat C, Bercovich D, Pikarsky E, Lerer I, Yaniv I, Abeliovich D, Peretz T (2009) Homozygosity of MSH2 c.1906 G-- > C germline mutation is associated with childhood colon cancer, astrocytoma and signs of Neurofibromatosis type I. Fam Cancer 8:187–194

Umar A, Boland CR, Terdiman JP, Syngal S, de la Chapelle A, Rüschoff J, Fishel R, Lindor NM, Burgart LJ, Hamelin R, Hamilton SR, Hiatt RA, Jass J, Lindblom A, Lynch HT, Peltomaki P, Ramsey SD, Rodriguez-Bigas MA, Vasen HF, Hawk ET, Barrett

JC, Freedman AN, Srivastava S (2004) Revised Bethesda Guidelines for hereditary nonpolyposis colorectal cancer (Lynch syndrome) and microsatellite instability. J Natl Cancer Inst 96:261–268

Viana-Pereira M, Lee A, Popov S, Bax DA, Al-Sarraj S, Bridges LR, Stávale JN, Hargrave D, Jones C, Reis RM (2011) Microsatellite instability in pediatric high grade glioma is associated with genomic profile and differential target gene inactivation. PLoS One 6:e20588

Vladimirova V, Denkhaus D, Soerensen N, Wagner S, Wolff JE, Pietsch T (2007) Low level of microsatellite instability in paediatric malignant astrocytomas. Neuropathol Appl Neurobiol 34:547–554

Wimmer K, Etzler J (2008) Constitutional mismatch repair-deficiency syndrome: have we so far seen only the tip of an iceberg? Hum Genet 124:105–122

Woerner SM, Kloor M, von Knebel Doeberitz M, Gebert JF (2006) Microsatellite instability in the development of DNA mismatch repair deficient tumors. Cancer Biomark 2:69–86

Wong YF, Cheung TH, Lo KW, Yim SF, Chan LK, Buhard O, Duval A, Chung TK, Hamelin R (2006) Detection of microsatellite instability in endometrial cancer: advantages of a panel of five mononucleotide repeats over the National Cancer Institute panel of markers. Carcinogenesis 27:951–955

Low-Grade Glioma in Children: Effects of Radiotherapy

23

Erin S. Murphy and Thomas E. Merchant

Contents

Abstract

Low-grade gliomas are a heterogeneous group of tumors that overall have a better prognosis than WHO grade III and IV tumors. However, these tumors can devastate a child because of progression in proximity to critical structures, or the long-term consequences of therapy. Observation after complete surgical resection is standard of care. Tumors may demonstrate an indolent natural history after incomplete resection, but progression-free survival at 5 years is only 56%. The choice of treatment remains controversial, particularly for younger children because of the anticipated adverse effects of therapy including neurocognitive dysfunction, endocrinopathy, hearing loss, vasculopathy, and malignant transformation. Advances in radiotherapy and thoughtful planning techniques seek to minimize these long-term sequelae and maintain a good quality of life for children with low-grade gliomas.

Introduction

Low-grade gliomas are a heterogeneous group of tumors located most commonly in the cerebellum followed by the cerebral hemispheres and by the deep midline structures such as the hypothalamus, visual pathways, brainstem, thalamus, lateral and 3 rd ventricles, and the corpus callosum. Low-grade gliomas make up approximately 26% of childhood central nervous system malignancies seen in the United States.

E.S. Murphy (✉)
Department of Radiation Oncology, Taussig Cancer Institute, 9500 Euclid Ave. T28, Cleveland, OH 44195, USA
e-mail: murphye3@ccf.org

T.E. Merchant
Division of Radiation Oncology, St. Jude Children's Research Hospital, 262 Danny Thomas Place, Mail Stop 220, Memphis, TN 38105-3678, USA

M.A. Hayat (ed.), *Pediatric Cancer, Volume 3: Diagnosis, Therapy, and Prognosis*, Pediatric Cancer 3,
DOI 10.1007/978-94-007-4528-5_23,

Observation after gross total resection is standard of care and can produce progression-free survival from 80% for Grade II tumors to more than 90% for Grade I tumors (Gajjar et al. 1997). Tumors may demonstrate an indolent natural history after incomplete resection, but progression-free survival at 5 years is only 56% as reported from the Children's Cancer Group/Pediatric Oncology Group low-grade glioma trial (Wisoff et al. 2011). Therefore neurologic symptoms or progression demonstrated on imaging, or risk of progression at a critical site necessitates treatment with either radiation or chemotherapy. The choice of treatment remains controversial, particularly for younger children because of the anticipated adverse effects of therapy including neurocognitive dysfunction, endocrinopathy, hearing loss, vasculopathy, and malignant transformation.

Radiotherapy

The use of radiotherapy is impacted by physician bias, patient age, tumor location and grade, risks associated with progression, severity of symptoms, and lack of randomized evidence. Studies demonstrate immediate adjuvant radiotherapy improves progression-free survival (Kidd et al. 2006; Pollack et al. 1995; van den Bent et al. 2005) and one suggests the added benefit of improved seizure control for early RT (van den Bent et al. 2005). Adjuvant radiotherapy after incomplete surgical resection results in a 10-year progression-free survival improvement from 40% to 82% (Pollack et al. 1995).

More controversial is the benefit of immediate radiotherapy on survival with one study showing that immediate radiotherapy offered a survival benefit (Fisher et al. 2001). A retrospective study demonstrated a trend for a survival benefit of radiotherapy for WHO grade I tumors and a significant survival benefit for WHO grade II tumors (Shaw et al. 1989). However, the majority of studies demonstrate no survival advantage to the addition of radiotherapy (Mishra et al. 2006; Pollack et al. 1995; van den Bent et al. 2005). Therefore after an incomplete resection, a course of observation is usually recommended for asymptomatic patients who are not at severe risk for neurologic compromise if the tumor progressed. Multiple chemotherapy regimens have been investigated to delay or avoid radiotherapy, particularly in younger patients (Gnekow et al. 2004; Massimino et al. 2010; Mishra et al. 2010; Packer et al. 1997). The addition of radiotherapy to chemotherapy has demonstrated a progression free survival benefit over chemotherapy alone (Fouladi et al. 2003). The ideal timing and sequence of radiotherapy and chemotherapy remains unknown.

WHO Grade I

WHO grade I astrocytomas include pilocytic astrocytoma (JPA), and subependymal giant cell astrocytoma and are generally characterized by well circumscribed lesions (Louis et al. 2007). JPAs are most commonly located in the cerebellum followed by the diencephalic region and only 3% have disseminated disease. Subependymal giant cell astrocytomas occur along the lining of the ventricles and are associated with tuberous sclerosis. The primary treatment for WHO grade I tumors is maximal safe resection. The 15 year survival rate for completely resected tumors has been reported at 90% (West et al. 1995). Radiation is recommended for symptomatic or progressive disease that is not resectable or for residual disease with the potential to grow and damage critical structures.

Tumor location is particularly important for this group of tumors. Studies have demonstrated that tumors of the infratentorial location are less likely to progress (Kidd et al. 2006). Extent of resection has prognostic significance and is often associated with location. Tumors in the deep tissues of the brain are less likely to be completely resected and therefore are likely to benefit from radiotherapy (West et al. 1995). From an English Children's Tumor Registry, children with deep-seated tumors treated with surgery alone did not demonstrate long-term survival whereas the addition of radiotherapy allowed for 15 year survival of 64% (West et al. 1995). The recent change in

WHO criteria now classifies ganglioglioma as a WHO grade I tumor. These tumors do not respond as well to radiation or chemotherapy as their pilocytic counterparts.

Optic Pathway Tumors

Radiation therapy is highly effective for optic pathway tumors with 10-year progression-free survival rates greater than 80% (Jenkin et al. 1993; Tao et al. 1997). Initial choice of therapy does not impact survival, but when radiotherapy is administered, progression-free survival at both 5 and 10 years is improved (Bloom et al. 1990; Gajjar et al. 1997; Jenkin et al. 1993). Many patients with optic pathway tumors present at a young age, with 25% before 18 months of age and 50% less than 5 years of age (Alvord and Lofton 1988; Janss et al. 1995). Following combination chemotherapy, progression has been noted at a median of 3 years from treatment (Packer et al. 1988). At time of progression second line chemotherapy, surgical resection, and radiation therapy need to be considered with a decision made by a multidisciplinary team.

WHO Grade II

WHO Grade II gliomas include the diffuse astrocytomas, pleomorphic xanthoastrocytoma, oligodendroglioma, oligoastrocytoma, and pilomyxoid astrocytoma (Louis et al. 2007). These tumors are more likely to demonstrate progression than WHO grade I tumors. From a group of 159 adult WHO II patients treated with surgery and RT (mostly at the time of progression), the 5-year overall and progression-free survival rates were 77.5% and 43.2% (Stander et al. 2004). In comparison, a report of 90 children with WHO grade II gliomas, describes 5-year overall and progression-free survival rates at 90% and 56%, respectively, with 10-year rates of 81% and 42%, respectively (Mishra et al. 2006). Of note, for patients older than 3 years without a gross total resection, administration of early radiation did not appear to influence progression-free or overall survival. The 10 year progression-free survival was 43% whether the patients received radiotherapy early or at the time of progression.

Long-Term Effects

Neurocognitive Effects

A group out of the Royal Manchester Children's Hospital, UK performed a study on 50 children with astrocytomas (Chadderton et al. 1995). The children that received radiotherapy performed significantly worse on measures of intelligence and information processing. In addition, there was a greater incidence of special education needs in the radiated group. The authors concluded that both supratentorial and posterior fossa radiotherapy is detrimental to neurocognitive abilities. Clinical factors including pre-therapy symptoms, surgical complications, and progression of disease may also lead to neurocognitive decline. A separate analysis of low-grade glioma patients found that the most significant predictor for change in IQ at 1 year post therapy was preoperative duration of increased intracranial pressure (Yule et al. 2001).

Patients with low-grade gliomas treated at the VU Medical Center in Amsterdam were compared to a cohort of low-grade hematologic malignancies and healthy individuals to differentiate between the effects of the tumor and treatment effects on cognitive function for patients (Klein et al. 2002). At a mean of 6 years after treatment, the tumor itself had the most detrimental effect on cognitive function and the impact of radiotherapy was significant when greater than 2 Gy per fraction is used. The use of anti-epileptic medications was strongly associated with disability in attentional and executive function. The group updated their analysis at 12 years from therapy and found that patients who received radiotherapy showed a progressive decline in attentional functioning, executive functioning, and information processing speed regardless of dose per fraction (Douw et al. 2009). These cognitive deficits were associated with white-matter hyperintensities and global cortical atrophy.

Vasculopathy

From the St. Jude experience using conformal radiotherapy, the predicted cumulative incidence of vasculopathy was 4.79% at 7 years (Merchant et al. 2009b). NF-1 status, sex and age were investigated as predictors for vasculopathy and only age less than 5 years was found to be significant. The risk at 6 years was 12.5% ± 12.6% for patients younger than 5 years of age (n = 8) compared with 3.8% ± 2.6% for those older than 5 years (n = 66) at the time of radiotherapy.

Sixty-nine children with optic pathway gliomas underwent radiation at Gustave Roussy Institute and had a minimum of 3 year follow up (Grill et al. 1999). Vasculopathy was defined by stroke, transient ischemic attack, or radiologically by ischemia on CT scans or MRI. Nineteen percent (13 out of 69) of patients developed radiation-induced vasculopathy at a median follow up of 7 years from radiotherapy. Only two patients were asymptomatic. Similar to the St. Jude experience, the children who developed vasculopathy were younger at the time of radiation. However, unlike the St. Jude report, the occurrence of cerebral vasculopathy was significantly more frequent in patients with NF-1 (11 out of 37) compared to those without (2 out of 32).

Neuroendocrine

There are two reports that discuss the impact of therapy on endocrine status specifically for children with optic pathway/hypothalamic low-grade gliomas (Brauner et al. 1990; Collet-Solberg et al. 1997). A French study evaluated 21 patients (mean age 5.4 years) with optic glioma before and/or after cranial irradiation (45–55 Gy) (Brauner et al. 1990). Of note only ten patients underwent endocrine evaluation prior to radiotherapy. Growth hormone deficiency was present in only one patient tested before radiation and in all patients after radiation. Precocious puberty occurred in 7 out of 21 cases, before radiation in five patients and after radiation in two patients. The authors concluded that the dose of cranial radiation used to treat optic glioma results in growth hormone deficiency within 2 years and recommend initiating human growth hormone therapy when the deficiency is documented.

A large retrospective review of 68 children (mean age at presentation of 5 years) who survived optic pathway/hypothalamic glioma was undertaken at the Children's Hospital of Pennsylvania (Collet-Solberg et al. 1997). Of 50 children with endocrine evaluations, 15 of the 19 with growth hormone deficiency received cranial radiation. However, 15 children treated with more than 15 Gy exhibited normal growth. Precocious puberty was diagnosed in 11 patients. Nine patients, all treated with cranial radiation, developed hypogonadotrophic hypogonadism. Hypothyroidism, hypoadrenalism, and diabetes insipidus were related to prior surgery. The proximity of these optic pathway/hypothalamic tumors to the hypothalamic-pituitary axis makes these children at increased risk for endocrinopathies.

The St. Jude phase II trial of three-dimensional conformal radiotherapy included a prospective evaluation of endocrine function both before and after radiotherapy for children with low-grade gliomas (Merchant et al. 2009a). This analysis provides results that can be translated to most children treated with modern techniques and a radiation dose of 54 Gy delivered at 1.8 Gy per fraction. The 10-year cumulative incidence of growth hormone replacement was 48.9%; of thyroid hormone replacement, 64.0%; of glucocorticoid replacement, 19.2%; and of gonadotropin-releasing hormone analog therapy, 34.2%. Of note, 24% of tested patients had growth hormone abnormalities prior to initiating radiotherapy.

Malignant Transformation

For adult WHO grade II gliomas, the rate of malignant progression has been reported at 33–42% at 5 years (Mehrkens et al. 2004; Stander et al. 2004). Broniscer et al., reported a 15 year cumulative incidence of malignant transformation of 6.7% from a group of grade II low-grade glioma patients treated at St. Jude with a median age at diagnosis of 13 (Broniscer et al. 2007).

Median time to malignant transformation was 5.1 years. It is important to note that no factors, including radiotherapy correlated with an increase risk of malignant transformation, although the number of patients was small.

Impact of Modern Radiotherapy

Radiotherapy techniques have improved over time. The St. Jude phase II trial of three-dimensional conformal radiotherapy resulted in excellent 10-year event-free and overall survival of 74% and 96%, respectively (Merchant et al. 2009b). The tumor volumes were based on MRI and a 1 cm clinical target volume (CTV) margin was used. Thirteen out of 78 patients developed treatment failure: Four with metastatic progression, one marginal failure, and eight infield failures (at a range of 18–86 months from start of radiotherapy). These patients were prospectively evaluated for impact of conformal radiotherapy on cognitive abilities, hearing, and endocrinopathies (Merchant et al. 2009a). It is important to note that patients with more aggressive surgery upfront (subtotal resection compared to biopsy), hydrocephalus, NF1, and younger age had lower baseline neurocognitive function prior to radiotherapy. Cognitive effects 5 years after conformal radiotherapy correlated with patient age, NF1 status, tumor location and volume, extent of resection, and radiation dose. The effect of age exceeded that of radiation dose, and patients younger than 5 years experienced the greatest decline in cognition. Patients not treated with chemotherapy prior to radiotherapy showed a trend toward higher scores on visual auditory learning. The mean cumulative incidence of hearing loss at 10 years did not exceed 5.7% at any frequency.

There is currently no prospective data available demonstrating the impact of proton therapy on long-term consequences of radiotherapy for pediatric low-grade gliomas. A dose-modeling project was performed using both protons and photons for common pediatric brain tumors including an optic pathway glioma (Merchant et al. 2008). The group was able to demonstrate that large normal tissue volumes such as supratentorial brain and temporal lobes received less intermediate and low dose radiation with protons. Modeled dose-volume effects on the Wechsler Individual Achievement Test for spelling predicted a significant benefit of protons over 3-D conformal photon therapy for the optic pathway glioma.

Stereotactic radiotherapy (SRT) has been prospectively studied for 50 pediatric patients with low-grade gliomas (Marcus et al. 2005). The trial utilized a margin of 2 mm on the preoperative tumor volume and a mean radiation dose of 52.2 Gy given at 1.8 Gy per fraction. Radiation was given at the time of progression after either surgery or chemotherapy. The progression-free and overall survival rate was 82.5% and 97.8% at 5 years, 65% and 82% at 8 years. Six patients had local progression. The authors concluded that limited margins using stereotactic immobilization and planning techniques can safely be used with the goal of minimizing late sequelae. Four children with optic glioma developed Moya Moya syndrome at 23, 40, 57, and 83 months after SRT and two children progressed to anaplastic gliomas at 3 and 7 years after SRT. The endocrine and neurocognitive results have not yet been reported.

References

Alvord EC Jr, Lofton S (1988) Gliomas of the optic nerve or chiasm: outcome by patients' age, tumor site, and treatment. J Neurosurg 68(1):85–98

Bloom HJ, Glees J, Bell J, Ashley SE, Gorman C (1990) The treatment and long-term prognosis of children with intracranial tumors: a study of 610 cases, 1950–1981. Int J Radiat Oncol Biol Phys 18(4):723–745

Brauner R, Malandry F, Rappaport R, Zucker JM, Kalifa C, Pierre-Kahn A, Bataini P, Dufier JL (1990) Growth and endocrine disorders in optic glioma. Eur J Pediatr 149(12):825–828

Broniscer A, Baker SJ, West AN, Fraser MM, Proko E, Kocak M, Dalton J, Zambetti GP, Ellison DW, Kun LE, Gajjar A, Gilbertson RJ, Fuller CE (2007) Clinical and molecular characteristics of malignant transformation of low-grade glioma in children. J Clin Oncol 25(6):682–689

Chadderton RD, West CG, Schuller S, Quirke DC, Gattamaneni R, Taylor R (1995) Radiotherapy in the treatment of low-grade astrocytomas. II. The physical and cognitive sequelae. Childs Nerv Syst 11(8): 443–448

Collet-Solberg PF, Sernyak H, Satin-Smith M, Katz LL, Sutton L, Molloy P, Moshang T Jr (1997) Endocrine outcome in long-term survivors of low-grade hypothalamic/chiasmatic glioma. Clin Endocrinol (Oxf) 47(1):79–85

Douw L, Klein M, Fagel SS, van den Heuvel J, Taphoorn MJ, Aaronson NK, Postma TJ, Vandertop WP, Mooij JJ, Boerman RH, Beute GN, Sluimer JD, Slotman BJ, Reijneveld JC, Heimans JJ (2009) Cognitive and radiological effects of radiotherapy in patients with low-grade glioma: long-term follow-up. Lancet Neurol 8(9):810–818

Fisher BJ, Leighton CC, Vujovic O, Macdonald DR, Stitt L (2001) Results of a policy of surveillance alone after surgical management of pediatric low grade gliomas. Int J Radiat Oncol Biol Phys 51(3):704–710

Fouladi M, Hunt DL, Pollack IF, Dueckers G, Burger PC, Becker LE, Yates AJ, Gilles FH, Davis RL, Boyett JM, Finlay JL (2003) Outcome of children with centrally reviewed low-grade gliomas treated with chemotherapy with or without radiotherapy on Children's Cancer Group high-grade glioma study CCG-945. Cancer 98(6):1243–1252

Gajjar A, Sanford RA, Heideman R, Jenkins JJ, Walter A, Li Y, Langston JW, Muhlbauer M, Boyett JM, Kun LE (1997) Low-grade astrocytoma: a decade of experience at St. Jude Children's Research Hospital. J Clin Oncol 15(8):2792–2799

Gnekow AK, Kortmann RD, Pietsch T, Emser A (2004) Low grade chiasmatic-hypothalamic glioma-carboplatin and vincristin chemotherapy effectively defers radiotherapy within a comprehensive treatment strategy – report from the multicenter treatment study for children and adolescents with a low grade glioma – HIT-LGG 1996 – of the Society of Pediatric Oncology and Hematology (GPOH). Klin Padiatr 216(6):331–342

Grill J, Couanet D, Cappelli C, Habrand JL, Rodriguez D, Sainte-Rose C, Kalifa C (1999) Radiation-induced cerebral vasculopathy in children with neurofibromatosis and optic pathway glioma. Ann Neurol 45(3):393–396

Janss AJ, Grundy R, Cnaan A, Savino PJ, Packer RJ, Zackai EH, Goldwein JW, Sutton LN, Radcliffe J, Molloy PT (1995) Optic pathway and hypothalamic/chiasmatic gliomas in children younger than age 5 years with a 6-year follow-up. Cancer 75(4):1051–1059

Jenkin D, Angyalfi S, Becker L, Berry M, Buncic R, Chan H, Doherty M, Drake J, Greenberg M, Hendrick B et al (1993) Optic glioma in children: surveillance, resection, or irradiation? Int J Radiat Oncol Biol Phys 25(2):215–225

Kidd EA, Mansur DB, Leonard JR, Michalski JM, Simpson JR, Perry A (2006) The efficacy of radiation therapy in the management of grade I astrocytomas. J Neurooncol 76(1):55–58

Klein M, Heimans JJ, Aaronson NK, van der Ploeg HM, Grit J, Muller M, Postma TJ, Mooij JJ, Boerman RH, Beute GN, Ossenkoppele GJ, van Imhoff GW, Dekker AW, Jolles J, Slotman BJ, Struikmans H, Taphoorn MJ (2002) Effect of radiotherapy and other treatment-related factors on mid-term to long-term cognitive sequelae in low-grade gliomas: a comparative study. Lancet 360(9343):1361–1368

Louis DN, Ohgaki H, Wiestler OD, Cavenee WK, Burger PC, Jouvet A, Scheithauer BW, Kleihues P (2007) The 2007 WHO classification of tumours of the central nervous system. Acta Neuropathol 114(2):97–109

Marcus KJ, Goumnerova L, Billett AL, Lavally B, Scott RM, Bishop K, Xu R, Young Poussaint T, Kieran M, Kooy H, Pomeroy SL, Tarbell NJ (2005) Stereotactic radiotherapy for localized low-grade gliomas in children: final results of a prospective trial. Int J Radiat Oncol Biol Phys 61(2):374–379

Massimino M, Spreafico F, Riva D, Biassoni V, Poggi G, Solero C, Gandola L, Genitori L, Modena P, Simonetti F, Potepan P, Casanova M, Meazza C, Clerici CA, Catania S, Sardi I, Giangaspero F (2010) A lower-dose, lower-toxicity cisplatin-etoposide regimen for childhood progressive low-grade glioma. J Neurooncol 100(1):65–71

Mehrkens JH, Kreth FW, Muacevic A, Ostertag CB (2004) Long term course of WHO grade II astrocytomas of the Insula of Reil after I-125 interstitial irradiation. J Neurol 251(12):1455–1464

Merchant TE, Hua CH, Shukla H, Ying X, Nill S, Oelfke U (2008) Proton versus photon radiotherapy for common pediatric brain tumors: comparison of models of dose characteristics and their relationship to cognitive function. Pediatr Blood Cancer 51(1):110–117

Merchant TE, Conklin HM, Wu S, Lustig RH, Xiong X (2009a) Late effects of conformal radiation therapy for pediatric patients with low-grade glioma: prospective evaluation of cognitive, endocrine, and hearing deficits. J Clin Oncol 27(22):3691–3697

Merchant TE, Kun LE, Wu S, Xiong X, Sanford RA, Boop FA (2009b) Phase II trial of conformal radiation therapy for pediatric low-grade glioma. J Clin Oncol 27(22):3598–3604

Mishra KK, Puri DR, Missett BT, Lamborn KR, Prados MD, Berger MS, Banerjee A, Gupta N, Wara WM, Haas-Kogan DA (2006) The role of up-front radiation therapy for incompletely resected pediatric WHO grade II low-grade gliomas. Neuro Oncol 8(2):166–174

Mishra KK, Squire S, Lamborn K, Banerjee A, Gupta N, Wara WM, Prados MD, Berger MS, Haas-Kogan DA (2010) Phase II TPDCV protocol for pediatric low-grade hypothalamic/chiasmatic gliomas: 15-year update. J Neurooncol 100(1):121–127

Packer RJ, Sutton LN, Bilaniuk LT, Radcliffe J, Rosenstock JG, Siegel KR, Bunin GR, Savino PJ, Bruce DA, Schut L (1988) Treatment of chiasmatic/hypothalamic gliomas of childhood with chemotherapy: an update. Ann Neurol 23(1):79–85

Packer RJ, Ater J, Allen J, Phillips P, Geyer R, Nicholson HS, Jakacki R, Kurczynski E, Needle M, Finlay J, Reaman G, Boyett JM (1997) Carboplatin and vincristine chemotherapy for children with newly diagnosed progressive low-grade gliomas. J Neurosurg 86(5):747–754

Pollack IF, Claassen D, al-Shboul Q, Janosky JE, Deutsch M (1995) Low-grade gliomas of the cerebral hemispheres in children: an analysis of 71 cases. J Neurosurg 82(4):536–547

Shaw EG, Daumas-Duport C, Scheithauer BW, Gilbertson DT, O'Fallon JR, Earle JD, Laws ER Jr, Okazaki H (1989) Radiation therapy in the management of low-grade supratentorial astrocytomas. J Neurosurg 70(6):853–861

Stander M, Peraud A, Leroch B, Kreth FW (2004) Prognostic impact of TP53 mutation status for adult patients with supratentorial World Health Organization Grade II astrocytoma or oligoastrocytoma: a long-term analysis. Cancer 101(5):1028–1035

Tao ML, Barnes PD, Billett AL, Leong T, Shrieve DC, Scott RM, Tarbell NJ (1997) Childhood optic chiasm gliomas: radiographic response following radiotherapy and long-term clinical outcome. Int J Radiat Oncol Biol Phys 39(3):579–587

van den Bent MJ, Afra D, de Witte O, Ben Hassel M, Schraub S, Hoang-Xuan K, Malmstrom PO, Collette L, Pierart M, Mirimanoff R, Karim AB (2005) Long-term efficacy of early versus delayed radiotherapy for low-grade astrocytoma and oligodendroglioma in adults: the EORTC 22845 randomised trial. Lancet 366(9490):985–990

West CG, Gattamaneni R, Blair V (1995) Radiotherapy in the treatment of low-grade astrocytomas. I. A survival analysis. Childs Nerv Syst 11(8):438–442

Wisoff JH, Sanford RA, Heier LA, Sposto R, Burger PC, Yates AJ, Holmes EJ, Kun LE (2011) Primary neurosurgery for pediatric low-grade gliomas: a prospective multi-institutional study from the Children's Oncology Group. Neurosurgery 68(6):1548–1554

Yule SM, Hide TA, Cranney M, Simpson E, Barrett A (2001) Low grade astrocytomas in the West of Scotland 1987–1996: treatment, outcome, and cognitive functioning. Arch Dis Child 84(1):61–64

Part V

Spinal Tumors

Pediatric Multiple Primary Cranio-Spinal Tumors Associated with Neurofibromatosis Type 2: Combined Therapeutical Strategies

24

Teresa Stachowicz-Stencel

Contents

T. Stachowicz-Stencel (✉)
Department of Pediatrics, Hematology, Oncology, and Endocrinology, Medical University of Gdansk, 7 Debinki Street, 80-211 Gdansk, Poland
e-mail: tsten@gumed.edu.pl

Abstract

Tumors of the central nervous system (CNS) represent approximately 20% of all pediatric neoplasms. Of these, 4–6% are primary spinal cord tumors. Multiple primary cranio-spinal tumors are often associated with inherited syndromes including neurofibromatosis type 2 (NF2). The principal clinical feature of NF2 is the existence of vestibular schwannomas, meningiomas, and ependymomas; therefore, NF2 is also called MISME (multiple inherited schwannomas, meningiomas, and ependymomas) syndrome. Consequently, a multidisciplinary approach is needed for these patients, and diagnosis and treatment should be performed in an appropriate oncological center with a neurosurgeon, otolaryngologist, neurologist, geneticist, ophthalmologist, pathologist, radiologist, audiologist, and experienced nursing staff. Magnetic resonance imaging of the brain and spinal canal with contrast is the method of choice for diagnosis of CNS tumors. Surgical procedures are often necessary to establish a diagnosis, perform complete or incomplete excision of the tumor mass, and to reduce intracranial pressure. Radiotherapy and chemotherapy are adjuvant treatment options.

Introduction

The incidence of tumors of the central nervous system (CNS) in children from 0 to 14 years old is 110–130 per one million per year. Primary

M.A. Hayat (ed.), *Pediatric Cancer, Volume 3: Diagnosis, Therapy, and Prognosis*, Pediatric Cancer 3,
DOI 10.1007/978-94-007-4528-5_24,

spinal cord tumors (PSCT) account for about 4–6% of all pediatric central nervous system tumors (Mottl and Koutecky 1997). According to the Central Brain Tumor Registry of the United States, PSCT occurs in 0.19 per 100,000 children, although the incidence varies with age and is 1.6-fold higher in patients aged 15–19 years than in those aged 0–4 years (CBTRUS 2004). There is a proven association between several inherited syndromes such as phacomatoses, neurofibromatosis, von Hippel-Lindau syndrome, and Li Fraumeni syndrome and CNS neoplasms.

Clinical Symptoms of Brain and Spinal Canal Tumors

The signs and symptoms of brain tumor in children are non-specific and very often misdiagnosed. In addition, they can vary depending on patient age and the site of origin and histology of the tumor. In tumors located in the midline or in the posterior fossa the most common symptoms are associated with increased intracranial pressure (ICP), including morning headache, morning vomiting, and visual disturbances. ICP may be caused by infiltration or compression of normal brain tissue or by obstruction of cerebrospinal fluid flow. In infancy, rapid head growth, bulging fontanel, and intellectual and motor regression are observed but the other symptoms of ICP may not be present. In older children the common signs are difficulties in school that were not observed before, fatigue, changes in behavior, irritability, headaches, anorexia, and somnolence. Depending on their location infratentorial tumors (brain stem and cerebellum) may present with impairment of balance and gait, cranial nerve abnormalities, and vision disturbances (diplopia or 6th nerve palsy, papilledema, or Parinaud syndrome). In smaller children diplopia may present as frequent blinking or intermittent strabismus. Papilledema may present as intermittent blurred vision. Nystagmus and gaze palsy may occur alone or in combination with deficits of cranial nerves V, VII, and IX suggesting brain stem infiltration. Supratentorial tumors cause headaches and subsequent seizures, hemiparesis, hyperreflexia, and clonus. Other non-specific symptoms are endocrine abnormalities due to effects on the hypothalamus or pituary gland and manifest as anorexia/bulimia, weight loss, diabetes insipidus, sexual precocity, or delayed puberty. Visual loss associated with compression of the optic chiasm/optic nerve may be observed in cases of hypothalamus localization.

The symptoms of PSCT depend on anatomical location (extradural or intradural) and pathology. The majority of tumors are extradural and metastatic. Intradural spinal tumors are subclassified as those located outside or inside the spinal cord parenchyma (extramedullary and intramedullary, respectively). The common symptoms of a primary spinal canal tumor are localized pain and weakness, which may precede other neurological symptoms. Extramedullary tumors can appear as a dural distention with pain that is characteristically aggravated by lying flat because of venous congestion. The manifestation often results from spinal nerve compression and weakening of the vertebral structure. Approximately 1% of intraspinal tumors present with hydrocephalus.

Neurofibromatosis Type 2

Multiple primary cranio-spinal tumors may be present in patients with NF2. The first recorded case of NF2 was described in 1882 by Wishart. NF2 is an inherited rare autosomal dominant multiple neoplasia syndrome that is characterized by the development of multiple benign cranial and spinal tumors (schwannomas, meningiomas, and ependymomas) with peripheral neuropathy, ophthalmological lesions (cataracts, epiretinal membranes, and retinal hamartomas) and cutaneous lesions (tumors of the skin, mainly schwannomas) (Asthagiri et al. 2009). Schwannomas, meningiomas, and ependymomas are characteristic features of NF2, and consequently NF2 is also called MISME (multiple inherited schwannomas, meningiomas, and ependymomas) syndrome. The disorder is present in one of 25,000 live births and approximately 10% of NF2 patients are under the age of 10 years (Asthagiri et al. 2009).

Among patients with NF2, 18% present with symptoms of the disease at the age of 15 years or less (Janse et al. 2001). Although most CNS tumors in NF2 are slow growing, they may grow faster during childhood and in this situation the prognosis is often poor (Moffat et al. 2003). The development of new tumors is likely in patients with NF2, even after surgery (Evans 2009). In such cases, a new management strategy and early diagnosis are necessary. There are four methods for establishing a diagnosis of NF2 but none of them is specific and sensitive enough for diagnosis in patients with a de novo mutation without a positive family history. One of the best methods seems to be the Manchester criteria, established by experts from Department of Medical Genetics, St Mary's Hospital, Manchester (Baser et al. 2002).

The Manchester diagnostic criteria of NF2 are as follows: bilateral cranial nerve (CN) VIII schwannomas observed on MRI or CT scan (no biopsy necessary) or first-degree relative with NF2 and either unilateral early-onset CN VIII schwannoma (age < 30 years) or any two of meningioma, glioma, schwannoma, or juvenile posterior subcapsular lenticular opacity (juvenile cortical cataract). In case of suspicion of NF2 the following criteria are used: early onset of unilateral CN VIII schwannomas on MRI or CT scan detected in patients younger than 30 years and one of the following: meningioma, glioma, schwannoma, juvenile posterior subcapsular lenticular opacity; or multiple meningiomas (>2) and unilateral CN VIII schwannoma or one of the following: glioma, schwannoma, or juvenile posterior subcapsular lenticular opacity (Gutmann et al. 1997). The recommendations for screening children of affected parents are as follows: ophthalmological examination once a year from infancy; neurological examination once a year from infancy; audiology with auditory brainstem evoke potentials yearly from infancy; genetic testing before symptoms-one test from 10 years of age; cranial MRI at 10–12 years of age; and spinal MRI every 2–3 years from 10 to 12 years of age. Cranial and spinal MRI before 10 years old is recommended in severely affected families.

Molecular Biology of Neurofibromatosis

The molecular basis of neurofibromatosis is currently of great interest to clinicians because of new possibilities in molecular diagnostics. The genes associated with neurofibromatosis, NF1 and NF2, were localized in 1987 and cloned at the beginning of the 1990s. However, there is still no commercial test that could be helpful in establishing a diagnosis. The main problem associated with the NF1 gene is its size and great number of rare mutations (Thomson et al. 2002). Tumors associated with NF2 are caused by inactivation of both alleles of the NF2 tumor-suppressor gene localized on chromosome 22q12 by mutation or allele loss (Asthagiri et al. 2009 and Evans 2009). Testing for such mutations is associated with huge costs, which has important implications for diagnostics.

Identification of the NF1 and NF2 genes and their products has led to further understanding of the process of tumorigenesis and many other pathways and processes occurring in the organism and cells. The products of the NF1 and NF2 genes – neurofibromin and merlin, also called schwannomin, respectively – play a role as a tumor suppressor genes or antioncogenes. Recent evidence suggests that between 20% and 30% of NF2 cases without a family history of the disease are mosaic for the underlying disease-causing mutation and that more than 50% of patients represent new mutations (Evans 2009). Such mutations cause loss of protein integrity and are responsible for the appearance of pathological symptoms.

With respect to NF2, the product of the merlin (schwannomin) gene is a protein that is normally associated with hialuronic receptor CD44 and other proteins such as spectrin, actin, and paxilin. Merlin is localized in the cell membrane-cytoskeletal interface and participates in the adhesion and extension of cells. The effects of merlin on protein organization, cytoskeletal architecture, and cell-cell adhesion influence the regulation of many signaling pathways necessary for protein translation, cell growth, and proliferation (Asthagiri et al. 2009 and Wiederhold et al. 2004). Although two human isoforms of merlin have been identified (I and II), only isoform I was found to be responsible for tumor suppression activity (Sherman et al. 1997). The activity of merlin is related to its phosphorylation status; phosphorylation at serine-518 by p21-activated kinase and cyclic AMP dependent-protein kinase A results in inactivation and relocation of merlin protein (Jin et al. 2006). Mouse models with inactivation of the NF2 gene in Schwann's cells or leptomeningeal cells developed schwannomas or meningiomas respectively, providing evidence that abnormal or deficient merlin function is responsible for disruption of tumor suppression (Asthagiri et al. 2009). Mutations in this protein, which may be inherited as a germline mutation from a parent or appear de novo, are responsible for tumorigenesis and expansion of tumor cells. This situation is especially observed in cases of neoplasms from Schwann's cells and meningiomas; somatic inactivation of both alleles of the NF2 gene is observed in more than 90% of sporadic schwannomas, 50% of meningiomas, and 5% of ependymomas (Seizinger et al. 1987).

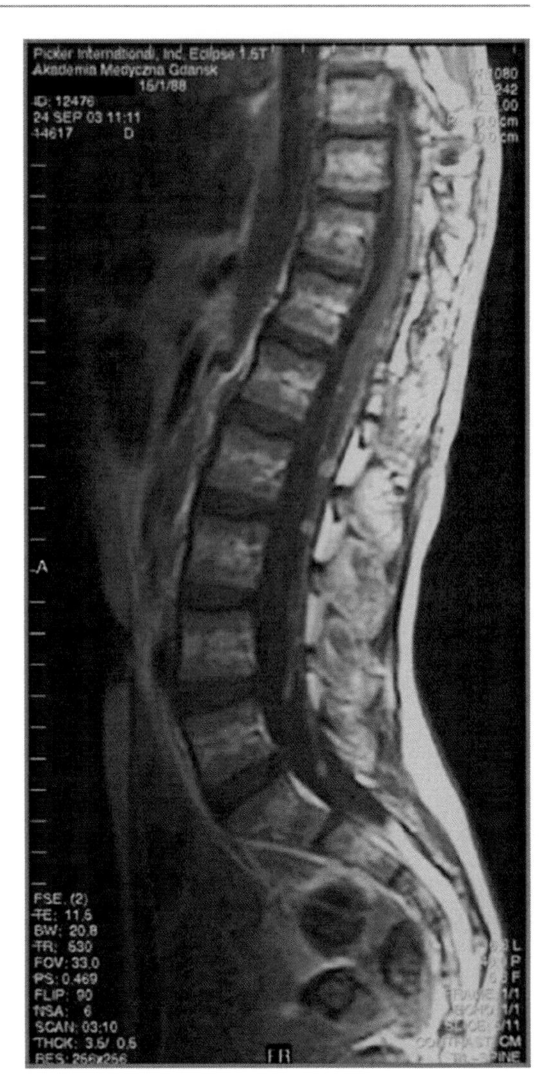

Fig. 24.1 Contrast-enhanced T1-weighted MR image: numerous intradural spinal canal nodules and small tumors in intervertebral foramen on the *right side* at level L5-S1

Diagnosis of CNS Tumors

Imaging

Radiological examination is necessary for patients with suspicion of NF2. Computed tomography (CT) is a readily available diagnostic tool that is helpful in recognition of calcifications and assessment of the skull. However, magnetic resonance imaging (MRI) with contrast is preferable and recommended as first line imaging in cases of brain and spinal canal tumors, especially those located in the posterior fossa (Figs.24.1 and 24.2.). Some types of inoperable tumors, such as diffuse pontine gliomas, tectal plate glioma, and chiasmatic/hypothalamic gliomas, may have characteristic findings in MRI that allow initiation of therapy without histopathological confirmation. For imaging of children, MRI has the advantage of avoiding radiation exposure, although it takes a long time to perform and requires general sedation.

Positron emission tomography (PET) is very useful in determining transformation of a lower grade tumor to a higher grade neoplasm, and also for differentiation of post-therapy (especially post-radiation) treatment effects from tumor progression (Vézina 2005). In infants with open fontanelles, ultrasonography should be the first line of non-invasive investigation.

Cerebrospinal Fluid Evaluation

Evaluation of cerebrospinal fluid (CSF) in patients with NF2 is essential. The current recommendations are as follows: cell count with cytocentrifuge for cytology of tumor cells, and determination of

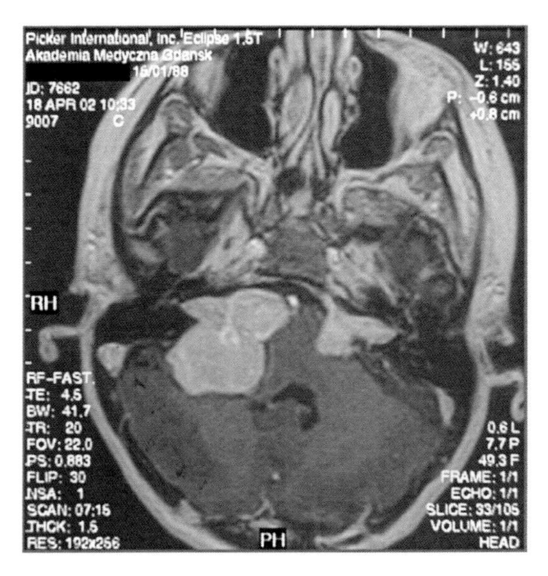

Fig. 24.2 In the posterior cranial fossa, bilateral pathological *solid* masses located in pontocerebellar cisterns, which extend to the auditory meatus; intensive contrast enhancement MR image—schwannomas of the VIII nerve

levels of glucose and protein, α-fetoprotein (AFP), and human chorionic gonadotropin (HCG). This test has additional value for tumors that are in proximity to the circulating CSF, such as medulloblastoma, ependymoma, and brain stem glioma. Elevated levels of HCG and AFP in CSF and serum may be observed in cases of germinal tumors.

Bone Marrow Biopsy and Other Studies

In cases of high malignancy or suspicion of dissemination outside the CNS, bone marrow biopsy, bone scan, and CT of the abdomen is recommended. Ophthalmologic evaluation, laryngological examination with audiogram, and laboratory tests should also be performed.

Misme Syndrome

Schwannomas

Schwannomas, also called neurilemmomas, are benign tumors that arise from Schwann's cells and are usually encapsulated. This kind of neoplasm, especially with peripheral localization, is mainly associated with NF1 and is only occasionally present in NF2, although in this situation the lesions are usually multiple. The most common locations of this kind of tumor are the head, the flexor surfaces of the upper and lower extremities, and the trunk.

Schwannomas can develop along the course of cranial, spinal, and peripheral nerves. They most often arise from the oculomotor, trigeminal, and facial nerves. Schwannomas of spinal nerves may result in discrete peripheral neuropathies (Fisher et al. 2007). This pathologic mass is often mobile along the axis of the nerve. Clinical symptoms may be present or the tumor may be asymptomatic, even for many years. Because the lesions grow very slowly, the neurological symptoms typically appear quite late, usually only when the tumor mass is large. Some of the clinical signs are dependent on anatomical location; for example, changes in the sciatic nerve may manifest as lower back pain. In cases of tumor compression on the nerve origin, the main complaint may be localized pain and paresthesia (Guerrissi 2009). Nonvestibular schwannomas occur in more than half of patients and are often diagnosed in patients with an earlier age of diagnosis of NF2. Cranial nerves III and V are most commonly involved, but the rare occurrence of jugular foramen schwannomas potentially impacting the glossopharyngeal, vagus, and/or spinal accessory nerves may lead to dysphagia, esophageal dysmotility, hoarseness, or aspiration. On the other hand, nonvestibular schwannomas in patients with NF2 tend to be more indolent and to grow slowly over time. This can complicate decisions regarding treatment, since the options include surgery, radiation therapy, and watchful waiting. In patients with NF2, a characteristic feature is schwannoma developing from the vestibular and, more rarely, the cochlear nerve. Bilateral vestibular schwannomas are the most common neoplasms in this group of patients and are found in 90–95% of cases. About 99% of them are benign, but their location makes them impossible to treat and for this reason they remain a major cause of mortality (Asthagiri et al. 2009). Devastation of vestibular fibers progresses slowly and the function of the vestibular nerve may be compensated by central cerebral mechanisms. As a result symptoms often occur only when the tumor mass is sufficiently large, usually about 3–4 cm. Tumors larger than 4 cm in size may be responsible for the development of hydrocephalus in the cerebral aqueduct and fourth ventricle effacement (Rogg et al. 2005). Hearing loss, often accompanied by tinnitus, occurs in around 60% of adults and up to 30% of children (Ruggieri et al. 2005). The hearing loss is often unrelated to the size and growth rate of the tumor and may stay stable for about 2 years, even when untreated (Masuda et al. 2004). Therefore, tumor size and growth rate are not predictive factors for hearing status. On the other hand, the vestibulocochlear nerve is quite sensitive to stretching and even tumors that are small in size may provoke symptoms earlier than compression on the other nerves, such as facial nerves. No connection between genotype and phenotype for hearing loss in NF2 has been found. The main diagnostic tool is MRI with gadolinium contrast, and the characteristic findings include T1 contrast enhancement. The management strategy in vestibular schwannoma (VS) is controversial. Because more than 50% of VS cases are stable in size, some clinicians recommend an initial "watch and wait, then rescan" strategy, completed with surgical resection and stereotactic radiotherapy (Moffat et al. 2003). However, others suggest that early removal of tumors smaller than 3 cm in diameter may preserve normal hearing in 30–65% of cases and normal function of the facial nerve in 75–92% (Brackmann et al. 2001). The management strategy for bilateral vestibular schwannomas may comprise of bilateral resection and eventual cochlear implantation in patients with an anatomically and physiologically undamaged cochlear nerve. It is very difficult to establish the proper time of implantation, which can be either at the first vestibular schwannoma removal with intent for future use or after the second tumor surgery.

Meningiomas

Meningiomas arising from arachnoidal cap cells are one of the most common tumors of the central nervous system in NF2 patients. Intracranial neoplasms are seen in 45–58% of patients (Patronas et al. 2001). They may also be present in the spinal cord (intradural extramedullary location) in about 20% of cases and outside the CNS (in the skin). These meningiomas are usually multiple and may be the first manifestation of the disease in young patients. Sporadic meningioma that is not associated with neurofibromatosis occurs more frequently in older individuals at an increasing frequency with age and typically appears as a single element.

Clinical symptoms are strictly correlated with the size and localization of the tumors. Meningiomas are usually characterized by their slow growth, and the actual number of patients with meningiomas may therefore be higher than reported. Autopsy studies reveal that 2.3% of the population has undiagnosed and asymptomatic meningiomas (Evans 1999). Because meningiomas are usually based in the arachnoid layer that covers the surface of the brain, the clinical signs may be caused by irritation of the cortex and manifest as seizures. Compression of the brain or cranial nerves is related to tumor size and causes symptoms such as headaches and various non-specific cerebral disturbances (focal weakness, lethargy, dysphasia, and somnolence). Depending of their location, these tumors may give rise to other symptoms that are not specific for meningiomas: for example, subfrontal tumors lead to apathy, changes in behavior, and urinary incontinence; tumors in the cavernous sinus are associated with cranial nerves deficits (often multiple); cerebellopontine angle tumors lead to damaged hearing; spinal cord defects cause localized pain and Brown-Sequard syndrome; and optic nerve tumors cause exophthalmos. In rare cases, meningiomas may obturate cerebral arteries and cause transient ischemic attack (TIA)-like episodes or tumors situated in ventricles may give rise to hydrocephalus.

The main diagnostic tools are imagining studies. CT examination reveals dural-based tumors, which are hyperenhanced after contrast injection. In addition, edema around the tumor and calcification may be visible. Multiple meningiomas, which often occur in NF2 patients, may make it difficult to differentiate primary lesions from metastases. MRI provides the best images of meningiomas, which are visible as homogenous enhancement in T1-weighted imaging. T2-weighted FLAIR (fluid-attenuated inversion recovery) may show edema and/or cysts. Involvement of the dura by tumor tissue is observed as an enhancing mass, usually well encapsulated. Relatively new diagnostic tools such as PET and magnetic resonance spectroscopy (MRS) are useful for predicting the in vivo aggressiveness of meningiomas (Lee et al. 2009).

The treatment of choice for benign meningoma remains surgical resection, which is safe and complete in most cases. Sometimes the tumor location makes complete resection impossible, for example in the optic nerve and skull base. In such cases the surgical procedure might be associated with severe neurological complication and morbidity. In such high-risk situations, stereotactic radiosurgery techniques may be considered as they provide very good focal control and minimal toxicity. These techniques are mostly used for small lesions (smaller than 3 cm) or for the local control of residual tumor. For this type of treatment the 5-year progression-free survival rate for patients with NF2 is 86%. No long-term follow up for malignant transformation induced by radiation was considered (Evans et al. 2006). The outcome associated with use of chemotherapy is disappointing.

Ependymomas

Ependymomas arise from ependymal cells through the central canal and cells of the ventriculus terminal in the filum terminale and account for about 10% of all CNS tumors in children. The majority (90%) of ependymomas are situated intracranially and only 10% are present in the spinal canal. For the purpose of this chapter we will focus on ependymomas in NF2 patients. In these cases, tumors are found mainly in the spinal canal and may be divided into three groups: intramedullary, myxopapillary, and metastases from an intracranial localization. About 50% of intraspinal ependymomas are localized at the cauda equina and 15% are multiple. Approximately 75% of spinal-cord tumors associated with NF2 have an intra-medullary location with the following order of frequency: cervical cord, thoracic region, and the conus (Dow et al. 2005).

These tumors are mostly found in NF2 patients with constitutional nonsense and frame shift mutations and appear as a low-grade ependymoma of grade II according to WHO classification (Patronas et al. 2001). Myxopapillary ependymoma, grade I, occurs mostly in the cauda equina region and is associated with certain chromosomal aberrations and molecular genetic changes related to both poor and good prognosis. It is generally considered that gain of chromosomes 9, 15q, and 18, and loss of chromosome 6 are associated with good prognosis (Korshunov et al. 2010), whereas gain of 1q25, overexpression of EGFR, hTERT expression, high levels of nucleolin, activation of the Notch pathway, or expression of Tenascin C are associated with poor prognosis (Puget et al. 2009).

In histological examination the low-grade tumors are well differentiated and characterized by their lack of mitosis and vascularity. Only 20% of cases are symptomatic, depending on the tumor size and location along the spinal canal. The typical clinical symptoms of intramedullary lesions are recumbent back pain in 56% of cases, weakness in 28%, and/or sensory disturbances in 16% (Chang et al. 2002). Loss of bladder and/or bowel function may also be present. Patients with ependymoma located in the conus and cauda equina may experience severe pain, flaccid paralysis of the legs, atrophy of the leg muscles, and foot drop.

The most reliable diagnostic method is MRI with contrast. The lesions are isointense or slightly hyperintense in T1-weighted images and hyperintense in T2-weighted images. This imaging allows estimation of other pathologies associated with the tumor such as edema, hemorrhage, cyst, syringomyelia, and cord atrophy. One of the specific MRI findings is the hemosiderin cap, which is characterized by low signal in T2-weighted images.

CT is not useful in evaluation of ependymoma in the spinal canal. In histopathological examination the ependymoma is revealed as a well-delineated moderately cellular tumor with round-oval nuclei. Perivascular pseudorosette and ependymal rosette are also observed. Most ependymomas can only be treated by total resection and this method remains the most important although different therapeutic approaches may be used depending on the tumor location and age of the patient. Total excision is recommended for intracranial non-anaplastic tumors, independent of age. Radiotherapy in doses of 45–50 Gy with boost on the tumor bed is the treatment of choice in children over 3 years old with intracranial localization in low-grade stage, for subtotal resection, and for any other location independent of the type of resection. Stereoradiosurgery is considered as an alternative therapy for small relapses or residual malignant tumors. Tumors in children under 3 years old without anaplasia, tumors located in the posterior fossa that were removed radically, tumors that were resected incompletely independent of localization, and all tumors with anaplasia are treated by chemotherapy with vincristine, etoposide, cisplatin, and cyclophosphamide. In patients over 3 years old with anaplastic tumors, independent of location and type of resection, the recommended therapy is induction chemotherapy with etoposide, ifosfamide, and doxorubicine, with subsequent radiotherapy and maintenance chemotherapy (cisplatin, lomustin, and vincristine) 2 weeks after finishing radiotherapy (Barszcz and Perek-Polnik 2006). After completion of treatment, MRI is indicated every 6 months for the first 5 years and once a year thereafter.

In conclusion, all of the tumors described above may occur as a separate element or simultaneously. The treatment strategy for a single neoplasm is well established, but in cases of coexistence of multiple, histologically different tumors the therapeutic approach must be considered individually for each tumor (Stachowicz-Stencel et al. 2011).

References

Asthagiri AR, Parry DM, Butman JA, Kim HJ, Tsilou ET, Zhuang Z, Lonser RR (2009) Neurofibromatosis type 2. Lancet 373:1974–1986

Barszcz S, Perek-Polnik M (2006) Ependymomas. In: Perek D, Roszkowski M (eds) Central nervous system tumours in children. Diagnostic and treatment, Ith edn. Fundacja Euronet, Warsaw, pp 133–150

Baser ME, Friedman JM, Wallace AJ, Ramsden RT, Joe H, Evans DG (2002) Evaluation of clinical diagnostic criteria for neurofibromatosis 2. Neurology 59:1759–1765

Brackmann DE, Fayad JN, Slattery WH 3rd, Friedman RA, Day JD, Hitselberger WE, Owens RM (2001) Early proactive management of vestibular schwannomas in neurofibromatosis type 2. Neurosurgery 49:274–283

CBTRUS, Central Brain Tumor Registry of the United States (2004–2005) Primary brain tumors in the United States, statistical report, 1997–2001, years data collected. Central Brain Tumor Registry of the United States, Chicago

Chang UK, Choe WJ, Chung SK, Chung CK, Kim HJ (2002) Surgical outcome and prognostic factors of spinal intramedullary ependymomas in adults. J Neurooncol 57:133–139

Dow G, Biggs N, Evans G, Gillespie J, Ramsden R, King A (2005) Spinal tumours in neurofibromatosos type 2. Is emerging knowledge of genotype predictive of natural history? J Neurosurg Spine 2:574–579

Evans DG (1999) Neurofibromatosis type 2: genetic and clinical features. Ear Nose Throat J 78:97–100

Evans DG (2009) Neurofibromatosis type 2 (NF2): a clinical and molecular review. Orphanet J Rare Dis 4:16

Evans DGR, Birch JM, Ramsden RT, Sharif S, Baser ME (2006) Malignant transformation and new primary tumours after therapeutic radiation for benign disease: substantial risks in certain tumour prone syndromes. J Med Genet 43:289–294

Fisher LM, Doherty JK, Lev NH, Slattery WH 3rd (2007) Distribution of nonvestibular cranial nerve schwannomas in neurofibromatosis 2. Otol Neurotol 28:1083–1190

Guerrissi JO (2009) Solitary benign schwannomas in major nerve systems of the head and neck. J Craniofac Surg 20:957–961

Gutmann DH, Aylsworth A, Carey JC, Korf B, Marks J, Pyeritz RE, Rubenstein A, Viskochil D (1997) The diagnostic evaluation and multidisciplinary management of neurofibromatosis 1 and neurofibromatosis 2. JAMA 278:51–57

Janse AJ, Tan WF, Majoie ChBLM, Bijlsma EK (2001) Neurofibromatosis type 2 diagnosed in the absence of vestibular schwannomas. A case report and guidelines for a screening protocol for childrenat risk. Eur J Pediatr 160:439–443

Jin H, Sperka T, Herrlich P, Morrison H (2006) Tumorigenic transformation by CPI-17 through inhibition of a merlin phosphatase. Nature 442:576–579

Korshunov A, Witt H, Hielscher T, Benner A, Remke M, Ryzhova M, Milde T, Bender S, Wittmann A, Schöttler A, Kulozik AE, Witt O, von Deimling A, Lichter P, Pfister S (2010) Molecular staging of intracranial ependymoma in children and adults. J Clin Oncol 28:3182–3190

Lee JW, Kang KW, Park SH, Lee SM, Paeng JC, Chung JK, Lee SM, Paeng JC, Chung JK, Lee MC, Lee DS (2009) (18)F-FDG PET in the assessment of tumor grade and prediction of tumor recurrence in intracranial meningioma. Eur J Nucl Med Mol Imaging 36:1574–1582

Masuda A, Fisher LM, Oppenheimer ML, Iqbal Z, Slattery WH (2004) Hearing changes after diagnosis in neurofibromatosis type 2. Otol Neurotol 25:150–154

Moffat DA, Quaranta N, Baguley DM, Hardy DG, Chang P (2003) Management strategies in neurofibromatosis type 2. Otology 260:12–18

Mottl H, Koutecky J (1997) Treatment of spinal cord tumors in children. Med Pediatr Oncol 29:293–295

Patronas NJ, Courcoutsakis N, Bromley CM, Katzman GL, MacCollin M, Parry DM (2001) Intramedullary and spinal canal tumors in patients with neurofibromatosis 2: MR imaging findings and correlation with genotype. Radiology 218:434–442

Puget S, Grill J, Valenti A, Bieche I, Dantas-Barbosa C, Kauffmann A, Dessen P, Lacroix L, Geoerger B, Job B, Dirven C, Varlet P, Peyre M, Dirks PB, Sainte-Rose C, Vassal G (2009) Candidate genes on chromosome 9q33-34 involved in the progression of the childhood ependymomas. J Clin Oncol 27:1884–1892

Rogg JM, Ahn SH, Tung GA, Reinert SE, Norén G (2005) Prevalence of hydrocephalus in 157 patients with vestibular schwannoma. Neuroradiology 47:344–351

Ruggieri M, Iannetti P, Polizzi A, La Mantia I, Spalice A, Giliberto O, Platania N, Gabriele AL, Albanese V, Pavone L (2005) Earliest clinical manifestations and natural history of neurofibramatosis type 2 (NF2) in childhood: a study of 24 patients. Neuropediatrics 36:21–34

Seizinger BR, Rouleau G, Ozelius LJ (1987) Common pathogenetic mechanism for three tumor types in bilateral acoustic neurofibromatosis. Science 236:317–319

Sherman L, Xu HM, Geist RT, Saporito-Irwin S, Howells N, Ponta H, Herrlich P, Gutmann DH (1997) Interdomain binding mediatestumor growth suppression by the NF2 gene product. Oncogene 15:2505–2509

Stachowicz-Stencel T, Synakiewicz A, Bien E, Adamkiewicz-Drozynska E, Wybieralska-Dubaniewicz M, Balcerska A (2011) Multiple primary cranio-spinal tumours in a 13-year-old female with neurofibromatosis type 2 management strategy. Childs Nerv Syst 27:175–178

Thomson SA, Fishbein L, Wallace MR (2002) Nf-1 mutations and molecular testing. J Child Neurol 17:555–561

Vézina LG (2005) Neuroradiology of childhood brain tumors: new challenges. J Neurooncol 75:243–252

Wiederhold T, Lee MF, James M, Neujahr R, Smith N, Murthy A, Hartwig J, Gusella JF, Ramesh V (2004) Magicin, a novel cytoskeletal protein associates with the NF2 tumor suppressor merlin and Grb2. Oncogene 23:8815–8825

Pediatric Intradural Lipoma of the Cervicothoracic Spinal Cord: Laminectomy and Duraplasty

25

Ahmet Metin Şanlı, Hayri Kertmen, and Bora Gürer

Contents

A.M. Şanlı (✉) • H. Kertmen • B. Gürer
Department of First Neurosurgery, Dışkapı Yıldırım Beyazıt Research and Education Hospital, Ankara 06580, Turkey
e-mail: ahmetmetinsanli@hotmail.com

Abstract

Spinal cord lipomas are rare lesions that represent less than 1% of all intraspinal tumors. Ninety percent of spinal lipomas are located in the lumbosacral area as components of spinal dysraphism, whereas non-dysraphic lipomas are almost always completely intradural. Pediatric intradural lipoma of the cervicothoracic spinal cord is a rare entity. To the best of our knowledge, up to now, only 41 cases have been presented in the literature. The typical neurological manifestation of this condition is a slowly progressing paresis. Magnetic resonance imaging is the test of the choice, having characteristic demonstration. Surgical treatment with bony decompression and subtotal resection gives satisfactory results. Aggressive resection may cause catastrophic results.

Introduction

Spinal cord lipomas are rare lesions that constitute less than 1% of all intraspinal tumors (Caram et al. 1957; Ehni and Love 1945; Giuffre 1966). They occur approximately once in every 4,000 births (La Marca et al. 1997). Ninety percent of spinal lipomas are located in the lumbosacral area as components of spinal dysraphism, and are evident at birth (Muraszko 1999). In contrast to the dysraphic variety, non-dysraphic lipomas are completely intradural and have no subcutaneous component (Blount and

M.A. Hayat (ed.), *Pediatric Cancer, Volume 3: Diagnosis, Therapy, and Prognosis*, Pediatric Cancer 3,
DOI 10.1007/978-94-007-4528-5_25,

Elton 2001; Wood et al. 1985). Especially, pediatric intradural lipoma of the cervicothoracic spinal cord is extremely rare clinical condition.

Embryology

At the third week of embryonic development, the edges of the developing neural plate elevate and form neural folds. As the neural folds approach each other in the midline, superficial ectoderm trails their leading edge. Cellular processes from opposite sides of neural cells make contact, recognition occurs, and cell adhesions close the tube. At this point the superficial ectoderm closes and separates by disjunction from the neural tube. Mesenchyme migrates into the space between the neural tube and the superficial ectoderm. This mesenchyme will generate vasculature of the spinal cord, and develop into the meninges and vertebral column (Bhatoe et al. 2005).

Lipomas develop when there is premature disjunction of the cutaneous ectoderm from the forming neural tube. The surrounding mesenchyme migrates into the developing neural tube below the cutaneous ectoderm. In this environmental condition, the mesenchyme, instead of differentiating into dura mater, changes into fat. This theory is called "developmental error theory". It is therefore not a true neoplasm, but a hamartoma or a malformation (Ammerman et al. 1976). This theory also explains the dorsal location of lipomas and may also explain spinal lipoma without dysraphism (Lee et al. 1995; Ammerman et al. 1976). Growth of lipoma displaces the normal spinal cord laterally and thus lipoma was located between dorsal roots.

The second hypothesis is "metaplasia theory". Connective tissue metaplasia may lead to deposition of fat within the dura (Ammerman et al. 1976). The third theory is "hamartomatous origin theory". The fat tissue can include peripheral nerve twig, dermoid cyst, skeleton muscle and lymphoid or renal tissue, which originate from ectoderm or mesoderm (Ammerman et al. 1976; Li et al. 2001). The fourth hypothesis is that adipocytes could arise from cells giving rise to the spinal vessels. In normal conditions, mesenchymal cells form the spinal vessels and these cells are perverted from forming adipocyte cells. However, if neural crest cells are defective, the inhibition fails and mesenchymal cells form adipocytes (Catala 1997). All of these share some basic aspects but none fully explain the exact genesis of the spinal lipoma. However, the "developmental error theory" is commonly accepted.

Pathology

Intradural spinal lipoma characteristically presents soft, yellow, fusiform tumor which seems to be intimately attached to the posterior aspect of the spinal cord. It is covered by pia mater or capsula. In general no plane cleavage can be found due to the involvement of several spinal cord segments (Sanli et al. 2010). Histologically, cells appear large, regular, polygonal, radiculated and optically empty with delicate cytoplasmic membranes and an unremarkable, eccentric nucleus consists with mature fat (Liebeskind et al. 1974). These cells are part of the body fat pool and may increase along with other fat deposits during periods of fat deposition.

In general, lipomas of the spinal canal are a mixture of highly vascularized lobulated fatty tissue that consist of mature fat cells separated by delicate connective tissue and interposed in the neural tissue (Lee et al. 1995). The nerve bundles are located predominantly at the periphery of specimens. This finding suggested secondary entrapment of adjacent nerve roots by the lipoma (Ammerman et al. 1976).

Most intradural lipoma of the cervicothoracic spinal cord are either intramedullar or subpial localization, whereas only one case is described as extramedullar location (Sanli et al. 2010). Microscopically, subpial lipomas represent either a benign neoplasm or hamartoma although their growth pattern suggests a true neoplasm (Khanna et al. 1999). Unless unusual components such as teratomas or dermoid cysts are immersed in a lipoma, these processes do not contain neoplastic cells or cysts which may grow. Some authors believe that spinal lipomas may be classified under hamartomas rather than true neoplasm because of their association with other malformations such as spina bifida and the histological evidence. Pathology of lipomas shows no evidence of malignancy or dedifferentiation (Lee et al. 1995).

Clinical Presentation

Non-dysraphic cervicothoracic lipomas are almost always completely have intradural localization, and such lipomas may also have intracranial extension into the posterior fossa (Sanli et al. 2010). The common characteristics of these patients are severe neurological dysfunction (mostly quadriparesis) and have no association with spinal dysraphism.

Spinal lipomas have been noted to become symptomatic, primarily during the first 5 years of life (Ehni and Love 1945; Giuffre 1966). Males and females are both equally affected. The typical neurological manifestation of this condition is a slowly progressive course of spastic paresis and pain (Giuffre 1966; Klekamp et al. 2001). Also, presenting with growth retardation, dysphagia, respiratory difficulty, sensory disturbance, gait problems and scoliosis have been described (Kai et al. 2003; Kogler et al. 1998; Naim-Ur-Rahman et al. 2006). It is postulated that slow growth of the lipoma allows accommodation within the spinal canal without compromise of function until a point is reached where further growth causes a rapid decline in function (Lee et al. 1995).

To our knowledge, Table 25.1 summarizes the various types of intradural lipomas found in the cervicothoracic spinal canal of 41 pediatric patients published between 1925 and 2010.

Diagnostic Studies

Plain Radiography

Vertebra plain radiographs can frequently be normal, but sometimes may show widening of the spinal canal, scalloping of the vertebral bodies, or destruction of the pedicle (Kogler et al. 1998). These findings can indicate a mass lesion, but are not specific for lipoma. Myelography is now rarely performed but will show a complete or partial block in the flow of contrast within the subarachnoid space (Liebeskind et al. 1974).

Computed Tomography

Spinal computed tomography (CT) scan can detect spinal cord lipomas as low-density mass lesions. Because of the low attenuation values of the lipomas (−70 to −130 Hounsfield Units), CT scan appearances are quite characteristic and diagnostic. A non-contrast CT scan allows definite diagnosis of these lesions because of low fat density (Naim-Ur-Rahman et al. 2006). Being quick and cost effective, CT scan can be used as a screening test whenever a spinal lipoma is suspected.

Magnetic Resonance Imaging

Spinal magnetic resonance imaging (MRI) is the investigation of choice because of the characteristic MRI appearance of fat and the significant delineation of the lesion and the surrounding soft tissue, neural structures and subcutaneous planes. Whole neuroaxis screening is mandatory in all cases of spinal dysraphism and in intradural lipamatous lesion, whenever suspected. Due to high proportion of fat, there is a short T1 relaxation time. Thus, lipomas have characteristic hyperintense appearances on T1 weighted images (T1WI). On T2 weighted images fat is hypointense or hyperintense. High T1 signal changes can also be seen in methemoglobin and sometimes in high protein containing structure and some stages of calcification (Kamel et al. 1999). Fat is distinguished by using the fat suppression effect from other lesions that are also hyperintense on T1 weighted images. In such cases, the high signal will characteristically drop when the fat suppression effect is added to the imaging sequence (Beall et al. 2007). Benign lipomas have relaxation parameters similar to those of subcutaneous fat. Liposarcomas and other fat related tumors have longer T1 relaxation times, rendering them less intense than subcutaneous

Table 25.1 Presented cases of pediatric intradural lipoma of the cervicothoracic spinal cord

Author and year	Age, sex	Presenting symptom	Location	Vertebra level	Surgery	Outcome
Elsberg (1925)	11 year, F	Paraparesis	Intradural	C8-T2	N/A	Slight improvement
Caram et al. (1957)	15 year, F	Paraparesis	Intramedullar	C5-T3	Biopsi	No change
Beaudoing et al. (1966)	6 month, F	Quadriparesis	Intradural	C1-2	N/A	Functional improvement
Hubert et al. (1972)	16 year, M	Arm paresis	Intradural	C1-4	N/A	Died
Rappaport et al. (1982)	4 month, M	Quadriparesis	Intradural	Post. fossa-cervical cord	Subtotal	Died
	10 month, F	Quadriparesis	Infilitrates SC	Post. fossa-cervical cord	Subtotal	Functional improvement
White and Fraser (1983)	11 year, F	Quadriparesis	Subpial	Post. fossa-T2	Subtotal	No change
de la Cruz and Pascual (1985)	14 month, F	Quadriparesis	Intramedullar	Cervical cord	Partial	Died
Wood et al. (1985)	5 month, M	Spastic paraparesis + HCP	Subpial	Post. fossa-T2	Subtotal	No change
	15 year, F	Back pain	Infilitrates SC	C3-T6	Subtotal	No change
Mori et al. (1986)	7 year, M	Quadriparesis	Subpial	Foramen magnum-C7	Subtotal	Slight improvement
Fan et al. (1989)	18 year, M	Quadriparesis + HCP	Subdural	Foramen magnum - C5	Subtotal	Functional improvement
Tsuchiya et al. (1989)	18 year, M	Paraparesis	Subpial	C5-T1	Biopsi	Functional improvement
Amormarn et al. (1992)	18 month, M	Apnea	Intradural	Post. fossa-cervical cord	Subtotal	No change
Donati et al. (1992)	2 year, M	Hypertonia	Intradural	Post. fossa-cervical cord	Subtotal	Slight improvement
Crols et al. (1993)	17 year, M	Spastic quadriparesis	Intramedullar	Post. fossa-cervical cord	Subtotal	Slight improvement
Naim-ur-Rahman et al. (1994)	9 month, F	Spastic quadriparesis	Intramedullar	Post. fossa-cervical cord	Subtotal	No change
Lee et al. (1995)	8 year, M	Quadriparesis	Intramedullar	C1-C7	Subtotal	Functional improvement
Wilson et al. (1996)	2.5 month, F	Quadriparesis	Intramedullar	Post. fossa-cervical cord	Partial	Functional improvement
Chaskis et al. (1997)	3 month, F	Quadriparesis	Intramedullar	Post. fossa-cervical cord	Subtotal	No change
Kogler et al. (1998)	2 year, M	Incidental	Intramedullar	Post. fossa-T4	Subtotal	Functional improvement

Plaza et al. (1999)	10day, M	Unilateral brachial plexus palsy	Intramedullar	C3-T3	Subtotal	Progression after surgery
LeFeuvre (2004)	18 year, F	Quadriparesis	Intradural	Post. fossa-cervical cord	Subtotal	Functional improvement
Castilla et al. (2002)	10 year, F	Cervical pain	Intradural	C7-T1	Partial	No change
Kai et al. (2003)	8 month, F	Quadriparesis + disphagia	Intramedullar	Post. fossa-cervical cord	Partial	Functional improvement
Kim et al. (2003)	6 month, F	Hemiparesis	Intramedullar	Foramen magnum-T1	Subtotal	Functional improvement
	7 month, M	Incidental	Subpial	T9-T12	Subtotal	No change
	12 year, M	Hemiparesis	Intramedullar	C6-T11	Subtotal	No change
Bhatoe et al. (2005)	6 year, M	Quadriparesis	Intramedullar	Post. fossa-cervical cord	Partial	No change
Naim-ur-Rahman et al. (2006)	3 year, F	Quadriparesis + respiratory difficulty	Intramedullar	Post. fossa-T3	Subtotal	Functional improvement
Muthusubramaniam et al. (2008)	16 year, M	Quadriparesis	Intramedullar	Post. fossa-cervical cord	Subtotal	Functional improvement
Chagla et al. (2008)	17 year, M	Quadriparesis	Intramedullar	Post. fossa-cervical cord	Subtotal	Functional improvement
Moghaddam et al. (2008)	18 year, F	Upper extremity paraparesis	Intradural	C3	Subtotal	Functional improvement
Mengual et al. (2009)	16 year, M	Hemiparesis	Intradural	Post. fossa-cervical cord	Subtotal	No change
Sanli (2010)	12 year, F	Quadriparesis	extramedullar	Post. fossa-T2	Partial	No change
Fleming et al. (2010)	2 month, M	Hemiparesis	Intramedullar	C2-T8	Partial	Functional improvement
	13 month, F	Incidental	Intramedullar	Foramen magnum-T1	Partial	No change
	2 year, F	Quadriparesis	Intramedullar	C7-T10	Biopsi	Functional improvement
	2 year, F	Hemiparesis	Intramedullar	C5-T8	Partial	Functional improvement
	4 year, M	Quadriparesis	Intramedullar	C7-T6	Partial	Functional improvement
Kabir et al. (2010)	17 year, F	Hemiparesis	Subpial	T2-T6	Subtotal	Functional improvement

fat on T1WI (Ehni and Love 1945; Patwardhan et al. 2000). Intraoperative ultrasonography can be very useful in confirming proper localization before the opening of dura. Intramedullary tumors such as astrocytomas and ependymomas are differential diagnoses, but their MRI appearances are quite different, with high intensity on T2WI and low intensity on T1WI and variable enhancement following contrast administration. The diagnosis of lipoma is, therefore, relatively easy with neuroradiological methods.

Managements

Conservative Treatment

Optimum management of these lesions remains controversial and there have been wide variations in their management; ranging from strict diet control to aggressive total removal of the lesion (Iwatsuki 2006). The fat of the lipoma is metabolically similar to body fat, so that some authors advocate weight loss and strict diet control. Endoh et al. (1998) and Akyuz et al. (2005) reported that lipoma may shrink spontaneously with loss of general body fat. But rapid growth was also possible despite scrupulous diet control (Aoki 1990). Thus, in patients with asymptomatic compression have no diagnosis, neurological function may be deteriorated during nonsurgical therapy.

Surgical Treatment

The operative management of the intradural lipoma involves histological diagnosis, preservation of neurological function, adequately neural decompression and maintenance of spinal stability. The need for prophylactic surgery in asymptomatic patients, especially in pediatric cases, has been a matter of debate. Most of the authors concur that prophylactic surgery for asymptomatic patients is not recommended for intradural spinal lipomas due to the benign course of such lesions. However, early surgery may prevent the deterioration of a permanent neurological deficit in symptomatic patients.

Surgical decompression is indicated for patients with severe compression of the spinal cord.

Arresting the progression of symptoms is a principle surgical goal for intradural lipomas. Kabir et al. (2010) reported a guideline for the management of intradural spinal lipomas:

1. Asymptomatic patients, patients with local symptoms only, e.g., pain and no neurological signs and symptoms, can be managed conservatively with regular clinical and radiological monitoring.
2. In obese patients, weight loss should be advocated.
3. Any patient with worsening or intractable local symptoms or onset of any neurological symptom or signs or having bowel or bladder symptoms should be considered for surgery. This is because in these patients a point may have been reached when the spinal cord cannot accommodate any more and there is no longer any physiological reserve. Neurological dysfunction than rapidly manifests itself unless decompression is done.
4. The aim of surgery should be decompression with preservation of neurological function.
5. The percentage of tumor debulked does not necessarily correlate with the clinical outcome. Good outcome has been reported with laminectomy and biopsy alone.
6. Aggressive debulking should therefore not to be attempted.
7. Duroplasty should be considered if primary dural closure without tension is not possible.
8. Further debulking may be considered if primary patients continue to deteriorate during follow-up.

Position, Incision and Spine Exposure

Intradural lipomas are almost always approached through a laminectomy exposure with the patient in the prone position. For cervical tumors the head is generally secured using a three-point clamp affixed to the skull. Because the skin and soft tissues typically appear normal, localization can be challenging. It is often useful to place a vitamin E capsule on the skin at the time the MRI is performed to allow skin marking for incision planning. Alternately intraoperative preincision plain X-ray films may be obtained and compared with preoperative images position of the incision optimally. Once the midline incision is made, a midline approach and subperiosteal dissection is carried out to free the muscle and soft tissue from the spinous process and lamina. The number of lamina removed depends on the size of the underlying lesion.

Dural Sac Decompression (Laminectomy)

The goal of the laminectomy is to achieve adequate visualization for decompression and to maintain spinal stability. Many neurosurgeons suggested that laminoplasty is less likely to cause a deformity than laminectomy, whereas other neurosurgeons have not been convinced of superiorly of laminoplasty. Laminectomy or laminoplasty both are preferred. In particular, laminectomy may provide better decompression and have a high success rate for neurological improvement (Papagelopoulos et al. 1997).

Few techniques may be used to remove the lamina; and whatever technique used, great care must be taken not to compress the underlying dura or neural tissue. First, many neurosurgeons use a high-speed drill to thin the lamina, then the very thin remaining lamina can be peeled from the dura with curette or a very small angled Kerrison rongeur. Second, a rongeur can be used to thin the lamina while avoiding the placement of the jaw beneath the lamina. Especially, the jaws are biting parallel to the dura mater and do not compress the underlying dura and neural tissue. The laminectomy should be begun from midline to lateral direction (to a line between lamina and facet joint) and from spinous process to ligamentum flavum.

The second stage of the laminectomy is the removal of the ligamentum flavum. After the duramater can just be seen through this longitudinal cut, a blunt instrument such as the tip of a dissector or nerve hook can be placed into this longitudinal division in the ligamentum flavum to further enlarge this opening in the direction of the fibers. After this vertical incision in the ligament has made, an angled Kerrison rongeur can be used to cut the remaining ligament, where it attaches to the lamina above and below (Fig.25.1-*left*).

Dural Opening and Tumor Resection

After laminas are removed, dural opening with vertical incision and retention sutures are placed and the lipoma is inspected under operating microscope (Fig. 25.1-*middle*). Larger tumors or those with a well-defined capsule may be needed internal debulking. Dissection planes around the tumor are sought microsurgically and, if found, are extended gradually around the tumor surface, because removal of the central tumor bulk [by CO_2 laser, the combination of bipolar cautery and suction, or cavitron ultrasonic aspirator (CUSA)] causes the tumor to collapse. Especially, bipolar coagulation should be kept to minimum. Normal cord structures must not be exposed to the heat of bipolar coagulation. It should be used strictly for tumor vessels. Vessels around the lipoma should be left untouched. In addition, The CUSA was found to be very helpful in debulking; also laser with its selective fat melting and evaporating properties has proved to be an another effective tool for this purpose. Infiltrate lipomas with poorly defined dissection planes can not be removed completely and biopsy is often the safest course action.

If the lipoma is located intramedullary, it may entirely be covered by normal spinal cord tissue and expand the spinal cord. Myelotomy must be made through the thinnest area of spinal cord tissue overlying the lipoma. A smaller number of intramedullary lipoma have a large dorsally exophytic component that was entirely covered by pia mater. When there is an exophytic component to the lipoma, maximum safe debulking is performed to preserve neurologic function (Sanli et al. 2010).

Subpial lipomas may be appeared encapsulated by a fine membrane which is continuous

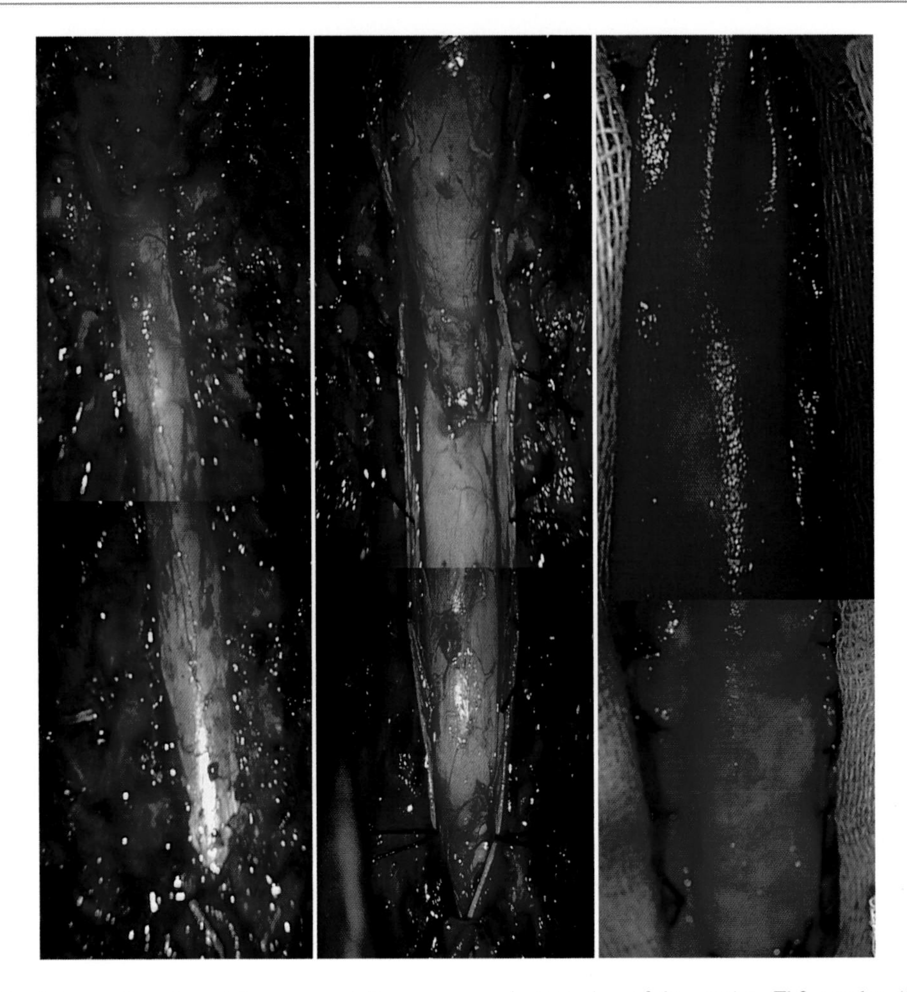

Fig. 25.1 Intraoprative view of the extramedullar cervicothoracic lipoma with intracranial extension. *Left*, surgical field after total laminectomy from occipital craniectomy (*top* of the page) to Th2 vertebra (*bottom*). *Middle*, operating microscopic view after opening the dura. *Right*, dural closure with duraplasty

pia mater of cord and the upper and the lower poles of the tumor can be separated from the cord over short lengths, whereas the superior and inferior tips of lipoma are well demarcated, but no definite plane or cleavage may be found. Moreover, the dorsal aspect of the cord is most frequently involved, but rarely there is extension to the lateral or anterolateral aspect of the cord (Sanli et al. 2010).

Dural Closure (Duraplasty)

The most important aspect after adequate tumor decompression is the closure of the dura to avoid cerebrospinal fluid (CSF) leakage. Sufficient excision of the tumor must be achieved to attain lax dural closure. The duramater must be closed primarily, if possible may be closed with interrupted, running or locking sutures (Fig.25.1-*right*).

If direct suturing is not possible, a fascial graft, cadaveric dura, bovine pericardium or other artificial dural substitutions may be used for this purpose. In addition, it is important to repair any dural tears to reducing the complication of CSF fistula. Several authors have emphasized the importance of water-tight reconstruction of the dura using a graft if necessary, and to make absolutely sure there is no impinging or constriction on the underlying neural tissue during dural or overlying muscle closure (La Marca et al. 1997; Mclone 1996). If suturing is not possible because of the location of the tear, a piece of fascia or muscle and fibrin glue may be used. Mclone (1996) highlighted the importance of supporting dural closure by establishing a secondary barrier with the overlying muscle and fascia. He also recommended a suturing technique to compress the skin and subcutaneous tissue against the paraspinous muscle to obliterate the space between the two.

Outcome

Based on our review of the literature, bony decompression and biopsy or subtotal resection may have satisfactory results. Aggressive debulking is not to be attempted. Because these tumors may lack a plane of cleavage and encase the neural tissues, total resection will result in unacceptable deficits. The dangers of total removal have long been recognized.

Elsberg (1925) discussed the dangers of total removal of these lesions with the description of a disastrous postoperative quadriplegia. In Ammerman's series (1976), the two patients who underwent total removal developed postoperative paraplegia. The other five patients who had a biopsy or subtotal removal either improved or had minimal deterioration. In the series of six patients described by Lee et al. (1995), who underwent 70% resection deteriorated neurologically during the immediate postoperative period. In contrast the patient who had 40% resection had neurological improvement postoperatively. Both these papers show that the degree of resection is not directly related to postoperative outcome. On the other hand, functional improvement was accomplished in less than 50% in all reported cervical lipomas with intracranial extension (Sanli et al. 2010). Aggressive resection is almost always associated with significant morbidity. Many surgeons advocate doing a decompression and wide dural opening and only biopsy (Foster 1966; Swanson and Barnett 1962).

Complications

Immediate Complications

In the literature despite the neurological complications, such complications range between 0%and 56% (average 25%) and are most commonly surgical hematoma infection, wound breakdown, CSF leakage and subcutaneous pseudomeningocele (Pierre-Kahn et al. 1997). CSF leakage is a well known complication at this surgery and in the literature rates as high as 20% have been reported with many patients requires an additional surgical procedure to repair the dura.

Late Complications

Delayed deformities such as cervical kyphosis, anterior subluxation, disabling scoliosis as a consequence of laminectomy have been reported. The incidence of deformity after multilevel laminectomy is related to the patient's age and spinal level of the laminectomy. In childhood, the incidence of spinal deformity following cervical laminectomy is higher than in adulthood (Yeh et al. 2001). The most important rationale for a laminoplasty is the preservation of spinal alignment. For avoiding postoperative cervical deformity, immobilization with a cervical collar for younger patients should be recommended for 3–6 months after multilevel laminectomy and serial x-rays of cervical spine. Spinal deformity following a multilevel laminectomy in the thoracic spine is rare. In conclusion, because the natural history of a lipoma in the cervical region is unknown, surgery for all types of lipoma may be recommended due to the progressive neurological symptoms. Surgery for these lesions may be limited to decompressive laminectomy and duraplasty if necessary. Even after adequate decompression these lesions may have a poor prognosis.

References

Akyuz M, Goksu E, Tuncer R (2005) Spontaneous decrease in the size of a residual thoracic intradural lipoma. Br J Neurosurg 19:53–55

Ammerman BJ, Henry JM, De Girolami U, Earle KM (1976) Intradural lipomas of the spinal cord: a clinicopathological correlation. J Neurosurg 44:331–336
Amormarn R, Faillace WJ, Clayman DM, Lu L, Prempree TJ (1992) Lipoma of cervical spinal cord and posterior, or fossa: case report. J Fla Med Assoc 79:27–30
Aoki N (1990) Rapid growth of intraspinal lipoma demonstrated by magnetic resonance imaging. Surg Neurol 34:107–110
Beall DP, Googe DJ, Emery RL, Thompson DB, Campbell SE, Ly JQ, DeLone D, Smirniotopoulos J, Lisanti C, Currie TJ (2007) Extramedullary intradural spinal tumors: a pictorial review. Curr Probl Diagn Radiol 36:185–198
Beaudoing A, Butin LP, Fischer G, Jaillard M, Bost M (1966) Subdural spinal lipomas in infants. Pediatrie 21:909–916
Bhatoe HS, Singh P, Chaturvedi A, Sahai K, Dutta V, Sahoo PK (2005) Nondysraphic intramedullary spinal cord lipomas: a review. Neurosurg Focus 18:ECP1
Blount JP, Elton S (2001) Spinal lipomas. Neurosurg Focus 10:e3
Caram PC, Scarcella G, Carton CA (1957) Intradural lipomas of the spinal cord; with particular emphasis on the "intramedullary" lipomas. J Neurosurg 14:28–42
Castilla JM, Martín-Velasco V, Rodríguez-Salazar A (2002) Intradural cervical lipoma without neurologic involvement; report of a case. Neurocirugia 13:54–58
Catala M (1997) Embryogenesis. Why do we need a new explanation for the emergence of spina bifida with lipoma? Childs Nerv Syst 13:336–340
Chagla AS, Balasubramanian S, Goel AH (2008) A massive cervicomedullary intramedullary spinal cord lipoma. J Clin Neurosci 15:817–820
Chaskis C, Michotte A, Gefray F, Vangeneugden J, Desprechins B, D'haens J (1997) Cervical intramedullary lipoma with intracranial extension in an infant. J Neurosurg 87:472
Crols R, Appel B, Klaes R (1993) Extensive cervical intradural and intramedullary lipoma and spina bifida occulta of C1: a case report. Clin Neurol Neurosurg 95:39–43
de la Cruz MM, Pascual CI (1985) Cervical intra-spinal cord lipoma in a 14-month-old girl. An Esp Pediatr 23:211–214
Donati F, Vassella F, Kaiser G, Blumberg A (1992) Intracranial lipomas. Neuropediatrics 23:32–38
Ehni G, Love JG (1945) Intraspinal lipomas: Report of cases, review of the literature, and clinical and pathologic study. Arch Neurol Psychiatry 53:1–28
Elsberg C (1925) In: Tumors of the spinal cord and the symptoms of irritation and compression of the spinal cord and nerve roots: pathology, symptomatology, diagnosis, and treatment, 1st edn. B. Paul Hoeber Inc, New York, pp 310–315
Endoh M, Iwasaki Y, Koyanagi I, Hida K, Abe H (1998) Spontaneous shrinkage of lumbosacral lipoma in conjunction with a general decrease in body fat: case report. Neurosurgery 43:150–151
Fan CF, Veerapen RJ, Tan CT (1989) Case report: subdural spinal lipoma with posterior fossa extension. Clin Radiol 40:91–94
Fleming KL, Davidson L, Gonzalez-Gomez I, McComb JG (2010) Nondysraphic pediatric intramedullary spinal cord lipomas: report of 5 cases. J Neurosurg Pediatr 5:172–178
Foster JJ (1966) Spinal intradural lipomas. A neurosurgical dilemma. Int Surg 46:480–486
Giuffrè R (1966) Intradural spinal lipomas: review of the literature (99cases) and report of an additional case. Acta Neurochir 14:69–95
Hubert JP, Monseu G, Stoupel N, Flament-Durand J (1972) Spinal lipoma. Anatomoclinical study. Acta Neurol Belg 72:338–346
Iwatsuki K (2006) Intradural cervical lipoma with parenchymal marginal fibrous tissue: case report. Neurosurgery 59:E208
Kabir SM, Thompson D, Rezajooi K, Casey AT (2010) Non-dysraphic intradural spinal cord lipoma: case series, literature review and guidelines for management. Acta Neurochir 152:1139–1144
Kai Y, Amano T, Inamura T, Matsushima T, Takamatsu M, Kai E, Fukui M (2003) An infant with an intradural lipomaof the cervical spine extending into the posterior fossa. J Clin Neurosci 10:127–130
Kamel HA, Brennan PR, Farrell MA (1999) Cervical epidural lipoblastomatosis: changing MR appearance after chemotherapy. Am J Neuroradiol 20:386–389
Khanna G, Mishra K, Agarwal S, Sharma S (1999) Congenital spinal lipomas-tumor versus hamartoma. Indian J Pediatr 66:940–944
Kim CH, Wang KC, Kim SK, Chung YN, Choi YL, Chi JG, Cho BK (2003) Spinal intramedullary lipoma: report of three cases. Spinal Cord 41:310–315
Klekamp J, Fusco M, Samii M (2001) Thoracic intradural extramedullary lipomas. Report of three cases and review of the literature. Acta Neurochir 143:767–773
Kogler A, Orsolic K, Kogler V (1998) Intramedullary lipoma of dorsocervicothoracic spinal cord with intracranial extension and hydrocephalus. Pediatr Neurosurg 28:257–260
La Marca F, Grant JA, Tomita T, McLone DG (1997) Spinal lipomas in children: outcome of 270 procedures. Pediatr Neurosurg 26:8–16
Lee M, Rezai AR, Abbott R, Coelho DH, Epstein FJ (1995) Intramedullary spinal cord lipomas. J Neurosurg 82:394–400
LeFeuvre DEJ, Semple PL, Peter JC (2004) Intradural cervical lipomas with intracranial extension: a managment strategy based on a case report and review of the literature. Br J Neurosurg 18:387–388
Li YC, Shin SH, Cho BK, Lee MS, Lee YJ, Hong SK, Wang KC (2001) Pathogenesis of lumbosacral lipoma: a test of the "premature dysjunction" theory. Pediatr Neurosurg 34:124–130
Liebeskind AL, Azar-Kia B, Batnitzky S, Schechter MM (1974) Intraspinal lipomas. Neuroradiology 7:198–200
Mclone DG (1996) Lipomyelomeningocele In: Cheek WR (ed) Atlas of pediatric neurosurgery, 1st edn. W.B. Saunders, Philadelphia, pp 11–15
Mengual MV, Lloret PM, Gonzalez AL, Simal JA, Garijio JAA (2009) Spinal cord lipoma without dysraphism in

the infancy that extends intracranially. Case report and rewiew of the literature. Surg Neurol 71:613–615

Moghaddam AM, Tanriöver N, Ulu MO, Muhammedrezai S, Akar Z (2008) Cervical intradural lipoma with associated hemivertebra formation at C6 level: a case report. Turk Neurosurg 18:187–190

Mori K, Kamimura Y, Uchida Y, Kurisaka M, Eguchi S (1986) Large intramedullary lipoma of the cervical cord and posterior fossa. Case report. J Neurosurg 64:974–976

Muraszko K (1999) Spinal dysraphism in the adult and pediatric populations. In: Grossman RG (ed) Principles of neurosurgery, 2nd edn. Lippincott-Raven, Philadelphia, pp 59–75

Muthusubramaniam V, Pande A, Vadevan MC, Ramamurth R (2008) Concomitant cervical and lumbar intradural intramedullary lipoma. Surg Neurol 69:314–317

Naim-ur-Rahman N, Salih M, Jamjoom AH, Jamjoom ZA (1994) Congenital intramedullary lipoma of the dorso-cervical spinal cord with intracranial extension: case report. Neurosurgery 34:1081–1083

Naim-ur-Rahman N, Shahat AH, Obaideen AM, Ahmed K, Ahmed S (2006) Intramedullary lipoma of the cervicodorsal spinal cord with intracranial extension: case report. Surg Neurol 65:486–489

Papagelopoulos PJ, Peterson HA, Ebersold MJ, Emmanuel PR, Choudhury SN, Quast LM (1997) Spinal column deformity and instability after lumbar or thoracolumbar laminectomy for intraspinal tumors in children and young adults. Spine 22:442–451

Patwardhan V, Patanakar T, Patkar D, Armao D, Mukherji SK (2000) MR imaging findings of intramedullary lipomas. Am J Roentgenol 174:1792–1793

Pierre-Kahn A, Zerah M, Renier D, Cinalli G, Sainte-Rose C, Lellouch-Tubiana A, Brunelle F, Le Merrer M, Giudicelli Y, Pichon J, Kleinknecht B, Nataf F (1997) Congenital lumbosacral lipomas. Childs Nerv Syst 13:298–334

Plaza MD, Santos J, Monzón L, Díaz P, Hernández J (1999) Cervico-dorsal intramedullary lipoma of neonatal presentation. Rev Neurol 28:483–485

Rappaport ZH, Tadmor R, Brand N (1982) Spinal intradural lipoma with intracranial extension. Childs Brain 9:411–418

Sanli AM, Türkoğlu E, Kahveci R, Sekerci Z (2010) Intradural lipoma of the cervicothoracic spinal cord with intracranial extension. Childs Nerv Syst 26:847–852

Swanson HS, Barnett JC (1962) Intradural lipomas in children. Pediatrics 29:911–926

Tsuchiya K, Michikawa M, Furuya A, Furukawa T, Tsukagoshi H (1989) Intradural spinal lipoma with enlarged intervertebral foramen. J Neurol Neurosurg Psychiatry 52:1308–1310

White RW, Fraser RAR (1983) Cervical spinal cord lipoma with extension into the posterior Fossa. Neurosurgery 12:460–462

Wilson JT, Shapiro RH, Wald SL (1996) Multiple intradural spinal lipomata with intracranial extension. Pediatr Neurosurg 24:5–7

Wood BP, Harwood-Nash DC, Berger P, Goske M (1985) Intradural spinal lipoma of the cervical cord. Am J Roentgenol 145:174–176

Yeh JS, Sgouros S, Walsh AR, Hockley AD (2001) Spinal sagittal malalignment following surgery for primary intramedullary tumours in children. Pediatr Neurosurg 35:318–324

Part VI

Miscellaneous Tumors

Pediatric Embryonal Tumors: Prognostic Role of Cyclin A and B1 Proteins

26

George A. Alexiou, Kalliopi Stefanaki, Amalia Patereli, and Neofytos Prodromou

Contents

Abstract

Embryonal brain tumors account for 20–25% of all brain neoplasms in children and represent the second most frequent group of pediatric brain tumors. Embryonal tumors include medulloblastoma, atypical teratoid/rhabdoid tumor and supratentorial primitive neuroectodermal tumor. These tumors are highly malignant and there is a significant long-term treatment related morbidity. Various biologic parameters have been related to outcome. Cyclins are a group of proteins which are periodically synthesized and degraded during the cell cycle. They affect progression in the cell cycle through activation of cyclin–dependent kinases forming heterodimers. This review focus on the prognostic role of the mytotic cyclins, namely cyclins A and B1, in pediatric embryonal tumors. Based on recent evidence there is a significant expression of cyclin A and cyclin B1 in embryonal tumors, whereas the expression patterns of these cyclins correlate with patient's prognosis.

Introduction

Embryonal brain tumors account for 20–25% of all brain neoplasms in children and represent the second most frequent group of pediatric brain tumors (Alexiou et al. 2011a). Embryonal tumors include medulloblastoma (MB), atypical teratoid/rhabdoid tumor (AT/RT) and supratentorial primitive neuroectodermal tumor (PNET).

G.A. Alexiou (✉) • N. Prodromou
Department of Neurosurgery, Children's Hospital "Agia Sofia", Athens, Greece
e-mail: alexiougrg@yahoo.gr

K. Stefanaki • A. Patereli
Department of Pathology, Children's Hospital "Agia Sofia", Athens, Greece

M.A. Hayat (ed.), *Pediatric Cancer, Volume 3: Diagnosis, Therapy, and Prognosis*, Pediatric Cancer 3,
DOI 10.1007/978-94-007-4528-5_26,

MB constitutes 40% of all cerebellar neoplasms; the most common brain tumor among children. The annual incidence of MB is approximately 0, 5/100,000 children younger than 15 years, with 70% of the tumors occurring in individuals less than 16 years. Nearly 75% of MB arise in the cerebellar vermis projecting in the fourth ventricle like gray/pink soft masses. The group of MB comprises (a) the classical (b) the desmoplastic/nodular (c) the MB with extensive nodularity (d) the anaplastic and (e) the large cell MB. Medullomyoblastoma and melanotic MB were considered patterns of differentiation, without any distinct genetic features to warrant designation as variants. Therefore, the descriptive terms MB with rhabdomyoblastic differentiation and MB with melanotic differentiation are proposed. These tumor usually have a worse prognosis (Alexiou et al. 2011b).

Atypical teratoid/rhabdoid tumors represent 1–2% of pediatric brain tumors and account for at least 10% of central nervous system (CNS) tumors in infants, due to the predominance in children younger than 3 years old. AT/RT is a highly malignant neoplasm, with a male preponderance, typically containing a variable percentage of rhabdoid cells, often composed of primitive neuroectodermal cells and showing divergent differentiation along epithelial, glial, neuronal and mesenchymal-like lines (MacDonald 2008). AT/RT is associated with inactivation of INI1/hSNF5/SMARCB1 gene in almost all cases. AT/RT can be located supratentorialy, especially in cerebral hemispheres and less frequently in the ventricular system, supraselar region and pineal gland. When infratentorial this tumor can be located mainly in the cerebellar hemispheres, the cerellopontine angle and the brain stem mostly in children younger than 2 years of age. No standard or effective therapy has been defined for the most patients (MacDonald 2008).

Central nervous system PNET is a heterogenous group of tumors occurring predominantly in children and adolescents, arising in the cerebral hemispheres, the brain stem and spinal cord. CNS PNETs are composed of undifferentiated or poorly differentiated cells, which may display divergent differentiation along neuronal, glial or ependymal cell lines. Features common to all CNS PNET are early onset and aggressive biological behaviour. Supratentorial PNET is an embryonal tumour composed of undifferentiated or poorly differentiated cells with the capacity for or with differentiation along neuronal, astrocytic, ependymal, muscular and melanocytic cell lines (Eberhart 2011). Tumors with only neuronal differentiation are termed cerebral neuroblastomas and if ganglion cells are also present, cerebral ganglioneuroblastomas.

The prognosis of patients with embryonal tumors has been substantially improved over the last decades (Northcott et al. 2011; de Haas et al. 2008; Patereli et al. 2010; Ellison et al. 2010). Although, stratification of tumors into risk groups based on parameters such as age, extent of disease at the time of diagnosis, and degree of surgical resection has been a major component of treatment for the past two decades, recent studies have identified the prognostic significance of various patterns of pathological and immunohistochemical features, as well as of several biological and clinical markers that hold promise to predict outcome (Northcott et al. 2011; de Haas et al. 2008; Patereli et al. 2010; Ellison et al. 2010). Northcott et al. (2011) reported on four disparate subgroups of MB with distinct demographics, clinical presentation, transcriptional profiles, genetic abnormalities, and clinical outcome. These groups were the WNT (wingless), SHH (sonic hedgehog), group C and group D. These MB subgroups could be reliably identified through immunohistochemistry. Cyclins are proteins controlling elements of the cell cycle. Cyclin overexpression has been reported in several human cancers (Musgrove et al. 2011). This review will focus on the prognostic role of cyclins A and B1 in pediatric embryonal tumors.

Cyclins

Cyclins are a group of proteins which are periodically synthesized and degraded during the cell cycle. They affect progression in the cell cycle through activation of cyclin–dependent kinases (CDKs) forming heterodimers. The CDKs are serine–threonine protein kinases and serve as the catalytic subunits of these heterodimers. CDKs themselves are regulated through association with several tumor suppressor gene products such as $p16^{INK4a}$, $p21^{WAF1}$ and $p27^{KIP1}$ (Tarn and Lai 2011). There are also proteins which are biochemically homologous to cyclins but are not associated with CDKs and CDKs which are not activated by cyclins.

The levels of CDKs remain constant through the cell cycle. However, the expression of cyclins varies during the cell cycle (Coqueret 2002). In mammalian cells, the cyclins can be divided into the G1 cyclins (D-type cyclins D1, D2, D3 and cyclin E), the S phase cyclins (cyclins A and E), and the mitotic cyclins (cyclins A and B). Accordingly, the cyclin-dependent kinases can be grouped in relation to their roles in the various phases of the cell cycle, that is, the G1 CDKs (CDK4, CDK6, and CDK2), the S phase CDKs (CDK2), and the M phase CDKs (CDK2 and CDK1) (Ivanchuk and Rutka 2004). Cyclins are important for the development and progression of several cancers including those of the breast, oesophagus, brain, bladder and lung. Cyclin D1 is overexpressed in breast, liver, lung and brain cancers (Musgrove et al. 2011). A growing body of evidence indicated that decreased p-27 expression and overexpression of G1 Cyclins, Cyclin D3 and Cyclin E, are correlated with aggressive histology and adverse prognosis in various malignant neoplasms (Lloyd et al. 1999). In medulloblastoma, Mendrzyk et al. (2005) reported that CDK6, which is activated by binding to D-type cyclins, proved to be a molecular marker that may facilitate the prognostic assessment of MB patients. Low levels of p-27 were associated with poor prognosis in gliomas. In MB p-27 level of expression may also have prognostic value (Adesina et al. 2000).

Cyclins A and B1

Cyclins A and B are known as mitotic cyclins. The complex cyclin-A-CDK2 is required for S phase progression and is important for the initiation and the maintenance of DNA synthesis. Cyclin B-CDC2 complex is required for entry into M-phase. Cells with a suppressed cyclin B1/CDC2 activity would be arrested in the G2 phase, whereas elevated cyclin B1/CDC2 activity favors mitosis entrance (Wang et al. 2000). Immunohistochemical overexpression of cyclins A and B1 in Hodgkin and Reed-Sternberg cells has been demonstrated to be a common feature of most classical Hodgkin lymphomas (Bai et al. 2004). Regarding cyclin A expression in brain tumors, Nakabayashi et al. demonstrated a significant difference between meningioma grades and cyclin A labeling indices. A linear positive correlation between the cyclin A labeling index and bromodeoxyuridine labeling index was also observed. In the multivariate analysis high cyclin A labeling index was a significant risk factor for meningioma recurrence (Nakabayashi et al. 2003) (Fig. 26.1).

In mammals two cyclin B proteins are found, B1 and B2 that associate with CDC2 and are essential components of the cell cycle regulatory machinery. Cyclin B1 is translocated to the nucleus from the cytoplasm, and has a pivotal role in cell proliferation since it governs entry into mitosis by regulating the G2/M checkpoint. Cyclin B1 is overexpressed in a variety of cancers compared to normal cells and tissues. Cyclin B1 immunoreactivity may be nuclear or cytoplasmic. In breast cancer only nuclear cyclin B1 was significantly associated with adverse clinical outcome, whereas the multivariate analyses demonstrated nuclear cyclin B1 as an independent marker. Cytoplasmic immunohistochemical expression of cyclin B1 may be a potential prognostic biomarker in squamous cell carcinomas of the head and neck (Hoffmann et al. 2011). The overexpression of cyclin B1 and CDC2 have also been correlated with survival in esophageal squamous cell carcinoma and hepatocellular carcinoma (Ito et al. 2000).

Concerning brain tumors, Allan et al. studied by immunohistochemistry the expression of cyclin A, B1 and Ki-67 in astrocytomas. The results of the study demonstrated that cyclin A had a good correlation with both astrocytoma grade and Ki-67 index. Both nuclear and cytoplasmic cyclin B1 expression correlated well with tumor grade but

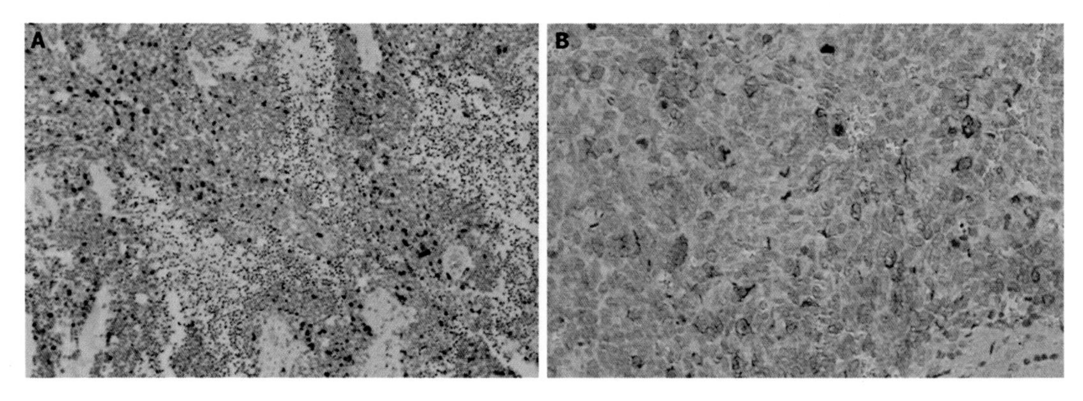

Fig. 26.1 (**a**) Expression of cyclin A in atypical teratoid/rhabdoid tumor (×200). (**b**) Expression of cyclin B1 in atypical teratoid/rhabdoid tumor (×400)

showed poor correlation with Ki-67 index (Allan et al. 2000). Chen et al. reported that high-grade gliomas tended to express higher CDC2/CyclinB1 protein levels than lower grade gliomas. The authors found that inhibition of CDC2 in turns inhibited proliferation of human malignant glioma cells *ex vivo* and suppressed tumor growth *in vivo* (Chen et al. 2008). Regarding embryonal tumors, Moschovi et al. studied the expression of cyclin A and cyclin B1 in resection specimens of 53 pediatric embryonal brain tumors using immunohistochemistry. In this study there were 42 cases of MB, 9 cases of AT/RTs and two cases of PNETs. Cyclin A expression was observed in all patients. Patients with cyclin A index more than 40% were associated with significant poorer survival. Cyclin B1 expression was detected in 62% of patients. In patients with Cyclin B1 index more than 15% there was a trend towards poorer survival (Moschovi et al. 2011). De Haas et al. analyzed immunohistochemically the expression of *MYC*, *LDHB* and *CCNB1* genes in MB patients and found to have a strong prognostic significant. Thus, cyclin B1 gene signature is able to predict survival in medulloblastoma patients (de Haas et al. 2008), On the contrary, Neben et al. found that cyclin B1 expression had no statistical significant effect on survival in medulloblastoma (Neben et al. 2004).

In conclusion, the expression patterns of cyclin A and cyclin B1 show promise for the prognostic assessment of pediatric embryonal tumors. Furthermore, combined with the known molecular and clinical variables, cyclins may provide additional information for patient's risk classification. The role of cyclins A and B1 expression in embryonal tumors thus warrants further investigation.

References

Adesina AM, Dunn ST, Moore WE, Nalbantoglu J (2000) Expression of p27kip1 and p53 in medulloblastoma: relationship with cell proliferation and survival. Pathol Res Pract 196:243–250

Alexiou GA, Moschovi M, Stefanaki K, Sfakianos G, Prodromou N (2011a) Epidemiology of pediatric brain tumors in Greece (1991–2008). Experience from the Agia Sofia Children's Hospital. Cen Eur Neurosurg 72:1–4

Alexiou GA, Stefanaki K, Moschovi M, Sfakianos G, Prodromou N (2011b) A 2 year-old boy with a posterior fossa tumor. Brain Pathol 21:469–472

Allan K, Jordan RC, Ang LC, Taylor M, Young B (2000) Overexpression of cyclin A and cyclin B1 proteins in astrocytomas. Arch Pathol Lab Med 124:216–220

Bai M, Tsanou E, Agnantis NJ, Kamina S, Grepi C, Stefanaki K, Rontogianni D, Galani V, Kanavaros P (2004) Proliferation profile of classical Hodgkin's lymphomas. Increased expression of the protein cyclin D2 in Hodgkin and Reed-Sternberg cells. Mod Pathol 17:1338–1345

Chen H, Huang Q, Dong J, Zhai DZ, Wang AD, Lan Q (2008) Overexpression of CDC2/CyclinB1 in gliomas, and CDC2 depletion inhibits proliferation of human glioma cells in vitro and in vivo. BMC Cancer 8:29

Coqueret O (2002) Linking cyclins to transcriptional control. Gene 299:35–55

de Haas T, Hasselt N, Troost D, Caron H, Popovic M, Zadravec-Zaletel L, Grajkowska W, Perek M, Osterheld MC, Ellison D, Baas F, Versteeg R, Kool M (2008) Molecular risk stratification of medulloblastoma patients based onimmunohistochemical analysis of MYC, LDHB, and CCNB1 expression. Clin Cancer Res 14:4154–4160

Eberhart CG (2011) Molecular diagnostics in embryonal brain tumors. Brain Pathol 21:96–104

Ellison DW, Kocak M, Dalton J, Megahed H, Lusher ME, Ryan SL, Zhao W, Nicholson SL, Taylor RE, Bailey S, Clifford SC (2010) Definition of disease-risk stratification groups in childhood medulloblastoma using combined clinical, pathologic, and molecular variables. J Clin Oncol 29:1400–1407

Hoffmann TK, Trellakis S, Okulicz K, Schuler P, Greve J, Arnolds J, Bergmann C, Bas M, Lang S, Lehnerdt G, Brandau S, Mattheis S, Scheckenbach K, Finn OJ, Whiteside TL, Sonkoly E (2011) Cyclin B1 expression and p53 status in squamous cell carcinomas of the head and neck. Anticancer Res 31:3151–3157

Ito Y, Takeda T, Sakon M, Monden M, Tsujimoto M, Matsuura N (2000) Expression and prognostic role of cyclin-dependent kinase 1 (cdc2) in hepatocellular carcinoma. Oncology 59:68–74

Ivanchuk SM, Rutka JT (2004) The cell cycle: accelerators, brakes, and checkpoints. Neurosurgery 54:692–699

Lloyd RV, Erickson LA, Jin L, Kulig E, Qian X, Cheville JC (1999) p27kip1: a multifunctional cyclin-dependent kinase inhibitor with prognostic significance in human cancers. Am J Pathol 154:313–323

MacDonald TJ (2008) Aggressive infantile embryonal tumors. J Child Neurol 23:1195–1204

Mendrzyk F, Radlwimmer B, Joos S, Kokocinski F, Benner A, Stange DE, Neben K, Fiegler H, Carter NP, Reifenberger G, Korshunov A, Lichter P (2005) Genomic and protein expression profiling identifies CDK6 as novel independent prognostic marker in medulloblastoma. J Clin Oncol 23:8853–8862

Moschovi M, Alexiou GA, Patereli A, Stefanaki K, Doussis-Anagnostopoulou I, Stofas A, Sfakianos G, Prodromou N (2011) Prognostic significance of cyclin A and B1 in pediatric embryonal tumors. J Neurooncol 103:699–704

Musgrove EA, Caldon CE, Barraclough J, Stone A, Sutherland RL (2011) Cyclin D as a therapeutic target in cancer. Nat Rev Cancer 11:558–572

Nakabayashi H, Shimizu K, Hara M (2003) Prognostic significance of cyclin a expression in meningiomas. Appl Immunohistochem Mol Morphol 11:9–14

Neben K, Korshunov A, Benner A, Wrobel G, Hahn M, Kokocinski F, Golanov A, Joos S, Lichter P (2004) Microarray-based screening for molecular markers in medulloblastoma revealed STK15 as independent predictor for survival. Cancer Res 64:3103–3111

Northcott PA, Korshunov A, Witt H, Hielscher T, Eberhart CG, Mack S, Bouffet E, Clifford SC, Hawkins CE, French P, Rutka JT, Pfister S, Taylor MD (2011) Medulloblastoma comprises four distinct molecular variants. J Clin Oncol 29:1408–1414

Patereli A, Alexiou GA, Stefanaki K, Moschovi M, Doussis-Anagnostopoulou I, Prodromou N, Karentzou O (2010) Expression of epidermal growth factor receptor and HER-2 in pediatric embryonal brain tumors. Pediatr Neurosurg 46:188–192

Tarn WY, Lai MC (2011) Translational control of cyclins. Cell Div 6:5

Wang TH, Wang HS, Soong YK (2000) Paclitaxel-induced cell death: where the cell cycle and apoptosis come together. Cancer 88:2619–2628

Intracranial Pediatric Ependymoma: Role of Cytogenetic Markers Using Comparative Genomic Hybridization and Fluorescent *In Situ* Hybridization

27

Annalisa Pezzolo

Contents

A. Pezzolo (✉)
Laboratory of Oncology, Department of Laboratory and Experimental Medicine, Instituto Giannina Gaslini, Largo G. Gaslini, 5, 16147 Genoa, Italy
e-mail: annalisapezzolo@ospedale-gaslini.ge.it

Abstract

Pediatric ependymoma are enigmatic tumors that continue to present a clinical management challenge despite advances in neurosurgery, neuroimaging techniques, and radiation therapy. Difficulty in predicting tumor behavior from clinical and histological factors has shifted the focus to the molecular biology of ependymoma in order to identify new correlates of disease outcome and novel therapeutic targets. The biologic behavior of intracranial ependymoma is unpredictable on the basis of current staging approaches. Patient age at diagnosis and tumor location has also been suggested as prognostic factors. Children below 3 years of age and infratentorial ependymoma have been associated with a poor outcome. Poor outcome and the unpredictable behavior of this tumor in children have turned attention to improving the knowledge of ependymoma biology. Nevertheless, an enhanced understanding of the biology of ependymoma remains crucial if we are to identify additional prognostic markers, discover molecular targets for novel or existing therapeutic agents in the clinic and allow adjuvant therapy to be tailored according to tumor-specific molecular characteristics. Progress in these areas could minimize the long term adverse effects of therapy and improve patient survival. Before the advent of detailed genomic analysis, karyotypic studies had found that pediatric ependymoma showed a spectrum of complexity ranging from single

M.A. Hayat (ed.), *Pediatric Cancer, Volume 3: Diagnosis, Therapy, and Prognosis*, Pediatric Cancer 3,
DOI 10.1007/978-94-007-4528-5_27,

rearrangements to structural and numerical aberrations. The most frequently used technique for high resolution genomic analysis of ependymoma to date has been comparative genomic hybridization (CGH) and fluorescent *in situ* hybridization (FISH). Recently, the advent of array-CGH has enabled the identification of genomic imbalances at a higher resolution than conventional metaphase CGH. Ependymoma with few and often partial chromosomal imbalances may confer a worse prognosis and are more likely to occur in younger children. At present, the explanations for this remain unclear. Genomic aberrations in ependymoma are powerful independent markers of disease progression and survival. By adding genetic markers to established clinical and histopathologic variables, outcome prediction can potentially be improved.

Introduction

Cytogenetics has had considerable impact on many fields of medical and basic sciences, including clinical genetics, hematology, and oncology. There are two major fields where the impact of cancer cytogenetic is highly significant. One is basic cancer research. The identification of chromosomal breakpoints involved in specific chromosome aberrations indicates the role of genes that through rearrangement, alter expression control, or inactivation which are of importance in tumorigenesis. This is often the first step towards the identification of tumor associated genes. The other major application of cytogenetics is in clinical oncology. The type of aberrations found in individual cancer patients may be useful in reaching a diagnosis, prognosis, and in assessing the consequences of therapy (Mitelman et al. 1997). Progress in understanding the clinical significance of cytogenetics in hematologic malignancies was made more quickly than in solid tumors. Nonetheless, in recent years significant progress has been made in solid tumor cytogenetics, and the increase in published solid tumor karyotypes has been significant. In addition to the classic banding techniques, two promising new molecular cytogenetics techniques (at the interface between molecular genetics and cytogenetics approaches) have been developed: fluorescent *in situ* hybridization (FISH) and comparative genomic hybridization (CGH). Both have contributed data that have added significantly to our understanding of cancer genetic mechanisms, and they promise to play an even more relevant role in future investigations. Step-by-step details of these techniques were recently presented by Hayat (2004–2005)

Molecular Cytogenetics Techniques

The FISH technique (Gray and Pinkel 1992) relies on hybridization with probes that identify a specific chromosomal structure (they may, for example, hybridize specifically with satellite centromeric sequences in one particular chromosome pair), unique sequence probes, or probes that react with multiple chromosomal sequences (e.g., chromosome-specific library probes). Chromosome painting with the latter probes may be used to identify structural rearrangements that have given rise to marker chromosomes. Hybridization with centromere-specific probes may be the method of choice to identify numerical chromosome aberrations. FISH is applicable to a variety of specimen types, including fresh or frozen tissues, cytological preparations, and formalin-fixed paraffin embedded (FFPE) tissue. A major advantage of FISH techniques is that they can be applied to both dividing and interphase cells, including archival material. It is possible to combine FISH with immunofluorescence, thus allowing to perform separate counts of immunopositive and negative cells. For example, this approach was required to demonstrate numerical chromosomal alterations in the CD30-positive Reed-Sternberg cells of Hodgkin's lymphoma (Nolte et al. 1996) and to demonstrate that NB associated endothelial micro-vessels can originate from primary NB *MYCN* amplified tumors (Pezzolo et al. 2007).

In comparison to classic metaphase cytogenetic (i.e., karyotyping), FISH has several advantages, first lack of requirements for mitotically active cells. Given that karyotype can be done only with cells capable of proliferating *in vitro*, there can be significant growth selection biases, including overgrowth of non neoplastic elements, particularly when analyzing benign or low-grade neoplasms. An example of this drawback was the virtual absence of any 1p or 19q deletions reported in early karyotypes of oligodendrogliomas, compared with 60–70% losses of these chromosomal arms detected in later studies utilizing loss of heterozygosity (LOH). On the other hand, FISH is not a genomic screening tool, because it is based on more targeted approach for alterations initially identified by global genome assessment by conventional cytogenetic, comparative genomic hybridization (CGH), or gene expression microarray chips.

A number of different probe types are currently available for FISH. Centromere enumerating probes (CEPs) were among the first to be developed and are ideal for detecting whole chromosome gains and losses, such as monosomy, trisomy, and other polysomies. Because these probes target highly repetitive 171 bp sequences of α-satellite DNA, they allow excellent hybridization efficiencies and typically yield large, bright signals. CEPs are very useful for detecting aneusomies, and are still among the best FISH probes available. The presence of similarly repetitive DNA sequences in subtelomeric regions has now led to the development of commercially available telomere probes for each chromosomal arm.

Another chromosome-specific probe is the whole chromosome paint (WCP), in which a cocktail of DNA fragments is created to target all the non repetitive DNA sequences in an entire chromosome. Because these fragments cover such a large region of DNA, they yield more diffuse signals in interphase nuclei and are primarily utilized on metaphase spreads for resolving complex structural alterations. However, some of the smaller, acrocentric chromosomes yield sufficiently discrete signals to permit their enumeration in interphase nuclei. Currently, some of the most versatile and commonly used FISH probes are the locus-specific (LSI) or gene specific probes. As the names imply, these probes target specific regions of interest and utilize single copy rather than repetitive DNA sequences. Therefore, in order to yield signals large enough to be detected in tissue sections, the probe typically needs to be at least 1 Kb in size. The largest FISH probes are often >1 Mb and most are into the 100–300 Kb range. Until recently, commercially available LSI probes have been very limited in scope. Therefore, cloning vectors have been exploited for creating homemade FISH probes, including cosmids, bacterial artificial chromosomes (BACs), P1 artificial chromosomes (PACs), and yeast artificial chromosomes (YACs). Whereas in the past, this required a rather lengthy and tedious screening of vector libraries with PCR primers, the recent human genome initiative and mapping of entire BAC libraries has enabled rapid internet screening, utilizing DNA sequences of interest, gene names, or physical maps of chromosomes (e.g., http://genome.ucsc.edu, http://gdbwww. gdb.org). Similarly, mapped BAC clones spread throughout the human genome at 1-Mb intervals, and have also become available (http://www.resgen.com). Therefore, it is now relatively simple to obtain a BAC clone localizing to virtually any region of interest, label the DNA with commercially available kits, and utilize it as a FISH probe.

A number of FISH protocols have been published and vary depending on individual preferences and specimen type. In general, simple protocols are preferable, because they require less manipulation, have fewer steps in which errors may be introduced, and are easier to troubleshoot. While the FISH protocol itself is often mastered quickly, interpretation of the results still requires specific experience. The major drawbacks are truncation artifacts, aneuploidy, auto fluorescence, and partial hybridization failure. Truncation artifact refers to the underestimation of target copy numbers due to incomplete DNA complements in transected nuclei. Therefore, it is important to include controls cut at the same thickness. We usually set cutoffs for deletion based on median percentages of control nuclei with < 2 signals plus 3 standard deviations. However, a number of other approaches have also been applied and are acceptable.

Aneuploidy and polyploidy are particularly common in malignant neoplasms and can result in confusing hybridization signal counts. The assessment of multiple targets is most informative in such situations. Although the simplest approach is to interpret absolute losses (< 2 copies) and gains (> 2 copies), one may opt to delineate "relative" losses and gains compared with a reference ploidy, obtained either by flow cytometry or the assessment of multiple chromosomes by FISH. For example, the finding of three copies would be considered a relative gain in a diploid tumor, normal in a triploid tumor, and a relative loss in a tetraploid tumor. Lastly, one may combine a centromere and locus-specific probe from a single chromosome and determine their ratios. For example, cells with 4 chromosome 9 centromeres, and two copies of the *p16* region on 9p21 would be interpreted as having polysomy 9 and a hemizygous *p16* deletion. A similar tumor with 4 centromeres and no *p16* signals would be interpreted as polysomy 9 with homozygous *p16* deletion. Similarly, cells with 6 copies of *EGFR* might be interpreted as low-level amplification if there were only 2 chromosome 7 centromeres (Fig. 27.1), but would represent polysomy 7 without gene amplification if there were 6 centromeres.

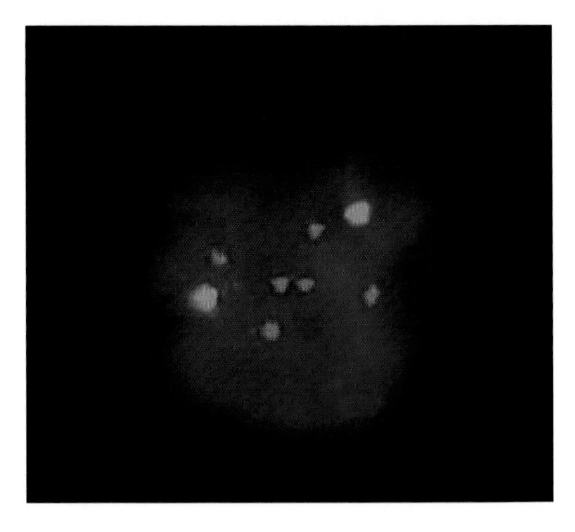

Fig. 27.1 Interphase FISH analysis of an ependymoma specimens with the probe for EGFR gene (*red signal*) and the probe specific for the centromere of chromosome 7 (*green signal*). The EGFR gene probe was labeled directly with TRITC, and the centromere of chromosome 7 probe was labeled directly with FITC. The nucleus was counterstained with DAPI, visualized using a triple-band bypass filter. The presence of 6 copies of *EGFR* gene and 2 chromosome 7 centromeres has been interpreted as a gain

The basic steps of FISH are similar to those of immunohistochemistry and include deparaffinization, pretreatment/target retrieval, denaturation of probe and target DNA, hybridization, post-hybridization washes, detection, and microscopy imaging. This is typically a 2-day assay, which requires roughly 3–4 h the first day and 30 min the second day. Similar to immunohistochemistry, microwave or heat-induced target retrieval often works better than chemical forms of pretreatment and significantly improves hybridization efficiency (Henke and Ayhan 1994). When this step is included, protein digestion may often be reduced or eliminated altogether. Nevertheless, optimal pretreatment and digestion varies from one specimen to another, depending on methods of fixation/processing. Lastly, a variety of amplification steps are available for cases with weak signals. However, we have rarely found this necessary and in our lab, we prefer the simpler protocol and cleaner background associated with directly labeled fluorochrome probes (e.g., FITC, TRITC), in contrast to indirectly labeled probes (e.g., digoxigenin, biotin) that require an additional step (e.g., fluorochrome-labeled secondary antibody) with or without further amplification.

The chromosomal CGH technique is based on the *in situ* hybridization of differently labeled total tumor DNA and normal reference DNA to normal male metaphase chromosomes (Kallionemi et al. 1992). This gives, in a single hybridization, an overview of DNA sequence copy number changes (losses, gains, amplifications) in a tumor specimen. Metaphase spreads are prepared from phytohemaglutinin-stimulated human peripheral blood lymphocytes from a normal healthy male. Test (tumor) DNA and reference (normal) DNA (obtained from lymphocytes of healthy donors) are labeled with different fluorophores, usually test DNA in green and reference DNA in red. These labeled DNAs are co hybridized to target metaphase chromosomes which are prepared from normal lymphocytes and spread on a glass slide. Hybridization is

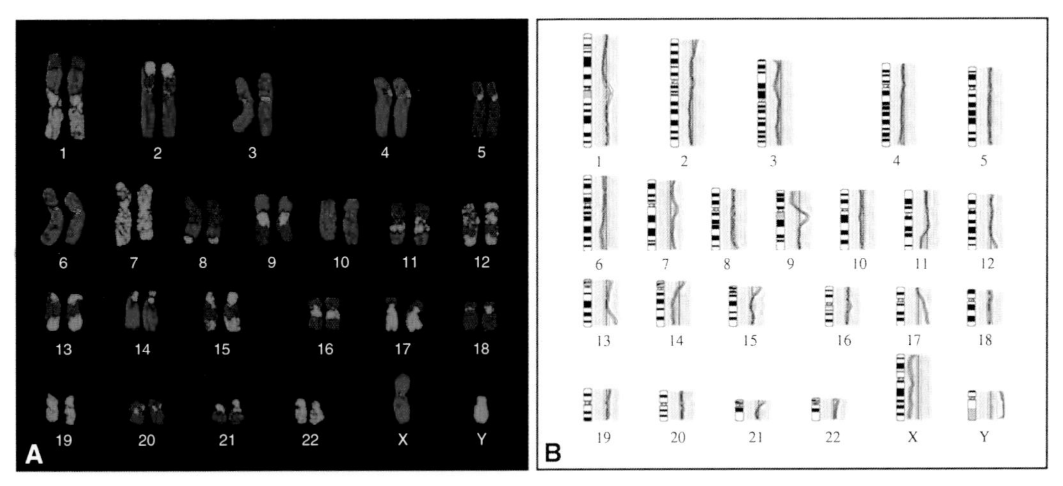

Rev ish enh (1q31.2-qter, 2p23-pter, 7, 8q24, 11q13, 12p13, 12q24, 13q22-qter, 15q23-q26, 17q11.2-qter, 19, 22) dim (1p22-p31, 2p11.2-p21, 2q11.2-qter, 3, 4, 6, 8q22-q23, 9p12-pter, 10, 11q21-qter, 14q11.2-qter, 21q22.1)

Fig. 27.2 Computer analysis of chromosomal CGH images of an ependymoma specimens. (**a**) The image of both *red* and *green* fluorochromes superimposed. Chromosomal regions that appear *green* have an increased in DNA copy number in the tumor compared to normal, whereas those that are *red* have a decrease number compared to normal. The *blue* areas represent chromosomal segments in which the DNA copy numbers are the same between the samples. (**b**) The final ratio profile is computed as the karyotype is being processed. Values to the left of the *black center line* indicate loss, whereas those to the *right* indicate gains. It can be seen from this profile that extra copies of chromosomes 1q31.2-qter, 2p23-pter, 7, 8q24, 11q13, 12p13, 12q13, 12q24, 13q22-qter, 15q23-q26, 17q11.2-qter, 19, 22; and deletions of chromosomes 1p22-p31, 2p11.2-p21, 2q11.2-qter, 3, 4, 6, 8q22-q23, 9p12-pter, 10, 11q21-qter, 14q11.2-qter, 21q22.1 are present in the tumor

captured under the fluorescence microscope and the ratio of the intensity of the green to the red fluorescence is analyzed along the axis of each chromosome with computer software. The ratio is higher than 1.0 in the region where the tumor has an increased number of DNA copies, and lower than 1.0 in the region where the tumor has a decreased number of DNA copies compared with normal DNA. The result may be seen as differential fluorescence staining of normal metaphase chromosomes with the intensity or color of the hybridization signals on particular chromosomes or chromosomal segments paralleling the copy number in the tumor (Fig. 27.2). If DNA is amplified in the green-labeled tumor DNA, more green-label than red-label will hybridize to homologous sites in the normal metaphase. If DNA is deleted in tumor less green signal will hybridize. The principal disadvantages compared with banding cytogenetic are that CGH gives no information about balanced rearrangements. Overall, the resolution at which copy number changes can be detected using these techniques are only slightly higher as compared to conventional karyotyping (43 Mb) and all experiments are labor intensive and time consuming. By replacing metaphase chromosomes with mapped DNA sequences or oligonucleotides arrayed onto glass slides as the hybridization targets, these limitations could be overcome. Following hybridization of differentially labeled test and reference genomic DNAs to the target sequences on the microarray, the slide is scanned to measure the fluorescence intensities at each target on the array. The normalized fluorescent ratio for the test and reference DNAs is then plotted against the position of the sequence along the chromosomes. Gains or losses across the genome are identified by values increased or decreased from a 1:1 ratio (log2 value of 0), and the detection resolution depends only on the size and the number of targets on an array and the position of these targets (their distribution) on the genome. This methodology was first described in 1997 and is termed matrix or array CGH. Array CGH was initially employed to analyze copy number changes in tumors with the aim to identify genes involved in the pathogenesis of cancers (Albertson and Pinkel 2003). This methodology has been optimized and applied to detect unbalanced constitutional rearrangements (Shaw-Smith et al. 2004). It has been proposed that in analogy with the introduction of chromosome karyotyping in the early 1960s, genomic arrays should now be implemented as a genetic diagnostic service, and several genetic centers already offer molecular karyotyping to patients (Friedman et al. 2006).

Several studies have shown the ability of molecular karyotyping to detect low-grade mosaicism with aneuploidy as low as 7% (Ballif et al. 2006). While in conventional karyotyping the chance to detect such low-grade mosaicism is dependent on the number of metaphases analyzed, in array CGH this depends on experimental outcome of the hybridization, that is the standard deviation of an array experiment as well as on the size and number of spotted target sequences (Le Caignec et al. 2006). The degree of mosaicism that can be detected can be established using mixtures of normal DNA versus abnormal DNA. To validate imbalances detected by array-CGH, follow-up analyses might be required. Whether or not alternative techniques are chosen to confirm a specific imbalance depends on the probability that a perceived imbalance is a true positive call. If this probability is low, small imbalances may be verified by independent molecular techniques including FISH, Q-PCR, MLPA or higher resolution arrays (de Vries et al. 2005). For deletions, all those techniques will be accurate. For small duplications, FISH should be quantitative, because the resolution of fluorescent microscopes may not separate the signals derived from a duplicon. Because both a deletion and a duplication may result from the unbalanced segregation of a balanced insertional translocation in one of the parents, it is mandatory to perform FISH on the parental metaphase spreads to exclude telomeric/insertional translocations or inversions.

Within one typical solid tumor karyogram there may be dozen of numeric and structural anomalies, and many differences between karyograms from the same specimen are generally the rule rather than the exception. Even though it has been more difficult to obtain analyzable spreads metaphase chromosomes from solid tumors in comparison to the hematologic malignancies, many cytogenetic alterations have been described in some tumor types which are already known to have clinical relevance, and it is certain that much more important data will continue to be gathered and analyzed in the future.

Tumors of the Nervous System

Tumors of the nervous system are, after leukemias and lymphoma, the neoplasms about which most extensive cytogenetics information is available: no less than 1,000 karyotypically abnormal cases have been published (Mitelman 1994). More than 90% of this information concerns tumors of the central nervous system. The pathology of these neoplasm is highly intricate, reflecting in many respects the complexities of the nervous system itself.

Brain Tumors in Children

Children with brain tumors have symptoms and therapeutic requirements that differ considerably from their adult counterparts. The most common childhood brain tumors are different from the most common adult brain tumors in that: (1) their locations are different, (2) they often behave differently than similar tumors in adults, and many have a better prognosis, (3) they are often treated differently from those in adults, particularly in very young children. Children who have brain tumors require special care because their body and brain are still developing. The young patients who receive state-of-the-art treatment from an experienced, multi-disciplinary pediatric healthcare team often has a better chance of survival and quality of life than their adult counterparts.

More brain tumors are found in children age 7 and younger than in older children, and they tend to be more common in boys than girls. These tumors are classified according to their histopathology based on the cell type of origin. Thus, astrocytoma, oligodendroglioma, and ependymoma are considered to derive from astrocytic, oligodendroglial and ependymal cells, respectively (Kleihues and Cavenee 2000). To our knowledge, the first studies utilizing FISH in normal and neoplastic brain specimens were those of Arnoldus et al. (1992). They showed that FISH was a sensitive method for detecting the aneusomies commonly reported by karyotyping and described the unusual phenomenon of somatic pairing for the chromosome 1 and 17 centromeres. Although we are still in the relatively early stages of genetic characterization of CNS tumors, subsequent studies have greatly expanded these initial findings, disclosing a number of relatively tumor-specific, progression-associated, and/or prognostically relevant alterations.

Ependymoma

Ependymoma represents ~ 7% of childhood brain tumors with half of the cases occurring in infants younger than 3 years of age (Massimino et al. 2004). They are the third most common pediatric CNS tumors. In contrast to adult ependymoma that shows predominantly a spinal location, ~ 90% of pediatric ependymoma cases develop intra-cranially, with most of them arising in infratentorial location (Massimino et al. 2004). The World Health Organization (WHO) classification distinguishes three major types of ependymal tumors: myxopapillary ependymoma and subependymoma (WHO grade I), classic ependymoma (WHO grade II), and anaplastic ependymoma (WHO grade III) (Wiestler et al. 2000). While WHO grade I tumors follow a benign course, grade II and III ependymoma show high propensity to recur (Massimino et al. 2004; Wiestler et al. 2000). Histopathological diagnosis and grading can be difficult, with frequent disagreements among neuropathologists. Furthermore, the impact of tumor histology on outcome remains controversial (Robertson et al. 1998). Thus far, histological classification has been an unreliable predictor of clinical behavior, and complete surgical resection remains the single most important predictor of relapse-free and overall survival (Robertson et al. 1998). Prognostic factors with an adverse impact on clinical outcome in pediatric ependymoma include young age at diagnosis (Pollack et al. 1995). Younger patients (< 3 years of age) with intracranial disease have a poorer outcome than older ones (Merchant 2002).

Ependymoma are slow-growing tumors that typically develop in the cerebral hemispheres, the posterior fossa, or the spinal cord of children and young adults. The 5-year progression-free survival ranges between 30% and 60%, with worse prognosis for those with residual disease after surgery, anaplastic histologic features, or age younger than 3 years. Surgery represents the main treatment, although radiotherapy also is a well-established strategy in disease control. Radiotherapy is the standard adjuvant treatment, at least for older children, while the use of adjuvant standard-dose chemotherapy has not resulted in significantly improved outcomes, and high-dose chemotherapy approaches to avoid radiation-therapy in young children have been disappointing (Zacharoulis et al. 2007). Ependymoma are tumors which can recur, but predictive factors of outcome in ependymoma are far from being well established with respect to age, localization, grading, and extent of resection. In contrast to the diffuse glioma, little is known regarding tumorigenic and progression-mediated events in ependymoma. There is, therefore, a need to identify biological factors to establish a correlation with tumor behavior.

Prognosis-Related Molecular Markers in Pediatric Ependymoma

In recent years, cytogenetics and molecular investigations have improved our understanding of the biology of cancer dramatically and defined clinically relevant molecular features. Reliable prognostic factors might permit tailored therapy, so that only patients with aggressive tumors would receive most intense treatments. A number of molecular markers have recently been developed to predict the response of ependymoma to certain types of therapy: DNA ploidy, loss of heterozygosity, and chromosomal aberrations detected by FISH and CGH (1q, 17p, 17q), as well as oncogenes/tumor suppressor genes (*TP53*, *PTEN*, *c-erbB2*, *MYCN*, *MYCC*) and their proteins, growth factor and hormonal receptors (PDGFRA, VEGF, EGFR, HER2, HER4, ErbB-2, hTERT, TrkC), cell cycle genes and cell adhesion molecules, as well as factors potentially related to therapeutic resistance (multi-drug resistance, DNA topoisomerase II alpha, metallothionein, P-glycoprotein, tenascin C).

Ependymoma represents a subset of glioma that occurs both sporadically and rarely, in association with neurofibromatosis type 2 (NF2). Much interest has been focused on *NF2* (22q12) and its gene product merlin (schwannomin), because alterations involving chromosome 22 have been well documented in ependymoma (Hirose et al. 2001; Lamszus et al. 2001). Given the increased frequency of intramedullary ependymoma in NF2 patients, it is interesting that several groups have reported an association between spinal tumor location and *NF2* mutations (Lamszus et al. 2001). This association has been confirmed using LSI probes for *NF2* and a related protein 4.1 family member, DAL-1. In contrast, *DAL-1* deletion is associated with intracranial ependymoma localization.

Therefore, there are currently multiple areas of interest, amenable to further clinic-pathologic FISH and CGH studies. Some work has been reported on the molecular biology and cytogenetics of these tumors. In ependymoma, abnormalities of chromosome 11 have been described; monosomy 11 was found in six cases (Sainati et al. 1992) and trisomy 11 was once reported. Rearrangements involving 11q13 were described in four pediatric ependymoma (Sainati et al. 1992). The locus q13 of chromosome 11 contains the oncogenes *BCT1*, *HST* and *INT2*, which are amplified in some human cancers. One of these genes is perhaps implicated in ependymoma.

Currently, however, molecular studies analyzing the genetic alterations in intracranial ependymoma have failed to identify the causative genes and to pinpoint unambiguously the clinically relevant genetic anomalies. Furthermore, ~ 70% of ependymoma in infants display an apparently normal karyotype and/or a normal comparative genomic hybridization (CGH) profile (Jeuken et al. 2002; Ward et al. 2001; Carter et al. 2002; Grill et al. 2002; Hirose et al. 2001; Zheng et al. 2000; Dyer et al. 2002) suggesting the possible presence of more subtle and so far undetected genomic abnormalities.

Using metaphase CGH analysis, several genetic aberrations have been detected in ependymoma involving gains and losses of several chromosomes that can vary in different studies but commonly include gains of 1q, 5, 7, 8, 9, 18, and 19, and losses of 3 and 6 (Dyer et al. 2002; Pezzolo et al. 2008). Importantly, the gain of 1q is a common finding associated with poor prognosis not only in ependymoma (Dyer et al. 2002; Mendrzyk et al. 2006) and medulloblastoma, but also in other pediatric tumors, including neuroblastoma, Wilms' tumor and Ewing's sarcoma. Currently, the gene(s) located on the region 1q25 that is gained in these malignancies has not been identified. Chromosome 7 gains were seen primarily in spinal, while gains of 1q and losses of 6q, 9 and 13 occurred preferentially in intracranial ependymoma (Hirose et al. 2001).

A CGH study showed clear and more remarkable cytogenetics differences between tumors that occurred in intracranial and spinal cord ependymoma (Hirose et al. 2001). First, there were far more copy number aberrations (CNAs) in spinal cord than in intracranial tumors. Secondly, the CNAs in these two groups were different. Spinal cord tumors featured a gain on chromosome 7. Other frequent CNAs seen in the spinal cord cases included gains on 2, 5, 9, 12, 15, 18, 20q, and X, and losses on 13q and 22q. All above-mentioned CNAs were far less frequent in the intracranial cases. On the other hand, cases of intracranial tumors, especially those of grade 3, had frequent gains on 1q and losses on 9;

these CNAs were nearly absent in the spinal cord tumors. Carter et al. (2002) confirmed this finding by analyzing 86 ependymoma from children and adults. It is well known that intracranial tumors frequently relapse (Robertson et al. 1998) and that spinal cord tumors rarely relapse after complete resection. These data suggest that intracranial and spinal cord ependymoma progress along substantially different pathways, although they comprise one histologic entity. Copy number aberrations frequently seen in other intracranial neuroepithelial tumors, gain on 7, losses on 1p/19q, and a loss on 10q were rare in intracranial ependymoma, which suggests that ependymoma develop through unique genetic modifications compared with astrocytoma and oligodendroglioma. The relationship of intracranial ependymoma grade to outcome is controversial. Nonetheless, there were indications that a gain on 1q and a loss on 9 were preferentially associated with histologic grade 3 among intracranial tumors; therefore, these CNAs might be indicators of outcome. The data also suggested that intramedullary spinal cord ependymoma and myxopapillary ependymoma were different genetic subgroups although both shared chromosome 7 gain. Loss on 22q, gains on 15q and 12 did not occur in myxopapillary tumors, while losses on chromosomes 1, 2, and 10 occurred solely in the myxopapillary group. Even though myxopapillary tumors grow slowly, they do have a greater potential for dissemination through the central canal than other spinal ependymoma. Thus, different CNAs in these two groups of spinal ependymoma may underlie differences in their clinical behavior.

Age-associated genetic alterations are also suspected, though the data are conflicting (von Haken et al. 1996; Reardon et al. 1999; Kramer et al. 1998). Remarkable cytogenetics differences in intracranial ependymoma occur in patients younger *vs* older than 3 years. CGH studies have defined at least three distinct genetic patterns among ependymoma patients (Dyer et al. 2002; Mendrzyk et al. 2006). The group of patients < 3 years of age showed few chromosomal changes compared with those > 3 years of age. A second group showed several chromosomal imbalances together with a non random gain or loss of chromosomes. A third group showed a balanced chromosome profile that occurred in tumors in children < 3 years of age, suggesting that these tumors developed by a different genetic pathway compared with tumors arising in older children. However, one study of pediatric ependymoma found that tumors in patients < 3 years of age were characterized by structural chromosome rearrangements (Pezzolo et al. 2008). In contrast, patients older than 3 years displayed both structural and numerical rearrangements, as well as a higher number of chromosomal imbalances (Pezzolo et al. 2008). These results suggest that chromosomal instability may be higher in tumors from patients older than 3 years and account for the higher number of CNAs detected in this group. In this study novel CNAs identified are the following: (1) 4q33-qter loss, (2) 10q25.2–q26.3 gain, (3) 3q23-qter losses, (4) 18q22.2 loss, and (5) 19p13.1–p13.3 gain. Among them, 10q25.2–q26.3 gain was detected exclusively in patients younger than 3 years, whereas 18q22.2 loss was significantly associated with patients over 3 years. Furthermore, 21q22-qter was an exclusive marker of the latter group. Additional CNAs with prognostic value were found to be 6p22-pter and 13q14.3-qter losses. Either 6p22-pter or 13q14.3-qter loss tested individually did not display any correlation with patient survival; however, the combined presence of 6p22-pter and 13q14.3-qter losses predicted significantly reduced survival (Pezzolo et al. 2008).

In the literature, six cases of abnormalities of chromosome 6 have been described in ependymoma as well as six cases with monosomy 6 and one case with a translocation involving 6q11. Moreover several cytogenetics and molecular genetic studies have revealed a variable frequency of deletions on 6q in ependymoma (Huang et al. 2003). Pediatric patients with anaplastic intracranial (supra- and infratentorial) ependymoma harboring the 6q25.3 deletion showed significantly longer overall survival than did patients of the same group without the aberration independent of the extent of resection. This supports the identified deletion on 6q25.3 as a candidate favorable prognostic parameter (Monoranu et al. 2008).

At least two independent studies have shown over expression of human telomere reverse transcriptase (*hTERT*, located at 5p15.33), which is a strong prognostic factor in ependymoma for poor survival (Mendrzyk et al. 2006; Tabori et al. 2006). In addition, inhibition of telomerase may be a future therapeutic target. Tumors need to maintain their telomeres in order to replicate chromosomes and thus reactivate the telomerase enzyme, whereas normal cells do not contain this active enzyme (Shay and Wright 2005). Inhibitors of tankyrase and telomerase have been successfully used in cell culture to induce shortening of telomeres such that tumor cells entered proliferation crisis and died (Seimiya et al. 2005). This novel therapeutic approach could be an effective anti cancer therapy. Moreover, ependymoma has shown frequent gains and amplification of *EGFR*, located at 7p11.2 (Mendrzyk et al. 2006). Over expression of *EGFR* was an independent prognostic marker of poor survival. Several agents targeting *EGFR* are currently in clinical trials, such as the tyrosine kinase inhibitors erlotinib and gefitinib, and the monoclonal anti-EGFR antibody C225 (cetuximab; Milano et al. 2008). The role of these agents in the treatment of EGFR-positive ependymoma, in combination with other chemotherapy and/or radiotherapy regimens, remains to be defined.

Recently, a number of studies investigated ependymoma by means of array-CGH and/or expression profiling using comparable technological platforms and identified differences in ependymoma subgroups and correlations with clinical parameters (Taylor et al. 2005; Suarez-Merino et al. 2005; Mendrzyk et al. 2006; Sowar et al. 2006). Integrated genomic and expression profiling allowed Modena et al. (2006) to identify genes whose expression is deregulated in intracranial ependymoma such as over-expression of the putative proto-oncogene *YAP1* (located at 11q22) and down-regulation of the *SULT4A1* gene (at 22q13.3). Moreover Modena et al. (2006) identified molecular signatures that correlate with tumor location, patient age at disease onset, and retrospective risk for relapse, and that warrant additional validation in independent larger series of samples. Supratentorial location of the tumor associated with chromosome 9p loss and gene expression profiling results identified three candidate genes located within chromosome 9p and down-regulated in supratentorial tumors, namely *FRAS1*-related extracellular matrix 1 (*FREM1*), *c9orf24*, and *KIAA1161* (Modena et al. 2006).

In summary, these data demonstrate that ependymoma with distinct clinical and pathologic characteristics are distinguished by specific molecular features, provide a solid basis for additional investigations into the genetics underlying ependymoma onset/progression, and might facilitate the development of specific molecular diagnostic procedures which could aid in clinical decision making. In conclusions FISH has become a useful clinical and research tool, which is still relatively underutilized. As with any technique, it has distinct advantages and disadvantages, though its main attraction for neuropathologists lies in its morphologic preservation and applicability to archival FFPE tissue. Given recent technical advances and a rapidly growing body of molecular cytogenetic literature, the role of FISH in diagnostic and investigative neuropathology laboratories will likely continue to grow in the near future. Array CGH is a technology that is rapidly evolving. Novel and increasingly higher resolution genome-wide screening tools are currently being developed. In addition to both clinical utility and validity, there is a cost/benefit relationship that influences the clinical introduction of novel technologies. These issues have been addressed elsewhere (Newman et al. 2007). These efforts will change our knowledge dramatically in the years to come. Our growing knowledge of the biology of pediatric brain tumors holds promise for finding new "molecular targeted" drugs that may augment, supplement or even replace conventional chemotherapy and radiotherapy.

References

Albertson DG, Pinkel D (2003) Genomic microarrays in human genetic disease and cancer. Hum Mol Genet 12:145–152

Arnoldus EPJ, Wolters LBT, Voormolen JHC, van Duinen SG, Raap AK, van der Ploeg M, Peters ACB (1992)

Interphase cytogenetics: a new tool for the study of genetic changes in brain tumors. J Neurosurg 76:997–1003

Ballif BC, Rorem EA, Sundin K, Lincicum M, Gaskin S, Coppinger J, Kashork CD, Shaffer LG, Bejjani BA (2006) Detection of low-level mosaicism by array CGH in routine diagnostic specimens. Am J Med Genet 140:2757–2767

Carter M, Nicholson J, Ross F, Crolla J, Allibone R, Balaji V, Perry R, Walker D, Gilbertson R, Ellison DW (2002) Genetic abnormalities detected in ependymomas by comparative genomic hybridization. Br J Cancer 86:929–939

de Vries BB, Pfundt R, Leisink M, Koolen DA, Vissers LE, Janssen IM, Reijmersdal S, Nillesen WM, Huys EH, Leeuw N, Smeets D, Sistermans EA, Feuth T, van Ravenswaaij-Arts CM, van Kessel AG, Schoenmakers EF, Brunner HG, Veltman JA (2005) Diagnostic genome profiling in mental retardation. Am J Hum Genet 77:606–616

Dyer S, Prebble E, Davison V, Davies P, Ramani P, Ellison D, Grundy R (2002) Genomic imbalances in pediatric intracranial ependymomas define clinically relevant groups. Am J Pathol 161:2133–2141

Friedman JM, Baross A, Delaney AD, Ally A, Arbour L, Armstrong L, Asano J, Bailey DK, Barber S, Birch P, Brown-John M, Cao M, Chan S, Charest DL, Farnoud N, Fernandes N, Flibotte S, Go A, Gibson WT, Holt RA, Jones SJ, Kennedy GC, Krzywinski M, Langlois S, Li HI, McGillivray BC, Nayar T, Pugh TJ, Rajcan-Separovic E, Schein JE, Schnerch A, Siddiqui A, Van Allen MI, Wilson G, Yong SL, Zahir F, Eydoux P, Marra MA (2006) Oligonucleotide microarray analysis of genomic imbalance in children with mental retardation. Am J Hum Genet 79:500–513

Gray JW, Pinkel D (1992) Molecular cytogenetics in human cancer diagnosis. Cancer 69:1536–1542

Grill J, Avet-Loiseau H, Lellouch-Tubiana A, Sévenet N, Terrier-Lacombe MJ, Vénuat AM, Doz F, Sainte-Rose C, Kalifa C, Vassal G (2002) Comparative genomic hybridization detects specific cytogenetic abnormalities in pediatric ependymomas and choroid plexus papillomas. Cancer Genet Cytogenet 136:121–125

Hayat MA (ed) (2004–2005) Immunohistochemistry and *in situ* hybridization of human carcinomas, vol 1–4. Elsevier/Academic, San Diego/London

Henke RP, Ayhan N (1994) Enhancement of hybridization efficiency in interphase cytogenetics on paraffin embedded tissue sections by microwave treatment. Anal Cell Pathol 6:319–325

Hirose Y, Aldape KD, Bollen A, James CD, Brat D, Lamborn KR, Berger MS, Feuerstein BG (2001) Chromosomal abnormalities subdivide ependymal tumors into clinically relevant groups. Am J Pathol 158:1137–1143

Huang B, Starostik P, Schraut H, Krauss J, Sorensen N, Roggendorf W (2003) Human ependymomas reveal frequent deletions on chromosomes 6 and 9. Acta Neuropathol 106:357–362

Jeuken JW, Sprenger SH, Gilhuis J, Teepen HL, Grotenhuis AJ, Wesseling P (2002) Correlation between localization, age, and chromosomal imbalances in ependymal tumours as detected by CGH. J Pathol 197:238–244

Kallionemi A, Kallionemi OP, Sudar D, Rutovitz D, Gray JW, Waldman F, Pinkel D (1992) Comparative genomic hybridization for molecular cytogenetic analysis of solid tumors. Science 258:818–821

Kleihues P, Cavenee WK (2000) WHO classification of tumors of the nervous system. IARC, Lyon, pp 6–82

Kramer DL, Parmiter AH, Rorke LB, Sutton LN, Biegel JA (1998) Molecular cytogenetic studies of pediatric ependymomas. J Neurooncol 37:25–33

Lamszus K, Lachenmayer L, Heinemann U, Kluwe L, Finckh U, Hoppner W, Stavrou D, Fillbrandt R, Westphal M (2001) Molecular genetic alterations on chromosomes 11 and 22 in ependymomas. Int J Cancer 91:803–808

Le Caignec C, Spits C, Sermon K, De Rycke M, Thienpont B, Debrock S, Staessen C, Moreau Y, Fryns JP, Van Steirteghem A, Liebaers I, Vermeesch JR (2006) Single-cell chromosomal imbalances detection by array CGH. Nucleic Acids Res 34:E68

Massimino M, Gandola L, Giangaspero F, Sandri A, Valagussa P, Perilongo G, Garrè ML, Ricardi U, Forni M, Genitori L, Scarzello G, Spreafico F, Barra S, Mascarin M, Pollo B, Gardiman M, Cama A, Navarria P, Brisigotti M, Collini P, Balter R, Fidani P, Stefanelli M, Burnelli R, Potepan P, Podda M, Sotti G, Madon E, AIEOP Pediatric Neuro-Oncology Group (2004) Hyperfractionated radiotherapy and chemotherapy for childhood ependymoma: final results of the first prospective AIEOP (Associazione Italiana di Ematologia-Oncologia Pediatrica) study. Int J Radiat Oncol Biol Phys 58:1336–1345

Mendrzyk F, Korshunov A, Benner A, Toedt G, Pfister S, Radlwimmer B, Lichter P (2006) Identification of gains on 1q and epidermal growth factor receptor over-expression as independent prognostic markers in intracranial ependymoma. Clin Cancer Res 12:2070–2079

Merchant TE (2002) Current management of childhood ependymoma. Oncology (Huntingt) 16:629–644

Milano G, Spano JP, Leyland-Jones B (2008) EGFR-targeting drugs in combination with cytotoxic agents: from bench to bedside, a contrasted reality. Br J Cancer 99:1–5

Mitelman F (1994) Catalog of chromosome aberrations in cancer, 5th edn. Wiley-Liss, New York

Mitelman F, Johansson B, Mandahl N, Mertens F (1997) Clinical significance of cytogenetic findings in solid tumors. Cancer Genet Cytogenet 95:1–8

Modena P, Lualdi E, Facchinetti F, Veltman J, Reid JF, Minardi S, Janssen I, Giangaspero F, Forni M, Finocchiaro G, Genitori L, Giordano F, Riccardi R, Schoenmakers EF, Massimino M, Sozzi G (2006) Identification of tumor-specific molecular signatures in intracranial ependymoma and association with clinical characteristics. J Clin Oncol 24:5223–5233

Monoranu CM, Huang B, Zangen LI, Rutkowski S, Vince GH, Gerber NU, Puppe B, Roggendorf W (2008) Correlation between 6q25.3 deletion status and survival in pediatric intracranial ependymomas. Cancer Genet Cytogenet 182:18–26

Newman WG, Hamilton S, Ayres J, Sanghera N, Smith A, Gaunt L, Davies LM, Clayton-Smith J (2007) Array comparative genomic hybridization for diagnosis of developmental delay-an exploratory cost-consequences analysis. Clin Genet 71:254–271

Nolte M, Werner M, Vonwasielewski R, Nietgen G, Wilkens L, Georgii A (1996) Detection of numerical karyotype changes in the giant cells of Hodgkins lymphomas by a combination of FISH and immunohistochemistry applied to paraffin sections. Histochem Cell Biol 105:401–404

Pezzolo A, Parodi F, Corrias MV, Cinti R, Gambini C, Pistoia V (2007) Tumor origin of endothelial cells in human neuroblastoma. J Clin Oncol 25:376–383

Pezzolo A, Capra V, Raso A, Moranti F, Parodi F, Gambini C, Nozza P, Giangaspero F, Cama A, Pistoia V, Garré ML (2008) Identification of novel chromosomal abnormalities and prognostic cytogenetics markers in intracranial pediatric ependymoma. Cancer Lett 261:235–243

Pollack IF, Gerszten PC, Martinez AJ, Lo KH, Shultz B, Albright AL, Janosky J, Deutsch M (1995) Intracranial ependymomas of childhood: long-term outcome and prognostic factors. Neurosurgery 37:655–667

Reardon DA, Entrekin RE, Sublett J, Ragsdale S, Li H, Boyett J, Kepner JL, Look AT (1999) Chromosome arm 6q loss is the most common recurrent autosomal alteration detected in primary pediatric ependymoma. Genes Chromosomes Cancer 24:230–237

Robertson PL, Zeltzer PM, Boyett JM, Rorke LB, Allen JC, Geyer JR, Stanley P, Li H, Albright AL, McGuire-Cullen P, Finlay JL, Stevens KR Jr, Milstein JM, Packer RJ, Wisoff J (1998) Survival and prognostic factors following radiation therapy and chemotherapy for ependymomas in children: a report of the Children's Cancer Group. J Neurosurg 88:695–703

Sainati L, Montali A, Putti MC, Giangaspero F, Rigobello L, Stella M, Zanesco L, Basso G (1992) Cytogenetic t(11;17)(q13;q21) in a pediatric ependymoma. is 11q13a recurring breakpoint in ependymoma? Cancer Genet Cytogenet 59:213–216

Seimiya H, Muramatsu Y, Ohishi T, Tsuruo T (2005) Tankyrase 1 as a target for telomere-directed molecular cancer therapeutics. Cancer Cell 7:25–37

Shaw-Smith C, Redon R, Rickman L, Rio M, Willatt L, Fiegler H, Firth H, Sanlaville D, Winter R, Colleaux L, Bobrow M, Carter NP (2004) Microarray based comparative genomic hybridization (array-CGH) detects submicroscopic chromosomal deletions and duplications in patients with learning disability/mental retardation and dysmorphic features. J Med Genet 41:241–248

Shay JW, Wright WE (2005) Mechanism-based combination telomerase inhibition therapy. Cancer Cell 7:1–2

Sowar K, Straessle J, Donson AM, Handler M, Foreman NK (2006) Predicting which children are at risk for ependymoma relapse. J Neurooncol 78:41–46

Suarez-Merino B, Hubank M, Revesz T, Harkness W, Hayward R, Thompson D, Darling JL, Thomas DG, Warr TJ (2005) Microarray analysis of pediatric ependymoma identifies a cluster of 112 candidate genes including four transcripts at 22q12.1-q13.3. Neuro Oncol 7:20–31

Tabori U, Ma J, Carter M, Zielenska M, Rutka J, Bouffet E, Bartels U, Malkin D, Hawkins C (2006) Human telomere reverse transcriptase expression predicts progression and in pediatric intracranial ependymoma. J Clin Oncol 24:1522–1528

Taylor MD, Poppleton H, Fuller C, Su X, Liu Y, Jensen P, Magdaleno S, Dalton J, Calabrese C, Board J, Macdonald T, Rutka J, Guha A, Gajjar A, Curran T, Gilbertson RJ (2005) Radial glia cells are candidate stem cells of ependymoma. Cancer Cell 8:323–335

von Haken MS, White EC, Daneshvar-Shyesther L, Sih S, Choi E, Kalra R, Cogen PH (1996) Molecular genetic analysis of chromosome arm 17p and chromosome arm 22q DNA sequences in sporadic pediatric ependymomas. Genes Chromosomes Cancer 17:37–44

Ward S, Harding B, Wilkins P, Harkness W, Hayward R, Darling JL, Thomas DG, Warr T (2001) Gain of 1q and loss of 22 are the most common changes detected by comparative genomic hybridization in pediatric ependymoma. Genes Chromosomes Cancer 32:59–66

Wiestler OD, Schiffer D, Coons SW (2000) Ependymal tumors. In: Kleihues P, Cavence WK (eds) World Health Organization (WHO) classification of tumors: pathology and genetics of tumors of the nervous system. IARC, Lyon, pp 71–82

Zacharoulis S, Levy A, Chi SN, Gardner S, Rosenblum M, Miller DC, Dunkel I, Diez B, Sposto R, Ji L, Asgharzadeh S, Hukin J, Belasco J, Dubowy R, Kellie S, Termuhlen A, Finlay J (2007) Outcome for young children newly diagnosed with ependymoma, treated with intensive induction chemotherapy followed by myeloablative chemotherapy and autologous stem cell rescue. Pediatr Blood Cancer 49:34–40

Zheng PP, Pang JC, Hui AB, Ng HK (2000) Comparative genomic hybridization detects losses of chromosomes 22 and 16 as the most common recurrent genetic alterations in primary ependymomas. Cancer Genet Cytogenet 122:18–25

Pediatric Hepatoblastoma. Complete Surgery and Ultrasound Monitoring

28

Daniela Iacob, Otilia Fufezan, and Alexandru Serban

Contents

D. Iacob (✉) • O. Fufezan
Third Pediatric Clinic, University of Medicine and Pharmacy, Cluj Napoca, Romania
e-mail: iacobdaniela777@gmail.com

A. Serban
Third Medical Clinic, University of Medicine and Pharmacy, Cluj Napoca, Romania

Abstract

Hepatoblastoma is the most common primary liver tumor of childhood. Most hepatoblastoma cases are sporadic, but others are associated with inherited conditions, suggesting the importance of genetic abnormalities in the pathogenesis and progression of this disease. A diverse range of cytogenetic alterations have been reported, as significant gains of genetic material, with various differences in the number and type of alterations between the different histologic components of hepatoblastoma. They could represent diagnostic marker, they may play a role in the tumorigenesis of hepatoblastoma and might become potential target for molecular therapeutics. An elevated serum alpha-fetoprotein is useful both at diagnosis of hepatoblastoma and in disease monitoring, by determining the success of surgical resection and/or response to adjuvant chemotherapy. Imaging has a significant role in the evaluation of hepatoblastoma, offering data about localization, resectability, and follow-up. Ultrasonography is the best initial imaging investigation of a child with a liver mass, allowing real-time investigation of the tumour. Complete surgical resection together with pre- and post-operative chemotherapy are the mainstay of treatment of hepatoblastoma. The potential down-staging effect of neoadjuvant chemotherapy on hepatoblastoma might facilitate remission and convert unresectable tumors into operable ones. Radical resection can be

M.A. Hayat (ed.), *Pediatric Cancer, Volume 3: Diagnosis, Therapy, and Prognosis*, Pediatric Cancer 3,
DOI 10.1007/978-94-007-4528-5_28,

obtained either conventionally by partial hepatectomy or with orthotopic liver transplant. Complete hepatectomy with living donor liver transplantation provides optimal surgical treatment in unresectable stage III and initial stage IV disease confined to the liver at resection. Referral to a transplant center during the first cycles of chemotherapy appears to offer the best opportunity for long-term survival.

Introduction

Hepatoblastoma (HB) is the most common liver tumor in children, representing 80% of all malignant liver neoplasms and 1% of all pediatric malignancies, having a peak incidence in the first 3 years of life. HB is an embryonic tumor that probably arises from a pluripotent stem cell occurring in the liver during embryonal life (Otte 2010). Congenital anomalies associated with HB include Beckwith-Weidemann syndrome and familial adenomatosis polyposis coli (Das et al. 2009). It was reported by Makin and Davenport (2010) that less than 10% of HB occur in the neonatal period. There is a predominance in boys (2:1) and an increased risk in low birth weight babies. It usually presents as an asymptomatic abdominal mass with systemic symptoms being less common. Serum alpha-fetoprotein (AFP) is elevated in 70–90% of patients with HB (Das et al. 2009). Surgical resection is the cornerstone of curative therapy for HB but less than 50% of tumours are resectable when diagnosed (Cacciavillano et al. 2004). Despite the importance of chemotherapy in the treatment of HB, complete removal of all viable tumour is still required for cure (Browne et al. 2008). Chemotherapy is administered as adjuvant therapy for completely resected tumours and it is also used both preoperatively and as an adjuvant, for tumours that are initially considered unresectable or when primary resection is hazardous (Cacciavillano et al. 2004). For those whose tumors are still not resectable after several cycles of chemotherapy, liver transplantation (LT) is recognized as the only option.

Ontogenesis and Oncogenesis

The complete hepatic organogenesis proceeds in a series of distinct phases, encompassing a priming phase, a phase of increasing specification, the growth of a liver bud, migration of hepatoblasts into the mesenchyme of the transverse septum, a phase of specific hepatic vascularisation, the expansion phase, terminal differentiation of the hepatocyte lineage, and the construction of the biliary tree. Early steps of liver development require an intricate network of several proliferation-specific transcription factors and a complex mesodermal–epithelial cell cross talk. The identification of specific histological HB morphotypes resulted in the widely used HB classification system and the system currently employed in SIOPEL (International Childhood Liver Tumours Strategy Group). One of the main merits of this classification now in use is that it recognizes that the histopathology of HB reflects distinct phases of liver cell development and maturation. In the differentiation of hepatoblasts to a mature hepatocyte phenotype a central regulator of this crucial step is the transcription factor, HNF4, belonging to the nuclear hormone receptor family (Zimmermann 2005).

In contrast to embryonal and foetal HB that consist of hepatocyte lineage cells with immature blastic features, several other types of liver cell tumours that develop in infants and children display a morphologically more mature phenotype. Tumours with cells resembling differentiated hepatocytes comprise macrotrabecular HB, and the recently described highly malignant transitional liver cell tumour (TLCT) that occurs in older children and young adolescents. TLCT is a highly aggressive lesion that usually presents with large neoplasms and high or very high serum AFP. The neoplastic cell lineage involved may reflect a differentiation window in the transition between immature and mature liver cells. Similar to many HB, TLCT in part express b-catenin.

It was reported by Zimmermann (2005) that biochemical and molecular biological abnormalities detected in HB are related to growth and regulation of the cell cycle. They include the up regulation of growth factors, alterations in the expression of factors affecting cell cycle progression and cycle checkpoints and also cytokinesis proteins such as Polo-like kinase-1 (the PLK1 oncogene) that is highly expressed in HB to indicate poor prognosis.

HB are characterised by complex alterations in signal transduction pathways. More prominent in HB are alterations of the b-catenin signalling pathway. Mutations in the b-catenin gene represent the most frequent molecular alteration in sporadic HB. It was reported by Nelson and Nusse (2004) that b-catenin is central to the convergence of the Wnt, b-catenin, and cadherin pathways, where it forms a signalling complex with axins, APC (adenomatous polyposis coli) tumour suppressor protein, glycogen synthase kinase 3b. Activating mutations of the b-catenin gene occur in at least 50% of HB, both in epithelial and mixed types. It was shown by Zimmermann (2005) that stabilised b-catenin can inhibit TNFa-induced apoptosis and affect growth responses.

The etiology of HB is unclear, but it occur in association with genetic disorders such as familial adenomatous polyposis, Beckwith-Wiedemann syndrome, hemihypertrophy and trisomy 18. The commonest cytogenetic abnormalities reported in HB are trisomy 2 and trisomy 20, and loss of heterozygosity at chromosome region 11p15 (Ma et al. 2000).

Analysing the genetic alterations of HB by using comparative genomic hybridization (CGH) and fluorescent in situ hybridization (FISH), Terracciano et al. (2003) reported that it is a chromosomally unstable tumor wherein gains are significantly more frequent than deletions. The most frequent alterations were gains of Xp and Xq.

Bacterial artificial chromosome array comparative genomic hybridization analysis of HB reveals a deletion in the 14q12 locus. A high frequency of copy gain was seen on chromosomes 1q, 2, 5p, 8 and 20. Frequent deletions were found at 6q, 17q and 1p with less frequent gains on 4p, 6p and 19p. Also, 14q12 deletion locus analyses using quantitative real-time polymerase chain reaction reveals copy number gain/amplification in the region immediately telomeric to the deleted locus, including copy number gain of FOXG1 in most of HB. This is associated with up-regulation of FOXG1 gene transcripts and increased protein expression. The dysregulation of expression of FOXG1 is seen in all histologic subtypes of HB and correlates with the loss of p21cip1 expression. This overexpression might be partly responsible for the maintenance of the undifferentiated state (Adesina et al. 2007).

Glypican 3 (GPC3) has been detected in hepatic stem cells and was identified as one of the most overexpressed genes in HB by microarray analysis. Fetal, embryonal, and small cell undifferentiated patterns were diffusely positive in almost all cases, whereas mesenchymal and teratoid patterns were nearly all negative. The high GPC3 expression suggests that it may play a role in the tumorigenesis of HB. Zynger et al. (2008) reported that in comparison to AFP, GPC3 may have a broader coverage of histologic subtypes and may exhibit stronger, more diffuse positivity. GPC3 might be a serum marker for the diagnosis and monitoring of tumor progression and a therapeutic target in patients with HB.

At transcription level serpin SERPINB3 (SB3) was positive in most cases of HB. By immunohistochemistry, SB3 expression was found mainly in the embryonic, blastemal, small cell undifferentiated (SCUD) components of HB. A direct correlation was observed between SB3 gene expression, the up-regulation of Myc and tumour extension. SB3 is over-expressed in HB, its expression being positively correlated with Myc expression and high tumour stage (Turato et al. 2011). The overexpression of Myc is currently considered as a negative clinical prognostic factor that predicts poor outcome, irrespective of therapeutic treatment, often characterised by tumour propagation and disease progression. The close relationship between SB3 and Myc expressions, with progressive intra-hepatic tumour extension and also with the SCUD variant of HB, allows to hypothesise that SB3 may intervene in defining the risk profile of children affected by HB. The association of SB3 expression with Myc expression, a high PRETEXT system and the SCUD variant of HB allow to assume that SB3 might help in defining the risk profile of children affected by HB (Turato et al. 2011).

Clinical Presentation and Laboratory Investigations

HB, more common in boys, typically presents in infants and young children less than 4 years old in the form of an asymptomatic abdominal mass in an otherwise healthy-appearing child. Delay in diagnosis has been associated with 65% of patients deemed unsuitable for surgery at diagnosis owing to extensive intrahepatic extension or the presence of extrahepatic disease (Dicken et al. 2004). Less common clinical presentations include anorexia, failure to thrive, abdominal pain, abdominal distension. HB can occasionally rupture and cause intra-abdominal bleeding and present findings of an acute abdomen. It was reported by von Schweinitz (2003) that extremely premature children have a significantly increased risk of developing a HB. In the newborn the clinical picture of the often extensive HB tumour may differ to HB in the typical age group of 6 months to 3 years. Metastases occur earlier and are often systemic, sometimes bypassing the lungs because of the fetal circulation. Neonatal HB do not seem to produce such excessive amounts of AFP as those in older children, whilst the natural blood concentrations are still high in this period of life. HB can be suspected antenatally by abdominal ultrasound and MR scan and may cause polyhydramnios and stillbirth. During labor and birth, tumour rupture with massive haemorrhage can occur (von Schweinitz 2003).

Most liver function studies in HB are usually normal. Serum AFP is a sensitive marker of active and viable HB. Browne et al. (2008) reported that more than 90% of HB patients exhibited abnormally high levels of serum AFP at presentation. When elevated at diagnosis, this serum tumour marker is an excellent aid in diagnosis, monitoring response to therapy and, very important, in the early detection of tumour recurrence. De Ioris et al. (2008) reported that a low serum AFP level (<100 ng/ml) at presentation is a poor prognostic factor. In infants under 6 months of age at diagnosis, the serum AFP level must be corrected for residual fetal AFP. A child presenting with a liver mass between 6 months and 3 years of age, a very high serum AFP level, and typical findings on imaging most often has HB (Otte 2010). About 65% of patients have thrombocytosis, including patients with platelet counts in excess of one million (Dicken et al. 2004).

The measurement of the serum AFP level has become the most reliable tool for assessing disease activity. Postoperatively, a failure of the serum AFP level to return to a normal level means an incomplete tumor resection, and a gradual increase of the serum AFP level to an abnormal range in patients who underwent a complete tumor resection indicates either tumor recurrence or the presence of distant metastasis. After surgery, it is crucial that serum AFP concentration has returned to normal before declaring the child in complete remission. This may take up to several weeks and a transitory rise in AFP can be observed shortly after surgery as a result of liver regeneration, especially in very young children. It was reported by Browne et al. (2008) that a rise or fall in the AFP level may indicate efficacy of treatment. In addition, AFP levels that do not decrease by 2 logs despite therapy have been found to have poor prognosis.

Ultrasound Diagnosis and Complementary Imagistic Methods

Imaging plays a significant role in the evaluation of HB. Advances in the imaging technologies have improved characterization, localization, determination of resectability and follow-up. The best initial, not invasive imaging investigation of a child with a liver mass is abdominal ultrasonography (USG). It identifies the origin of the mass, determines the structure and extent of the lesion, establish whether it is a solitary or a multifocal tumor (Fig. 28.1). On USG, it usually appears as a solitary lesion, although it can be multifocal. Das et al. (2009) reported that the lesion has well defined margins and shows minimal increased echogenicity Doppler USG studies are of particular value in children, allowing real-time investigation of the tumour and its relation to the main hepatic veins and portal branches, including an assessment of their patency or possible invasion by tumour.

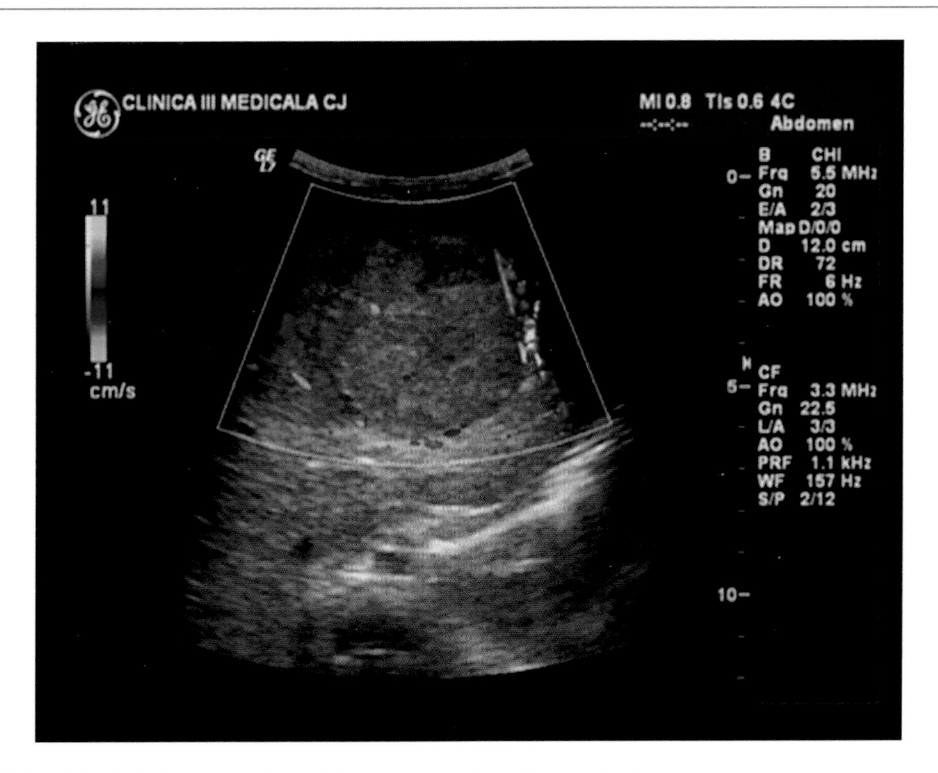

Fig. 28.1 Abdominal ultrasound – hepatoblastoma – color Doppler examination

The surgeon is encouraged to be present during Doppler USG studies to facilitate the immediate discussion with the radiologist (Czauderna et al. 2005). With increasing use of prenatal USG screening, many tumours are detected before birth; therefore, perinatal emergency situations can be avoided.

Interventional radiology has an increasingly important role in both the diagnosis and management of pediatric oncology patients. Image guided percutaneous biopsy or aspiration is frequently performed in the workup for the primary diagnosis and for management of sequelae of oncologic therapy. It was reported by Bittles and Hoffer (2007) that percutaneous biopsy has been shown to be minimally invasive, highly accurate and with a low complication rate. Color Doppler USG is used to avoid vessels.

In order to classify the tumour in the PRETEXT system, the patient must undergo imaging with spiral CT followed by contrast administration (including an angio-computed tomography reconstruction of hepatic vessels, when necessary) and/or magnetic resonance imaging (MRI) with gadolinium (Otte 2010).

CT plays an important role in the initial detection, staging, and assessment of surgical resectability. CT is also used for monitoring response to preoperative chemotherapy and for evaluating tumor recurrence after surgery. On CT, HB typically presents as a heterogeneously enhancing focal solid mass and less commonly as multifocal lesions or as a diffuse infiltrative mass. Associated calcification and area of cystic changes due to necrosis can also be seen. Evaluation of intravascular tumor extension typically into the inferior vena cava and distant metastasis into lungs can also be evaluated with CT (Arellano et al. 2011).

MRI appearance of HB varies with histology. The epithelial subtype is seen as a homogeneous mass, hypointense on T1-weighted imaging (WI) and hyperintense on T2WI. The mixed subtype is more heterogeneous in signal intensity. Malignant neovascularization, stretching of vessels, pooling of contrast media, and invasion or encasement of branches of portal vein or hepatic artery may be seen on angiography. With the gaining popularity of segmental resection, imaging has a pivotal role to play in delineation of the segmental anatomy of liver before surgery. USG and MRI are the preferred techniques as they are free of ionizing radiation and are usually complementary to CT. Multidetector CT (MDCT) is particularly helpful in the assessment of segmental volume prior to resection of liver tumours. Moreover, MDCT is extremely fast, which obviates the need for anaesthesia (Das et al. 2009).

Diffusion weighted (DW) magnetic resonance imaging (MRI) is a non-invasive method, which is capable of investigating the structure of biologic tissues at a microscopic level and may be used for in vivo tissue characterization. Reduced apparent diffusion coefficient (ADC) values have been reported for most malignant tumours and high ADC values for most benign ones. DW imaging can be used for reliable discrimination of benign and malignant pediatric abdominal mass lesions based on considerable differences in the ADC values and signal intensity changes. DW imaging can be used in HB detection, prediction and monitoring tumour response to treatment. Moreover, DW imaging can improve the diagnostic accuracy of biopsies by sampling more cellular areas instead of areas with necrosis for biopsy specimens used in the pathologic examination (Kocaoglu et al. 2010).

Positron emission tomography/computerized tomography (PET/CT) scan provides both functional and anatomical information in a single diagnostic test. The FDG avidity was demonstrated in all abdominal tumors, making it a very sensitive diagnostic modality. This may decrease with effective chemotherapy and/or maturation of the tumor. Although PET has been gaining popularity as a tool in the detection of tumor recurrences worldwide, it has been shown by Wong et al. (2004) that PET may not be useful in HB patients, and caution must be taken in the interpretation of positive results.

Pathologic Features, Liver Biopsy and Staging

Hepatoblastoma is an embryonal neoplasm composed of malignant epithelial tissue with variable differentiation, most often with embryonal or fetal components. Histologically, HB can be divided into six types based on patterns of differentiation including pure fetal epithelial, combined fetal and embryonal epithelial, macrotrabecular, small cell undifferentiated, mixed epithelial and mesenchymal, and mixed epithelial and mesenchymal with teratoid features. The least differentiated is the small cell undifferentiated (SCUD) pattern. In neonates, the relatively differentiated, pure fetal histology seems to predominate compared with older children. However metastases may occur early and are often systemic (cerebral, bone, placenta), bypassing the lungs presumably due to the fetal circulation (von Schweinitz 2003). Most commonly, HB present in the right lobe of liver with an average diameter of 10–12 cm. On cut section, the epithelial type is homogeneous whereas the mixed type is heterogeneous (Fig. 28.2). Definitive diagnosis of hepatoblastoma is by histology. Staining for AFP is positive in the majority of cases. The tumoral cells show positive immunolabel grouped into parcels for Hep par 1 and focally for AFP (Fig. 28.3a,b), as reported by Iacob et al. (2010).

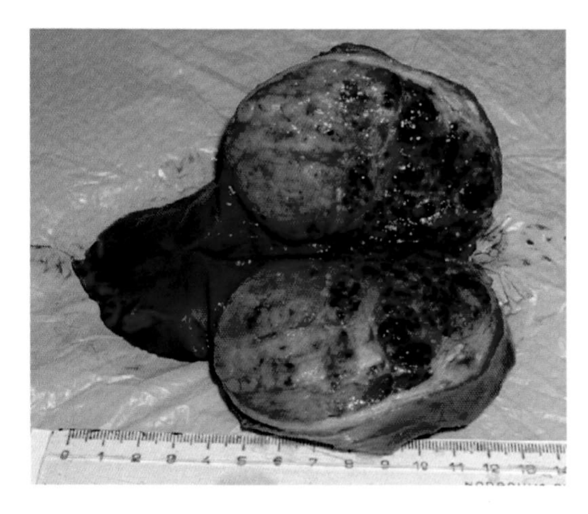

Fig. 28.2 Macroscopic aspect in section of resected mixt hepatoblastoma with hemorrhages

Biopsy of the primary hepatic tumour is mandatory in children (a) under 6 months of age, because of the wide differential diagnosis of liver masses and the possible confounding impact of an elevated serum AFP at this age; (b) over 3 years, because of the risk of misdiagnosing

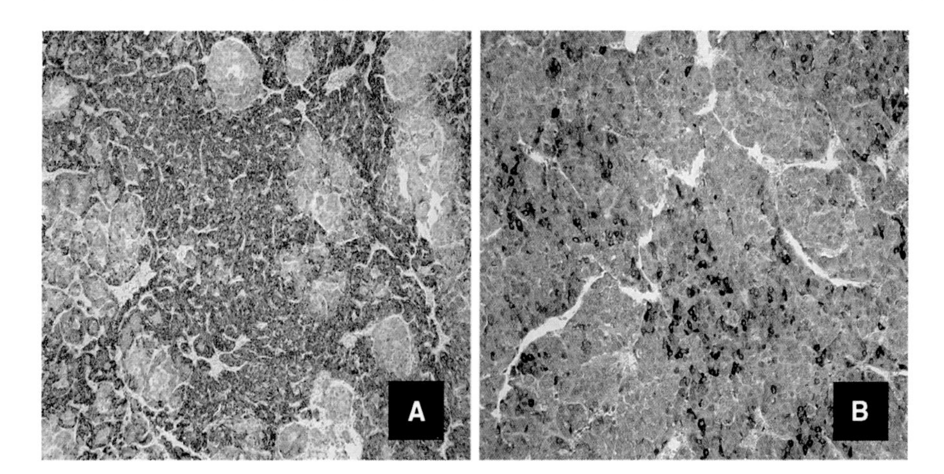

Fig. 28.3 (**a**) Microscopic aspect – Hep par 1 shows islands of positive tumoral cells close to an area of negative tumoral cells. 100×. (**b**) Microscopic aspect – positive alpha-fetoprotein in some of the tumoral cells. 100×

hepatocellular carcinoma. In children between 6 months and 3 years of age with findings suggesting HB (imagistic evidence of an intrahepatic mass, elevated AFP, thrombocytosis), biopsy is only strongly recommended, as pathological material would be available after tumour resection.

Minor complications are rare, including bleeding from the biopsy site, abdominal pain. Due to the risk of formation of adhesions between the tumour and the abdominal wall when an open biopsy is taken, a percutaneous, image-guided biopsy (by USG or CT) and passing through normal liver tissue is recommended (Czauderna et al. 2005).

Fine needle aspiration cytology (FNAC) allows the recognition of cytomorphological features of pediatric focal liver lesions.

The Liver Tumor Strategy Group (SIOPEL) of the International Society of Pediatric Oncology (SIOP) developed a PRE-Treatment EXTension staging system (PRETEXT), based on imaging at presentation which has been used in the first SIOPEL study trial and all the subsequent ones. The hepatic tumor is classified into one of the four categories depending on the number of sections free of tumor. Patients are staged according to the PRETEXT system at diagnosis, during neoadjuvant chemotherapy and before surgery. The main aim of PRETEXT grouping was to determine whether it would be possible, pre-operatively, to identify the patients in whom complete tumour resection might be performed by partial hepatectomy. This system is rather different from those developed by the Children's Cancer Study Group (CCSG) and the German Cooperative Pediatric Liver Tumor Study in which the stage of disease is determined at the initial surgical intervention, undertaken at diagnosis and before chemotherapy (Czauderna et al. 2005).

The PRETEXT grouping system was revised in 2005 to improve the original definition, to clarify the definitions of criteria for extrahepatic extension of tumor and to add new criteria for patients with caudate lobe involvement, tumor rupture, ascites, direct extension of tumor to the stomach or diaphragm, tumor focality, lymph node and vascular involvement and distant metastases (Otte 2010). The inclusion of additional criteria allows risk stratification in SIOPEL studies. Patients are considered high-risk with any of the following: serum AFP level <100 ng/ml, PRETEXT IV, extension beyond the liver in the abdomen, distant metastases, intraperitoneal hemorrhage, involvement of hepatic veins, vena cava or portal vein.

Prognostic Factors

The PRETEXT system has very good reproducibility and an excellent predictive value as regards prognosis. This system has been validated in the

SIOPEL-1 study (Czauderna et al. 2005). It was reported by Perilongo et al. (2004) that in multivariate analysis the PRETEXT category was the only statistically significant prognostic factor for 5-year overall survival.

Patients of older age, with a multifocal tumour, high PRETEXT, involvement of major liver vessels and AFP < 100 ng/ml are less likely to be cured by resection; these findings at presentation should lead to refer early in a transplantation centre to optimize the timing of the procedure. Multivariate analysis performed separately for primary liver transplant group showed that venous invasion was the only statistically significant adverse prognostic factor (Czauderna et al. 2005).

Lung metastases at presentation was an important negative prognostic factor in SIOPEL1 for the 5-year event-free survival rate. A resected tumor with small vessel vascular invasion and a multifocal disseminated pattern of growth was associated with tumor-related mortality. It was reported by Davies et al. (2004) that the identification of a SCUD pattern in the preoperative biopsy, as well as in the resected tumor, should alert the oncologist of an aggressive tumor, this cytologic pattern being predictive of a high mortality rate.

In PRETEXT III tumors there was no significant difference in survival rate between resection margins less than 1 cm and ≥1 cm. In patients presented with synchronous pulmonary metastatic disease, where survival was significantly worse, analysis confirmed that margins less than 1 cm did not significantly affect survival after controlling for pulmonary metastatic disease (Dicken et al. 2004). It was shown that there was no significant difference in local tumor recurrence with microscopic positive versus negative margins. Given the very good chemotherapy response rates (80%), the presence of microscopic residual disease does not necessarily portend a poor prognosis with respect to local tumor recurrence, nor does it imply the need for heroic chemotherapy or surgical salvage procedures, as shown by Dicken et al. (2004).

It was reported by De Ioris et al. (2008) that patients with HB and low serum AFP at diagnosis are a high-risk subgroup with extensive disease at diagnosis, poor response to chemotherapy and a poor outcome. An AFP of <100 ng/ml at diagnosis was significantly associated with a reduced overall survival, as was the presence of metastases. However, PRETEXT Group IV and the presence of extrahepatic disease showed no association with overall survival (Perilongo et al. 2004).

Other important prognostic factor at diagnosis and in response to therapy include the magnitude of the decrease in AFP and the histologically-documented complete response to therapy (Perilongo et al. 2004).

Nuclear accumulation of β-catenin is an adverse prognostic factor for survival of patients with HB. Loss of carcinoembryonic antigen-related cell adhesion molecule 1 (CEACAM1) expression in HB cells may promote hematogeneous metastasis. Loss of CEACAM1 expression is a significant risk factor for metachronous pulmonary metastases and vascular invasion. Univariate analysis showed that the CEACAM1 expression of tumor cells, vascular invasion, and size of the largest hepatic tumor >10 cm were significant prognostic factors (Tsukada et al. 2009).

Treatment

Complete surgical resection and pre- or post-operative chemotherapy are the mainstay of treatment of HB. Radical resection can be obtained either conventionally by partial hepatectomy or with orthotopic liver transplant. The International Society of Paediatric Oncology (SIOPEL) group recommended preoperative chemotherapy for childhood HB. In SIOPEL-1, all patients were treated preoperatively with four courses of cisplatin and doxorubicin (PLADO); surgical resection was followed by two more courses of chemotherapy. If the tumor was judged unresectable by imaging after four courses of chemotherapy, surgical resection was delayed until after the sixth course. If the tumor remained localized to the liver but was still unresectable, liver transplantation was recommended as the primary operative procedure (Czauderna et al. 2005).

In the SIOPEL 1 study, 28% of patients were downstaged by PRETEXT criteria after preoperative chemotherapy, there was tumour shrinkage in >90% of patients, resulting in less extensive liver resections than were initially anticipated (Czauderna et al. 2005).

The SIOPEL-2 pilot study was designed to test the efficacy and toxicity of two chemotherapy regimens, one for patients with HB confined to the liver and involving no more then three hepatic sections: standard-risk HB (SR-HB), and one for HB extending into all four sections and/or with lung metastases, or intra-abdominal extrahepatic spread, or tumor rupture at presentation, or with serum AFP < 100 units at presentation: high-risk HR (HR- HB) (Perilongo et al. 2004). Those with SR-HB were treated with four courses of cisplatin monotherapy, delayed surgery, and then two more courses of cisplatin. Patients with HR-HB were given cisplatin alternating with carboplatin and doxorubicin, pre- and postoperatively. For SR-HB patients, and HR-HB patients, the 3-year progression-free survival rates were 89% and 48%, respectively. For SR-HB patients, the efficacy of cisplatin monotherapy and the cisplatin/doxorubicin combination are compared in a prospective randomized trial (SIOPEL-3 study) (Perilongo et al. 2004). For HR-HB patients, intensified chemotherapy with cisplatin, doxorubicin and carboplatin is being investigated in a SIOPEL-4 study (Otte 2010).

Chemotherapy for low AFP patients should be revised.

North American study groups (the Children's Cancer Study Group CCSG), the Pediatric Oncology Group, and the Intergroup Hepatoma Study promoted immediate surgery for localised tumours. The German/Austrian Pediatric Oncology Group (GPOG) have suggested that there is little to be gained from prolonging chemotherapy beyond the planned treatment regimen because of the risk of developing tumour cell chemoresistance. At present, the SIOPEL and the German hepatoblastoma groups recommend no attempt at primary surgery for liver tumours (Czauderna et al. 2005).

Intraoperative ultrasound is useful in locating the major vessels. It was reported by Otte (2010) that extensive liver resections (up to 80% of the liver mass) can be tolerated by young children with HB and hepatic regeneration can be complete within 3 months, despite the administration of toxic agents since they usually have no underlying liver disease and excellent hepatic reserve.

Complete tumor resection can be easily achieved with a partial hepatectomy when the intrahepatic extent is limited to one or two sections (PRETEXT I and II). When the tumor involves three sections (PRETEXT III), preoperative neoadjuvant chemotherapy can make lesions initially considered unresectable become resectable with a trisegmentectomy (Otte 2010). In centrally located HB, resection of Couinaud's segments 4, 5 and 8 (central hepatectomy) can be performed by expert surgeons (Guérin, et al. 2010).

It was reported by Cacciavillano et al. (2004) the following response criteria, based on serum AFP and imaging techniques, such as ultrasonography, computed tomography, radiography: (a) complete response (CR): complete disappearance of tumour and a negative serum AFP; (b) partial response (PR): any tumour volume shrinkage associated with a decreasing serum AFP >1 log below the baseline measurement; (c) stable disease (SD): no change in tumour volume and/or <1 log drop in serum AFP concentration; (d) progressive disease (PD): an unequivocal increase in tumour size in one or more dimensions, or an unequivocal increase in the serum AFP concentration even without any clinical (physical and/or radiological) evidence of tumour regrowth.

Measuring tumour volume and serum AFP kinetics accurately reflects HB responsiveness to induction therapy. Treatment toxicities may be reduced by earlier resection (potentially after cycle 2 of induction therapy) and tailoring of chemotherapeutic regimens (Lovvorn et al. 2010). There is a different and unique biologic response between HB of right or left lobe origin. When compared with right lobe tumors, response kinetics of left lobe tumors seemed slower as measured by serum AFP decay and tumour volume. Right lobe tumors may be slightly more chemosensitive and perhaps require less overall treatment than left lobe tumors.

The principal toxicities of HB treatment include ototoxicity, chronic renal insufficiency and neurocognitive deficits. Evaluation of long-term treatment toxicity require after completion of therapy a check up every 1–3 months for the first year. After surviving 2 years off therapy, children are evaluated annually with physical examination, serum AFP, blood counts and routine chemistries, an annual audiology examination, and a screening for speech and learning difficulties (Lovvorn et al. 2010).

Data from the SIOPEL 1 study and global experience have shown excellent results with primary orthotopic liver transplant compared with those obtained by rescue transplant performed for relapse or incomplete tumour resection (87% versus 30% long-term, disease-free patient survival), as reported by Czauderna et al. (2005). Liver transplant is a reasonable option if lung metastases have been eradicated by chemotherapy.

Guidelines for early referral of patients with HB to a liver transplant unit are: (a) multifocal PRETEXT 4 HB; (b) large, solitary PRETEXT 4 HB, involving all four sectors of the liver; (c) unifocal, centrally-located tumours involving main hilar structures or all three main hepatic veins (Czauderna et al. 2005).

It was reported by Casas-Melley et al. (2007) that patients should be referred for evaluation at a transplant center if after the initial three courses of chemotherapy they continue to show evidence of unresectable tumor. There should also be early referral if the patient shows poor response to initial chemotherapy such as less than 1 to 2 log decrease in AFP level. It is imperative that early complete surgical resection with adjuvant chemotherapy is instituted before the development of chemotherapeutic resistance. Effectiveness of pretransplantation chemotherapy was defined as a drop of more than 99% in peak AFP levels. Decline in peak AFP of more than 99% was also associated with better survival. Posttransplantation chemotherapy reduce tumor recurrence and improves survival rate (Browne et al. 2008).

Pediatric Liver Unresectable Tumor Observatory (PLUTO) database, developed by the SIOPEL strategy group, will allow to find out the prognostic significance of vascular invasion, optimal timing of transplantation, optimal amount and timing of pretransplant (neoadjuvant) and posttransplant (adjuvant) chemotherapy. It will also offer data concerning the value of liver transplantation in children presenting with a relapse after partial liver resection, the potential role of transplantation in children who initially present with metastatic disease that resolves on neoadjuvant chemotherapy, and the amount of immunosuppression needed following transplantation (Otte 2010).

All patients need extensive metastatic workup before transplant, including computed tomography (CT) scan of the head, chest, abdomen and pelvis. After orthotopic liver transplant the patients have to be followed closely with AFP levels monthly and CT scan every 3 months for the first year and every 6 months after 1 year. Additional CT scans have to be done if there is any elevation of the AFP level (Casas-Melley et al. 2007).

Overall disease-free survival at 6 years post-transplant was reported as 82% for primary transplants and 30% for rescue transplants (Otte 2010). For primary transplants, the only parameter significantly related to overall survival was macroscopic venous invasion. In a review of database concerning liver transplantation in children transplanted for unresectable or recurrent HB the 1, 5, and 10-year survival were 79%, 69%, and 66% respectively (Otte 2010).

Major intraoperative complications of liver resection for HB such as severe bleeding, air embolism, and unrecognized bile duct injury are infrequent and operative mortality is very low, even after extended hepatectomies, since children with HB have no underlying liver disease. Persistence of viable extrahepatic tumor deposits after chemotherapy, not amenable to surgical resection, is the only absolute contraindication for liver transplantation. Macroscopic venous invasion (portal vein, hepatic veins, vena cava) is not a contraindication if complete resection of the invaded venous structures can be accomplished. Venous extent was associated with a significantly shorter survival. Timing of liver transplantation should not be delayed in excess of a few weeks after the last course of chemotherapy (Otte 2010).

Complete hepatectomy with living donor liver transplantation provides optimal surgical treatment in unresectable stage III and initial stage IV disease confined to the liver at resection. Children tolerate complete hepatectomy, transplantation, and postoperative chemotherapy well. Referral to a transplant center during the first three cycles of chemotherapy appears to offers the best opportunity for long-term survival (Casas-Melley et al. 2007).

Conclusion

Although uncommon, most of the pediatric liver tumors are malignant. Patient age, clinical signs and symptoms, and AFP levels are critical discriminators in the evaluation of HB. Histopathological evaluation remains essential for final diagnosis, characterization, and treatment planning. Imaging has to determine the character of HB, accurate staging, and follow-up after treatment. The preferred techniques are USG and MRI as they are free of ionizing radiation and are usually complementary to CT. For follow-up, USG is the initial technique of choice. CT and MRI may be used to investigate the extent of HB and its metastases, to refine the differential diagnosis and to follow-up after chemotherapy or surgery. Imaging methods are promising for better surgical outcomes and offer greater sensitivity for diagnosing residual or relapsed disease.

The principle of management remains the initial chemotherapy followed by surgical resection. The actual choice of regimen is governed by PRETEXT stage, with two broad risk groups ("high" or "standard" risk) and the subsequent chemotherapy is based on cisplatin (or carboplatin) and doxorubicin. Shrinkage of the tumour with reduction in AFP levels usually occurs and is then followed by tumour resection after 6–8 weeks, followed by a further course of chemotherapy. If imaging shows that the tumour are unresectable then consideration should be given to liver transplantation to achieve local disease control. Aggressive management of HB patients with preoperative chemotherapy, complete resection including total hepatectomy, orthotopic liver transplant and adjuvant chemotherapy will offer the best chance for long-term survival. Factors associated with an improvement in long-term posttransplantation survival were enhanced pretransplantation tumor sensitivity to chemotherapy, demonstrated by a greater than 99% drop in AFP levels in response to chemotherapy, and the administration of chemotherapy after transplantation.

Research directions for the future will be to create additional molecular classifications to define risk groups at the biological level.

References

Adesina AM, Nguyen Y, Guanaratne P, Pulliam J, Lopez-Terrada D, Margolin J, Finegold M (2007) FOXG1 is overexpressed in hepatoblastoma. Hum Pathol 38:400–409

Arellano CMR, Kritsaneepaiboon S, Lee EY (2011) CT Imaging findings of malignant neoplasms arising in the epigastric region in children. Clin Imaging 35:10–20

Bittles MA, Hoffer FA (2007) Interventional radiology and the care of the pediatric oncology patient. Surg Oncol 16:229–233

Browne M, Sher D, Grant D, Deluca E, Alonso E, Whitington PF, Superina RA (2008) Survival after liver transplantation for hepatoblastoma: a 2-center experience. J Pediatr Surg 43:1973–1981

Cacciavillano WD, Brugieres L, Childs M, Shafford E, Brock P, Pritchard J, Mailbach R, Scopinaro M, Perilongo G (2004) Phase II study of high-dose cyclophosphamide in relapsing and/or resistant hepatoblastoma in children: a study from the SIOPEL group. Eur J Cancer 40:2274–2279

Casas-Melley AT, Malatack J, Consolini D, Mann K, Raab C, Flynn L, Woolfrey P, Menendez J, Dunn SP (2007) Successful liver transplant for unresectable hepatoblastoma. J Pediatr Surg 42:184–187

Czauderna P, Otte JB, Aronson DC, Gauthier F, Mackinlay G, Roebuck D, Plaschkes J, Perilongo G (2005) Guidelines for surgical treatment of hepatoblastoma in the modern era – Recommendations from the Childhood Liver Tumour Strategy Group of the International Society of Paediatric Oncology (SIOPEL). Eur J Cancer 41:1031–1036

Das CJ, Dhingra S, Gupta AK, Iyer V, Agarwala S (2009) Imaging of paediatric liver tumours with pathological correlation. Clin Radiol 64:1015–1025

Davies JQ, de la Hall PM, Kaschula ROC, Sinclair-Smith CC, Hartley P, Rode H, Millar AJW (2004) Hepatoblastoma – evolution of management and outcome and significance of histology of the resected

tumor. A 31-year experience with 40 cases. J Pediatr Surg 39:1321–1327
De Ioris M, Brugieres L, Zimmermann A, Keeling J, Brock P, Maibach R, Pritchard J, Shafford L, Zsiros J, Czaudzerna P, Perilongo G (2008) Hepatoblastoma with a low serum alpha-fetoprotein level at diagnosis: the SIOPEL group experience. Eur J Cancer 44:545–550
Dicken BJ, Bigam DL, Lees GM (2004) Association between surgical margins and long-term outcome in advanced hepatoblastoma. J Pediatr Surg 39:721–725
Guérin F, Gauthier F, Martelli H, Fabre M, Baujard C, Franchi S, Branchereau S (2010) Outcome of central hepatectomy for hepatoblastomas. J Pediatr Surg 45:555–563
Iacob D, Serban A, Fufezan O, Badea R, Iancu C, Mitre C, Neamtu S (2010) Mixed hepatoblastoma in child. Case report. Med Ultrason 2:157–162
Kocaoglu M, Bulakbasi N, Sanal HT, Kismet E, Caliskan B, Akgun V, Tayfun C (2010) Pediatric abdominal masses: diagnostic accuracy of diffusion weighted MRI. Magn Reson Imaging 28:629–636
Lovvorn HN III, Ayers D, Zhao Z, Hilmes M, Prasad P, Shinall MC Jr, Berch B, Neblett WW III, O'Neill JA Jr (2010) Defining hepatoblastoma responsiveness to induction therapy as measured by tumor volume and serum α-fetoprotein kinetics. J Pediatr Surg 45:121–129
Ma SK, Cheung ANY, Choy C, Chan GCF, Ha SY, Ching LM, Wan TSK, Chan LC (2000) Cytogenetic characterization of childhood hepatoblastoma. Cancer Genet Cytogenet 119:32–36
Makin E, Davenport M (2010) Fetal and neonatal liver tumours. Early Hum Dev 86:637–642
Nelson WJ, Nusse R (2004) Convergence of Wnt, beta-catenin, and cadherin pathways. Science 303:1483–1487
Otte JB (2010) Progress in the surgical treatment of malignant liver tumors in children. Cancer Treat Rev 36:360–371
Perilongo G, Shafford E, Maibach R, Aronson D, Brugieres L, Brock P, Childs M, Czauderna P, MacKinlay G, Otte JB, Pritchard J, Rondelli R, Scopinaro M, Staalman C, Plaschkes J (2004) Risk-adapted treatment for childhood hepatoblastoma: final report of the second study of the International Society of Paediatric Oncology—SIOPEL 2. Eur J Cancer 40:411–421
Terracciano LM, Bernasconi B, Ruck P, Stallmach T, Briner J, Sauter G, Moch H, Vecchione R, Pollice L, Pettinato G, Gurtl B, Ratschek M, De Krijger R, Tornillo L, Bruder E (2003) Comparative genomic hybridization analysis of hepatoblastoma reveals high frequency of X-chromosome gains and similarities between epithelial and stromal components. Hum Pathol 34(9):864–871
Tsukada M, Wakai T, Matsuda Y, Korita PV, Shirai Y, Ajioka Y, Hatakeyama K, Kubota M (2009) Loss of carcinoembryonic antigen-related cell adhesion molecule 1 expression predicts metachronous pulmonary metastasis and poor survival in patients with hepatoblastoma. J Pediatr Surg 44:1522–1528
Turato C, Buendia MA, Fabre M, Redon MJ, Branchereau S, Quarta S, Ruvoletto M, Perilongo G, Grotzer MA, Gatta A, Pontisso P (2011) Over-expression of SERPINB3 in hepatoblastoma: a possible insight into the genesis of this tumour? Eur J Cancer. doi:10.1016/j.ejca.2011.06.004
von Schweinitz D (2003) Neonatal liver tumours. Semin Neonatol 8:403–410
Wong KKY, Lan LCL, Lin SCL, Tam PKH (2004) The use of positron emission tomography in detecting hepatoblastoma recurrence – a cautionary tale. J Pediatr Surg 39:1779–1781
Zimmermann A (2005) The emerging family of hepatoblastoma tumours: from ontogenesis to oncogenesis. Eur J Cancer 41:1503–1514
Zynger DL, Gupta A, Luan C, Chou PM, Yang GY, Yang XJ (2008) Expression of glypican 3 in hepatoblastoma: an immunohistochemical study of 65 cases. Hum Pathol 39:224–230

Treatment of Pineal Region Tumors in Childhood

29

Ali Varan, Nejat Akalan, and Faruk Zorlu

Contents

A. Varan (✉)
Department of Pediatric Oncology, Institute of Oncology, Hacettepe University, 06100 Ankara, Turkey
e-mail: hupog@tr.net

N. Akalan
Department of Neurosurgery, Faculty of Medicine, Hacettepe University, 06100 Ankara, Turkey

F. Zorlu
Department of Radiation Oncology, Faculty of Medicine, Hacettepe University, 06100 Ankara, Turkey

Abstract

Treatment options for pineal tumors include surgery as the first-line therapy, radiotherapy, and chemotherapy. Since the pineal gland is deeply seated, total resection is not always possible. Histopathologic examination is important for treatment planning, such as for determining whether radiotherapy is indicated. Chemotherapy has greatly improved overall pineal tumor survival rates, and therefore should be used for all malignant pineal tumors, with cisplatin, etoposide, and CCNU being the most preferred agents.

Introduction

Overall, pineal tumors account for < 1% of all brain tumors, and these tumors are rare malignancies in children. This rate varies according to geographic area, with a higher reported incidence in northeast Asia (~ 12%; Cho et al. 1998) and Japan. The Surveillance, Epidemiology, and End Results program of the National Cancer Institute of USA reported an 0.8% incidence of pineal tumors among the 77,264 registered central nervous system tumors (Al-Hussaini et al. 2009; Nomura 2001). In Turkey, this rate is 2.4% (Yazıcı et al. 2009), although the number of actual incidents reported is quite low. Most pineal region tumors are germ cell tumors (50–70%), followed by pineal parenchymal tumors (20–30%). Pineoblastomas and pineocytomas are the primary parenchymal tumors, followed by glial

M.A. Hayat (ed.), *Pediatric Cancer, Volume 3: Diagnosis, Therapy, and Prognosis*, Pediatric Cancer 3,
DOI 10.1007/978-94-007-4528-5_29,

tumors (including low- or high-grade astrocytic tumors). Atypical teratoid rhabdoid tumors (ATRT), ependymomas, meningiomas, and metastatic tumors are rarely detected.

Treatment

Multidisciplinary approaches are used to treat pineal tumors. Surgery, radiotherapy, and chemotherapy have been used alone or in combination, depending on tumor histopathology.

Surgery

Surgery is the most important component of brain tumor treatment. Resection provides tumor sample for an accurate diagnosis, restores deteriorated clinical signs and symptoms mostly due to hydrocephalus and neural tissue compression and offers fastest and most effective cytoreduction. Pineal gland resides extracerebrally almost at the center of the brain offering multiple trajectories for approach through natural planes without comprising any nervous tissue, including supratentorial and infratentorial routes. Moreover, enlarged ventricles associated with pineal tumors enable to utilize endoscopic techniques for treatment. The choice of the most appropriate approach depends on the size, texture and growth pattern of a given pineal tumor which can be appreciated with magnetic resonance imaging (MRI). The central and deep localization among vital structures carry substantial morbidity, especially when the aim is a total removal. Certain histopathological types of tumors known to be highly sensitive to adjuvant therapy like germinomas can be handled with biopsy alone, provided that increased intracranial pressure is normalized. Most preferred approach is endoscopic third ventriculostomy with tumor biopsy which enables to treat accompanying hydrocephalus and tissue diagnosis at the same setting (Oi et al. 2000; Gangemi et al. 2001). This conservative approach is most suitable for germ cell tumors where high levels of tumor markers such as α-fetoprotein or β-human corionic gonadotropin (hCG) can preoperatively be detected (Kanamori et al. 2008). Nevertheless, tumors with high proliferation index or which are relatively benign and germ cell tumors with focal compression require surgical excision. Total pineal tumoral resection should be done whenever possible, with total or gross total resection improving survival in pineoblastomas (Gilheeney et al. 2008). If total resection is not possible, then tissue diagnosis or subtotal resection should be considered (Tamaki and Yin 2000; Knierim and Yamada 2003; Konovalov and Pitskhelauri 2003; Shin et al. 1998).

Radiotherapy

Radiotherapy is the second primary treatment modality for most brain tumors. While benign tumors do not require radiotherapy, malignant tumors do. The dosage, treatment plan, and techniques used vary with the tumor type (Habrand and De Crevoisier 2001). A few reports have indicated that single fraction stereotactic radiosurgery can be used safely and effectively for all pineal tumors (Lekovic et al. 2007; Reyns et al. 2006), and this procedure has been mostly applied to pineocytomas and pineolomas, where better results were obtained with small-sized tumors. Fractionated radiosurgery is also being investigated.

Pineoblastomas and Primitive Neuroectodermal Tumors

Pineoblastomas are embryonal primitive neuroectodermal tumors (PNET) and should be treated similar to PNETs (Jakacki 1999; Gilheeney et al. 2008; Habrand and De Crevoisier 2001). Craniospinal imaging should be performed and, regardless of spinal seeding, pineoblastomas should be treated with craniospinal radiotherapy. Whole cranial doses should be 35 Gy, boost doses to the pineal gland should be 20–25 Gy, and 30–35 Gy should be given to the spinal axis.

Pineocytomas

Pineocytomas are slowly growing tumors derived from pineal parenchymal cells. The general approach for this tumor type is treatment with radiotherapy without chemotherapy (30–50 Gy). Better results are obtained with gross total resection than with subtotal resection or radiotherapy alone (Clark et al. 2010).

Germ Cell Tumors

All patients with germ cell tumors should be treated with radiotherapy (Habrand and De Crevoisier 2001; Kyritsis 2010). Dysgerminom can be treated by radiotherapy alone, as it is the most radiosensitive tumor. Some centers add chemotherapy to the radiotherapy, since germ cell tumors have a high recurrence rate. Radiotherapy doses should be 30–35 Gy to the whole cranium (Douglas et al. 2006). For dysgerminomas, irradiation of either the whole cranial or pineal tumoral area is effective; the decision of which is performed is based on institutional preference. For nondysgerminomatous tumors, the whole cranium should be irradiated and a boost should be given to the tumor bed, with tumoral doses of 50–54 Gy. Radiotherapy is a prognostic factor in intracranial germ cell tumors, with patients treated without radiotherapy having a poorer prognosis (Calaminus et al. 2004).

Astrocytic Tumors

Low-grade (WHO grade I-II) astrocytic tumors can be followed up without treatment (Habrand and De Crevoisier 2001). If there is recurrent disease or severe symptoms, tumors should be treated with cranial 30–35 Gy radiotherapy. High-grade astrocytic tumors (WHO grade III-IV) should be treated with cranial 30–35 Gy radiotherapy and a boost to the tumoral region of 50–54 Gy. All high-grade tumors should also be treated with chemotherapy.

Chemotherapy

Chemotherapy is an effective treatment modality for pineal region tumors. Germ cell tumors and embryonal brain tumors such as pineoblastomas are sensitive to chemotherapy. Survival increases with chemotherapy use.

Germ Cell Tumors

For germ cell tumors, cisplatin (CDDP)- and etoposide-based protocols are commonly used. Since the early 1970s, single or two chemotherapeutic agents have been used. Although vincristine, adriamycin, and actinomycin-D have previously been used as chemotherapeutics, the results were not satisfactory, with survival rates of < 50%. The addition of cisplatin (Einhorn and Donohue 1977) increased survival rates to > 80%. The most common chemotherapy protocol for this tumor subset is a cisplatin, etoposide, and bleomycin (BEP) regimen (Yazıcı et al. 2009). Cisplatin doses are 100–120 mg/m^2 in 1 day or 20 mg/m^2 for 5 day, depending on the center. The cisplatin dose used is an important prognostic factor for survival. Total doses of < 400 mg/m^2 are associated with poorer prognosis than higher doses ($p = 0.002$) (Calaminus et al. 2004). Some centers prefer to use carboplatin (400–500 mg/m^2 for 1 or 2 days) instead of cisplatin (Douglas et al. 2006). A common etoposide dose is 100–120 mg/m^2 for 3 days, and a common bleomycin dose is15 units/m^2 for 1 day. These cycles are repeated every 3 weeks, with four or six cycles. Ifosfamide combined with cisplatin has been used in some protocols, with alternating cycles (Kanamori et al. 2008).

Germinomas should be treated with a similar chemotherapeutic regimen, although some centers treat these tumors with radiotherapy alone. The Children's Oncology Group (COG) has stratified treatment according to risk (Kretschmar et al. 2007). Low-risk patients have pure germinomas as well as normal AFP and hCG (< 50 mIU/ml) levels. High-risk patients have mixed germinomas as well as elevated AFP and HCG levels. Patients were treated with CDDP (20 mg/m^2/day for 5 days) and etoposide (100 mg/m^2/day for 5 days), and the treatment was alternated every 3 weeks with vincristine (1.5 mg/m^2 on days 1, 8, and 15) and cyclophosphamide (1 g/m^2 for 2 days). In high-risk patients, the CDDP and cyclophosphamide doses were doubled. Using this protocol, the high-risk group had the best results for overall survival. Methotrexate and paclitaxel have also been used in different combinations (Kyritsis 2010). Methotrexate was preferred at either low doses of 100–300 mg/m^2 or a high dose of 1 g/m^2.

Pineoblastomas and Primitive Neuroectodermal Tumors

Pineoblastomas and primitive neuroectodermal tumors of the pineal area should be treated similar to other embryonal brain tumors. In the early 1960s and 1970s, the only treatment available was surgery, typically followed by radiotherapy. Subsequent addition of chemotherapeutic agents improved survival rates slightly. During this time, studies that compared radiotherapy alone to radiotherapy plus chemotherapy were performed, with the combined treatment modality being superior to radiotherapy alone. Afterwards, chemotherapeutic strategies were intensively investigated in patients.

Traditionally, a single agent or 2- or 3-drug combined regimen has been used for these tumor types. In the beginning of the chemotherapy era, commonly used treatments included lomustine (CCNU), vincristine, prednisone, procarbazine, cisplatin or carboplatin, and etoposide (Cuccia et al. 2006; Gilheeney et al. 2008). Vincristine and cyclophosphamide were successful agents, and CCNU was used in the earliest randomized studies. Common protocols included CCNU at 100 mg/m^2 on day 1, vincristine at 1.5 mg/m^2 weekly, and procarbazine at 100 mg/m^2 1–14 days, in 6-week intervals (PCV) (Cuccia et al. 2006; Gilheeney et al. 2008; Yazıcı et al. 2009). Cisplatin, carboplatin, and etoposide were used in phase II studies in the 1990s, and cisplatin, etoposide, CCNU, and cyclophosphamide have been preferred in COG protocols (Jakacki 1999). High-dose methotrexate (5 g/m^2) combined with other drugs was tested in German HIT studies (Hinkes et al. 2007), which used ifosfamide, etoposide, cisplatin, methotrexate, and cytarabine in the induction period, and CCNU, cisplatin, and vincristine in the maintenance protocol. All young children died in this protocol, and the results were not satisfactory.

High-dose chemotherapy with autologous stem-cell rescue has been attempted as both a first-line treatment and as a relapse protocol (Gururangan et al. 2003; Jakacki 1999). Although the first-line protocol results were better than relapse results, similar outcomes can be obtained with cisplatin + etoposide protocols. As a relapse protocol, the outcome is actually worse; the toxicity is very high due to previous combined chemoradiotherapy regimens.

Astrocytic Tumors

Low-grade astrocytic tumors do not require post-surgical treatment unless the disease shows recurrence or (rarely) has seeding metastasis. In these situation, radiotherapy should be the first choice, followed by chemotherapy. High-grade astrocytic tumors are mostly fatal, and require both radio- and chemotherapy. A cisplatin, etoposide, and vincristine combination or CCNU-based protocol can be given. PCV was used in early years, with results similar to astocytomes located in other regions (Finlay et al. 1995). A combination of carboplatin + vincristine was preferred by Packer et al. (1993). In the last decade, temozolomide (150–200 mg/m^2 for 5 days every 28 days) has been used in adult patients as a first-line protocol as well as in children, although there is little available data for the latter (Barone et al. 2006). In recent report, pineal ATRT was successfully treated with temozolomide after recurrence (Wang et al. 2009). The advantage of this agent is that it is used orally. Temozolomide has been combined with erlotinib or lomustine in phase I studies (Barone et al. 2006); however, adequate data and prospective studies are lacking for temozolomide and other new agents. None of these protocols is specific for pineal astrocytic tumors, as all were studied in general brain astrocytic tumors.

Ependymomas, ependymoblastomas, and ATRTs are rare tumor types of the pineal region that should be treated with radiotherapy. Chemotherapy should be added for embryonal tumors such as ATRTs and ependymoblastomas. The protocol used is the same as for other primitive neuroectodermal tumors. Ependymomas generally do not require chemotherapy, except in the case of recurrence. CDDP, etoposide, or PCV protocols can be used in such instances.

Prognosis

Prognosis depends on the presence of metastases, histopathology, tumor size, and degree of surgery. Germ cell tumors have a better prognosis than the other tumor types, and the worst prognosis is seen in atypical teratoid rhabdoid tumors. Seeding and extraneural metastases negatively affect the prognosis, except in the case of germ cell tumors that respond well to chemotherapy even with extraneural metastases. However, the blood-brain barrier generally prevents extraneural metastasis. If the tumor is large, the risk of complications is high and management is difficult. The degree of surgical resection is important in terms of prognosis for all brain tumors, with total resection being ideal.

Late Effects

The primary location of the tumor and the treatment modalities used can cause acute or late effects (Knierim and Yamada 2003; Konovalov and Pitskhelauri 2003; Shin et al. 1998; Tamaki and Yin 2000; Yazıcı et al. 2009). Surgery or tumoral cell invasion can damage the normal pineal gland or adjacent tissues, resulting in deafness, parinoud syndrome, ataxia, or epilepsy. Radiotherapy specifically inhibits the pituitary-hypothalamic axis. Side effects include endocrinopathies such as hypothyroidism, micropenis due to low FSH level, and diabetes insipidus. Chemotherapy can cause nephrotoxicitiy.

References

Al-Hussaini M, Sultan I, Abuirmileh N, Jaradat I, Qaddoumi I (2009) Pineal gland tumors: experience from the SEER database. J Neurooncol 94:351–358

Barone G, Maurizi P, Tamburrini G, Riccardi R (2006) Role of temozolomide in pediatric brain tumors. Childs Nerv Syst 22:652–661

Calaminus G, Bamberg M, Jürgens H, Kortmann RD, Sörensen N, Wiestler OD, Göbel U (2004) Impact of surgery, chemotherapy and irradiation on long term outcome of intracranial malignant non-germinomatous germ cell tumors: results of the German Cooperative trial MAKEI 89. Klin Padiatr 216:141–149

Cho BK, Wang KC, Nam DH, Kim DG, Jung HW, Kim HJ, Han DH, Choi KS (1998) Pineal tumors: experience with 48 cases over 10 years. Childs Nerv Syst 14:53–58

Clark AJ, Ivan ME, Sughrue ME, Yang I, Aranda D, Han SJ, Kane AJ, Parsa AT (2010) Tumor control after surgery and radiotherapy for pineocytoma. J Neurosurg 113:319–324

Cuccia V, Rodriguez F, Palma F, Zuccaro G (2006) Pinealoblastomas in children. Childs Nerv Syst 22:577–585

Douglas JG, Rockhill JK, Olson JM, Ellenbogen RG, Geyer JR (2006) Cisplatin-based chemotherapy followed by focal reduced-dose irradiation for pediatric primary central nervous system germinomas. J Pediatr Hematol Oncol 28:36–39

Einhorn LH, Donohue J (1977) Cis-diamminedichloroplatinum, vinblastine, and bleomycin combination chemotherapy in disseminated testicular cancer. Ann Intern Med 87:293–298

Finlay JL, Boyett JM, Yates AJ, Wisoff JH, Milstein JM, Geyer JR, Bertolone SJ, McGuire P, Cherlow JM, Tefft M, Turski PA, Wara WM, Edwards M, Sutton LN, Berger MS, Epstein F, Ayers G, Allen JC, Packer RJ, for the Childrens Cancer Group (1995) Randomized phase III trial in childhood high-grade astrocytoma comparing vincristine, lomustine, and prednisone with the eight-drugs-in-1-day regimen. J Clin Oncol 13:112–123

Gangemi M, Maiuri F, Colella G, Buonamassa S (2001) Endoscopic surgery for pineal region tumors. Minim Invasive Neurosurg 44:70–73

Gilheeney SW, Saad A, Chi S, Turner C, Ullrich NJ, Goumnerova L, Scott RM, Marcus K, Lehman L, De Girolami U, Kieran MW (2008) Outcome of pediatric pineoblastoma after surgery, radiation and chemotherapy. J Neurooncol 89:89–95

Gururangan S, McLaughlin C, Quinn J, Rich J, Reardon D, Halperin EC, Herndon J II, Fuchs H, George T, Provenzale J, Watral M, Mclendon RE, Friedman A, Friedman HS, Kurtzberg J, Vredenbergh J, Martin PL (2003) High-dose chemotherapy with autologous stem-cell rescue in children and adults with newly diagnosed pineoblastomas. J Clin Oncol 21:2187–2191

Habrand JL, De Crevoisier R (2001) Radiation therapy in the management of childhood brain tumors. Childs Nerv Syst 17:121–133
Hinkes BG, von Hoff K, Deinlein F, Warmuth-Metz M, Soerensen N, Timmermann B, Mittler U, Urban C, Bode U, Pietsch T, Schlegel PG, Kortmann RD, Kuehl J, Rutkowski S (2007) Childhood pineoblastoma: experiences from the prospective multicenter trials HIT-SKK87, HIT-SKK92 and HIT91. J Neurooncol 81:217–223
Jakacki RI (1999) Pineal and nonpineal supratentorial primitive neuroectodermal tumors. Childs Nerv Syst 15:586–591
Kanamori M, Kumabe T, Tominaga T (2008) Is histological diagnosis necessary to start treatment for germ cell tumors in the pineal region? J Clin Neurosci 15:978–987
Knierim DS, Yamada S (2003) Pineal tumors and associated lesions: the effect of ethnicity on tumor type and treatment. Pediatr Neurosurg 38:307–323
Konovalov AN, Pitskhelauri DI (2003) Principles of treatment of the pineal region tumors. Surg Neurol 59:250–268
Kretschmar C, Kleinberg L, Greenberg M, Burger P, Holmes E, Wharam M (2007) Pre-radiation chemotherapy with response-based radiation therapy in children with central nervous system germ cell tumors: a report from the Children's Oncology Group. Pediatr Blood Cancer 48:285–291
Kyritsis AP (2010) Management of primary intracranial germ cell tumors. J Neurooncol 96:143–149
Lekovic GP, Gonzalez LF, Shetter AG, Porter RW, Smith KA, Brachman D, Spetzler RF (2007) Role of gamma knife surgery in the management of pineal region tumors. Neurosurg Focus 23:E12
Nomura K (2001) Epidemiology of germ cell tumors in Asia of pineal region tumor. J Neurooncol 54:211–217
Oi S, Shibata M, Tominaga J, Honda Y, Shinoda M, Takei F, Tsugane R, Matsuzawa K, Sato O (2000) Efficacy of neuroendoscopic procedures in minimally invasive preferential management of pineal region tumors: a prospective study. J Neurosurg 93:245–253
Packer RJ, Lange B, Ater J, Nicholson HS, Allen J, Walker R, Prados M, Jakacki R, Reaman G, Needles MN, Phillips PC, Ryan J, Boyett JM, Geyer R, Finlay J (1993) Carboplatin and vincristine for recurrent and newly diagnosed low-grade gliomas of childhood. J Clin Oncol 11:850–856
Reyns N, Hayashi M, Chinot O, Manera L, Péragut JC, Blond S, Régis J (2006) The role of gamma knife radiosurgery in the treatment of pineal parenchymal tumours. Acta Neurochir 148:5–11
Shin HJ, Cho BK, Jung HW, Wang KC (1998) Pediatric pineal tumors: need for a direct surgical approach and complications of the occipital transtentorial approach. Childs Nerv Syst 14:174–178
Tamaki N, Yin D (2000) Therapeutic strategies and surgical results for pineal region tumors. J Clin Neurosci 7:125–128
Wang CH, Hsu TR, Wong TT, Chang KP (2009) Efficacy of temozolomide for recurrent embryonal brain tumors in children. Childs Nerv Syst 25:535–541
Yazıcı N, Varan A, Söylemezoğlu F, Zorlu F, Kutluk T, Akyüz C, Büyükpamukçu M (2009) Pineal region tumors in children: a single center experience. Neuropediatrics 40:15–21

Benign Testicular Tumors in Children: Testicular Preserving Surgery

30

Rajendra Nerli, Aseem Shukla, and Murigendra Hiremath

Contents

Abstract

Testicular tumors in children are rare and represent only 1% of all pediatric solid tumors. The incidence, histologic distribution and prognosis of testicular tumors in children differ greatly from those seen in the adult population. In comparison to tumors in adults, childhood testicular tumors are more likely to be benign, and those that are malignant are associated with a much lower incidence of metastases. As a result, a less aggressive approach to the management of these tumors in children has evolved. Concerns regarding surgical morbidity and preservation of testicular function have warranted a distinct approach to the treatment of prepubertal testicular tumors. Benign testicular tumors can be managed safely and effectively with testis-sparing excision. Localized malignant tumors can be managed with excision alone.

Introduction

Testicular tumors in children are uncommon and account for 1–2% of all pediatric solid tumors. The annual incidence of these tumors in boys younger than 15 years in the United States is 1 per 100,000 (Young et al. 1986). Incidence wise testicular tumors are far more common in adults than in children. For this reason alone, management of pediatric testicular tumors has been based on experience in adults. Indeed, testicular tumors in adults and children are similar in many ways.

R. Nerli (✉) • M. Hiremath
Department of Pediatric Urology,
KLE University's J N Medical College,
KLES Kidney Foundation, KLES Dr. Prabhakar Kore
Hospital and MRC, Belgaum 590010, India
e-mail: rajendranerli@yahoo.in

A. Shukla
Department of Urologic Surgery, Pediatric Division,
University of Minnesota, 420 Delaware Street S. E.,
MMC 394, Minneapolis, MN 590010, USA

M.A. Hayat (ed.), *Pediatric Cancer, Volume 3: Diagnosis, Therapy, and Prognosis*, Pediatric Cancer 3,
DOI 10.1007/978-94-007-4528-5_30,

The tumors usually present with a testicular mass in both the age groups and are initially treated with excision of the primary tumor. In both children and adults, malignant testicular tumors are particularly sensitive to platinum-based chemotherapy, which has revolutionized the management of testicular cancer throughout the age spectrum (Einhorn and Williams 1980; Flamant et al. 1990). However, there are important differences between testicular tumors occurring in children and those occurring in adults. These differences involve tumor histopathology, malignant potential, and pattern of metastatic spread. Benign lesions represent a greater percentage of cases in children than in adults. The American Academy of Pediatrics prepubertal testis tumor registry reported that benign tumors accounted for 38% of cases (Ross et al. 2002). Large series from single institutions report a higher percentage of benign lesions, thus suggesting that these entities were underreported to the tumor registry (Metcalfe et al. 2003; Shukla et al. 2004). A recent multicenter report found that 74% of primary testicular tumors in prepubertal children were benign (Pohl et al. 2004). The patients themselves are also dissimilar, with different concerns regarding surgical morbidity and preservation of testicular function.

Epidemiology

There is a bimodal age distribution for the incidence of testicular tumors in children. The incidence of childhood testicular tumors peaks at 2 years of age (Li and Fraumeni 1972; Haas and Schmidt 1995), tapers after 4 years of age, but then begins to rise again at puberty. In 1984, Weissbach and associates looked into the prevalence of various histologic types among adult and pediatric testicular tumors. They studied 1062 adult tumors from the Bonn registry and 1169 pediatric tumors from a review of the literature. They observed that seminomas and mixed germ cell tumors (MGCT) accounted for 89% of cases in the adults, with stromal tumors accounting for 8% and yolk sac tumors and teratomas accounting for 1% each. In contrast, 49% of tumors in children were yolk sac tumors, 29% were of stromal origin, 13% were teratomas and only 9% were seminomas or mixed germ cell tumors . The study had included adolescents among the pediatric tumors. However, when patients were divided along the line of puberty, virtually none of the prepubertal tumors were either seminomas or mixed germ cell tumors.

Pathology

Classification of prepubertal testicular tumors
Germ cell tumors
Yolk sac
Teratoma
Mixed germ cell
Seminoma
Gonadal stromal tumors
Leydig cell
Sertoli cell
Juvenile granulosa cell
Mixed
Gonadoblastoma
Tumors of supporting tissues
Fibroma
Leiomyoma
Hemangioma
Lymphomas and leukemias
Tumor-like lesions
Epidermoid cysts
Hyperplastic nodule secondary to congenital adrenal hyperplasia
Secondary tumors
Tumors of the adnexa

From Kay (1993)

Non–germ cell and germ cell neoplasms arise from the celomic epithelium and primordial germ cells, respectively. It is postulated that the totipotent germ cells can evolve into seminoma or embryonal carcinoma. Embryonal carcinoma is capable of differentiating into embryonic structures such as mature or immature teratomas and into extraembryonic structures such as endodermal sinus tumors and choriocarcinoma. Seminoma or dysgerminoma is a primitive germ cell neoplasm that lacks the capacity for further differentiation. These tumors are unusual in childhood except when related to gonadal dysgenesis.

Teratomas

Teratomas are the most common benign tumors in prepubertal patients. The median age of prepubertal teratoma presentation is 13 months, with several cases reported as presenting during the neonatal period (Grady et al. 1997; Levy et al. 1994). Histologically, teratomas consist of tissues representing the three germinal layers: endoderm, mesoderm, and ectoderm. Due to their benign behaviour, the true incidence of teratomas is probably under-reported in both tumor registries and large reviews. In fact, it represents by far the most common testicular tumor seen in our series (Nerli et al. 2010) and reported similarly by other authors (Rushton and Belman 1993). Although the diagnosis of teratoma is established only on Histopathological examination, one can suspect teratoma in a prepubertal child with a testicular mass, with no endocrinal manifestations or an elevated serum AFP levels, particularly when pre-operative sonography demonstrates a circumscribed, partly cystic intratesticular lesion. Prepubertal teratomas do not stain positively for AFP and elevated serum AFP levels have not been reported with this tumor (Rushton et al. 1990; Mostofi et al. 1987) . The characteristic appearance of sonolucent cystic areas with intervening septa and solid areas seen with most teratomas contrasts with the appearance of other intra-testicular tumors in children, which are typically solid except for the rare cystic granulose-cell tumor and simple cysts. Another helpful sonographic finding is the presence of calcification in the tumor, representing bone or a psammoma body. Metastasis from a teratoma in prepubertal children has not been reported (Brosman 1985; Weissbach et al. 1984).

Epidermoid and Simple Cysts

Epidermoid cysts are rare and account for 14% of all testicular tumors in children (Pohl et al. 2004). Epidermoid cysts are composed entirely of keratin-producing epithelium. They are to be distinguished from dermoid cysts, which contain skin and skin appendages, and from teratomas, which contain derivatives of other germ cell layers. Epidermoid cysts are universally benign in prepubertal children. The ultrasonographic findings of a complex heterogenous mass may suggest a diagnosis of an epidermoid cyst. However sonographic findings may be variable and may mimic those of teratomas (Ross et al. 2002). Simple cysts of the testis are rare benign lesions reported both in children and adults (Altadonna et al. 1988). The diagnosis can be made by the characteristic sonographic finding of an intra-testicular anechoic mass with sharply defined walls.

Stromal Tumors

Stromal tumors include Leydig cell, Sertoli cell, juvenile granulosa, and mixed or undifferentiated tumors. These tumors are of nongerminal origin and account for a higher proportion of testicular tumors in children. Stromal testis tumors are rare in children, and there are no large series to guide their management. Leydig cell tumors are universally benign in children (Coppes et al. 1994; Thomas et al. 2001) but hormonally active, secreting testosterone. Biochemical evaluation, including determinations of serum testosterone and urine 17-ketosteroid excretion allows the differentiation of Leydig cell tumor from other hormonally active lesions of the testis. They usually present with precocious puberty in children aged 5–10 years. Most patients present with virilisation. Persistence of androgenic effects following excision may be due to existence of a contralateral tumor, though uncommon in children. These tumors are difficult to detect on physical examination and an ultrasound may be necessary to rule out a contralateral tumor. Sertoli cell tumors account for only 2% of primary prepubertal testicular tumors. They are well circumscribed, lobulated and cysts are common. Sertoli cell tumors are usually hormonally inactive in children (Cortez and Kaplan 1993; Kolon and Hochman 1997). Although all reported cases to date in children younger than 5 years have been benign, there have been a few cases of malignant Sertoli cell tumors in older children (Cortez and Kaplan 1993; Kolon and Hochman 1997).

Juvenile Granulosa Cell Tumor

Testicular juvenile granulosa cell tumors are stromal tumors bearing a light microscopic resemblance to ovarian juvenile granulosa cell tumors. However, the histologic origin of this tumor in the testes is unclear. Granulosa cell tumors occur almost exclusively in the first year of life and most often in the first 6 months. Several cases have been described in association with ambiguous genitalia (Young et al. 1985). These tumors are hormonally inactive and benign. Although these children should undergo chromosomal analysis, no treatment or metastatic evaluation is required beyond excision (Thomas et al. 2001). Histologically mixed or undifferentiated stromal tumors consist of areas of gonadal stromal neoplasia and undifferentiated regions of spindle cells, which may exhibit a high mitotic rate. These stromal tumors have an epidemiology similar to that of granulose cell tumors (Thomas et al. 2001). Although some of these tumors have histologic characteristics commonly associated with malignancy, most are benign. Shukla et al. reported on testis sparing enucleation of a granulosa cell tumor with a 5 year recurrence free follow-up (Shukla et al. 2004).

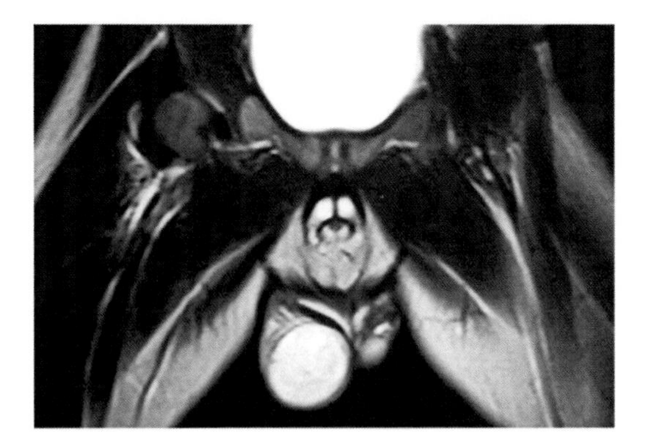

Fig. 30.1 MRI showing right testicular tumor

Clinical Presentation and Evaluation

Most children present with a testicular mass or swelling, noted by the parents, child or a health care provider. These masses are typically hard and painless to palpate and need to be differentiated from masses arising from the epididymis and other extra-testicular tissues. Acute abdominal pain can be the initial symptom with torsion of an abdominal undescended testicle containing a tumor. Some children with hormonally active tumors may have small intratesticular lesions that are not palpable on physical examination. Disorders that must be excluded are epididymitis, hydrocele, hernia, and spermatic cord torsion.

Testicular ultrasound is routinely performed for the evaluation of testicular masses in children. Color Doppler ultrasound has been reported to be more effective than gray-scale ultrasound in detecting intratesticular neoplasms in the pediatric population (Luker and Siegel 1994). There are no sonographic features that can reliably distinguish benign and malignant tumors, but the finding of anechoic cystic lesions can suggest a benign lesion, such as a simple cyst, cystic dysplasia, teratoma, or cystic granulosa cell tumor. The ultrasound findings of epidermoid cyst are also unique. There is a heterogeneous intratesticular mass with concentric rings of alternating hypoechoic and hyperechoic layers that give rise to an "onion-skin" appearance. This corresponds to the multiple layers of keratin debris within the lesion. The mass is surrounded by a hypoechoic or echogenic rim and the absence of flow on color Doppler sonography (Langer et al. 1999). Ultrasound can also assess whether there is enough normal testis parenchyma remaining to warrant salvage. If a child is identified with a cystic lesion on ultrasound and the serum AFP level is normal, the surgeon can plan for a testis-sparing procedure (Rushton et al. 1990; Grunert et al. 1992; Valla 2001; Metcalfe et al. 2003; Shukla et al. 2004). MRI (Fig. 30.1) may detect small functioning Leydig cell tumors not evident on ultrasound (Kaufman et al. 1990).

Tumor markers that are typically used in the evaluation and management of adult testis tumors include human chorionic gonadotropin (HCG) and α-fetoprotein (AFP). Although HCG is elaborated in a significant number of MGCT, this tumor type is vanishingly rare in prepubertal patients. Therefore, HCG is not a helpful marker in the prepubertal population. On the other hand, AFP levels are elevated in 90% of patients with yolk sac tumors and can be helpful in the preoperative distinction between yolk sac and other tumors (almost all of which are benign). One caveat is that AFP levels are quite high in healthy infants. Although highly variable, AFP levels are approximately 50,000 ng/mL in newborns, dropping to 10,000 ng/mL by age 2 weeks, 300 ng/mL by age 2 months, and 12 ng/mL by age 6 months. 10 Therefore, AFP levels among patients with yolk sac tumors and benign tumors overlap during the first 6 months of life, making AFP less helpful in distinguishing tumor types in young infants (Grady et al. 1997; Ross and Kay 2004). In addition to ultrasound, measurement of serum AFP can help identify tumors amenable to a testis-sparing procedure.

Many, if not most, prepubertal tumors are benign, the metastatic evaluation may be deferred until a histologic diagnosis of the primary tumor is obtained. A preoperative metastatic evaluation may be undertaken only in children older than 6 months who have elevated AFP levels and are likely harbor yolk sac tumors. Staging is based on both tumor markers and pathologic findings. AFP levels are determined at diagnosis and monitored after radical inguinal orchiectomy to determine whether an appropriate half-life decline has occurred. CT of the retroperitoneum and chest is obtained to exclude metastatic lesions. CT imaging of the retroperitoneum can identify most patients who have lymph node metastases, but there is a 15–20% false-negative rate (Pizzocara et al. 1987; Weiner et al. 1994).

Surgical Treatment

The standard initial treatment for a malignant testicular tumor in an adult, is an inguinal orchiectomy with early control of the vessels. However there has been a major change in the management of pre-pubertal testicular tumors. Except for tumors in children older than 6 months of age with elevated AFP levels (who are most likely to harbor yolk sac tumors), the initial surgical management of a prepubertal testicular tumor is excisional biopsy with frozen section analysis. This strategy is supported by the fact that, compared with adult tumors, for which inguinal orchiectomy is standard surgical management, a high percentage of prepubertal tumors are benign. In addition, the desire to preserve testicular tissue may be more compelling in a child who has yet to experience puberty.

The principles of cancer surgery must be adhered to strictly whenever a testis is explored for tumor. The affected testis should be explored (Fig. 30.2) through an high inguinal incision. The cord and the accompanying blood vessels are occluded with a non-crushing vascular clamps at the level of the internal ring. An transverse incision is made on the testis and the tumor is either excised or enucleated out. The excised tissue is sent for frozen section examination. If the frozen section reveals a or suspicious/malignant lesion, the entire testis is removed. However if the tumor is of benign histology, the remaining testis is closed with absorbable suture and returned to the scrotum.

Orchiectomy is known to cause harm to the patient both cosmetically and psychologically. It is also known that the treated testis, can recover to a size equal to the normal contralateral testis after enucleation of tumors. The aim of testis-sparing surgery has been preservation of testicular function that includes both appropriate androgen production and fertility. Secondary hormonal derangement can be corrected and fertility maintained with testis-sparing primary treatment. A worry exists regarding impairment of blood testis barrier following surgical testicular violation and therefore increase the risk of autoimmune reaction against spermatozoa. A recent report stated that autoimmunity against spermatic antigen is apparent in adults only (Mirilas and De Almeida 1999). Antisperm antibodies was negative in two cases at 5 years after both radical orchiectomy and a partial orchiectomy (Nonomura et al. 2001).

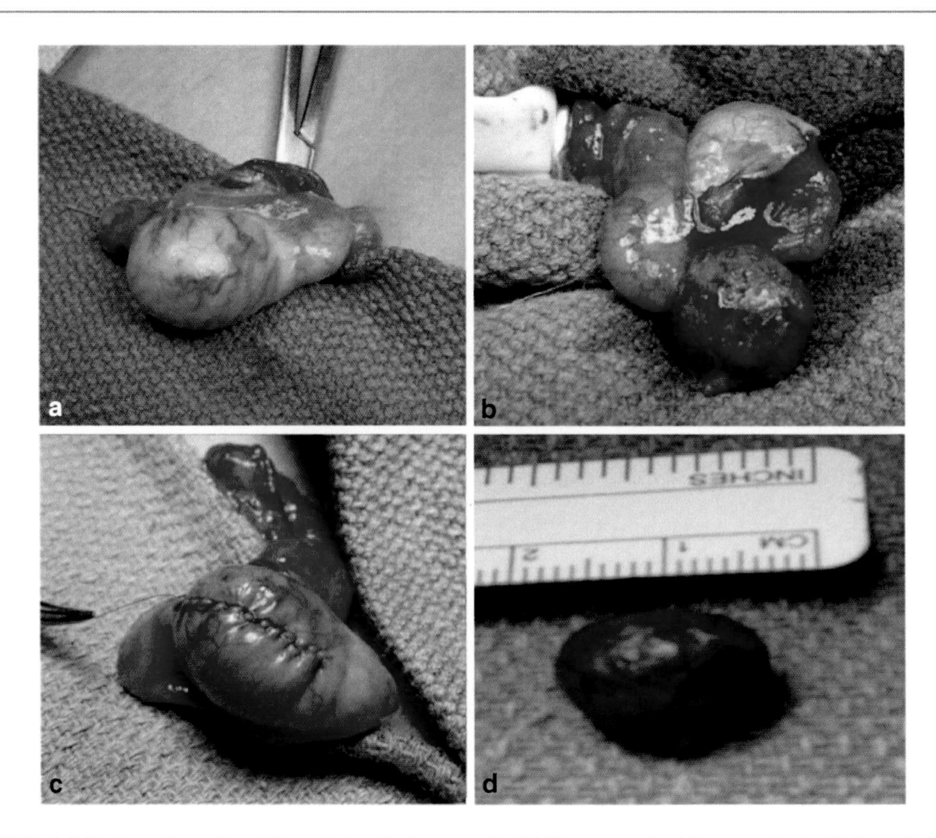

Fig. 30.2 (**a**) Right testis explored through inguinal approach. (**b**) Transverse incision over the testis is made and the tumor excised. (**c**) The incision over the testis closed with absorbable suture. (**d**) The excised tumor specimen

Summary

Prepubertal testicular tumors are distinct from those seen in the adults in relation to incidence, histology and prognosis. Testicular tumors in children are rare and form 1% of all pediatric solid tumors. In the prepubertal Testis Tumor Registry of the Urologic section of the American Academy of Pediatrics, the majority of primary testis tumors were yolk sac tumors, followed by teratomas and stromal tumors. Because teratomas and most stromal tumors are benign in children, it would follow that fewer than two thirds of prepubertal testicular tumors are malignant, compared with 90% of tumors in adults. Except for tumors in children older than 6 months with elevated α fetoprotein levels (who most likely harbour yolk sac tumors) the initial surgical management of a prepubertal testicular tumor is excisional biopsy with frozen section analysis. For children with epidermoid cysts and prepubertal children with teratomas, no radiologic studies or follow-up for the development of metastatic disease is required.

References

Altadonna V, Snyde HM, Rosenberg HK (1988) Simple cysts of the testis in children: preoperative diagnosis by ultrasound and excision with testicular preservation. J Urol 140:1505–1507

Brosman SA (1985) Tumors: male genital tract. In: Kelalis PP, King LR, Belman AB (eds) Clinical pediatric urology, 2nd edn. WB Saunders, Philadelphia, pp 1202–1219

Coppes MJ, Rackley R, Kay R (1994) Primary testicular and paratesticular tumors of childhood. Med Pediatr Oncol 22:329–340

Cortez JC, Kaplan GW (1993) Gonadal stromal tumors, gonadoblastomas, epidermoid cysts, and secondary tumors of the testis in children. Urol Clin North Am 20:15–26

Einhorn LH, Williams SD (1980) Chemotherapy of disseminated testicular cancer. Cancer 46:1339–1344
Flamant F, Baranzelli MD, Kalifa C, Lemerle J (1990) Treatment of malignant germ cell tumors in children: experience of the Institut Gustave Roussy and the French Society of Pediatric Oncology. Crit Rev Oncol Hematol 10:99–110
Grady R, Ross JH, Kay R (1997) Epidemiological features of testicular teratoma in a prepubertal population. J Urol 158(3 pt 2):1191–1192
Grunert RT, Van Every MJ, Uehling DT (1992) Bilateral epidermoid cysts of the testicle. J Urol 147:1599–1601
Haas RJ, Schmidt P (1995) Testicular germ cell tumors in childhood and adolescence. World J Urol 13:203–208
Kaufman E, Akiya F, Foucar E, Grambort F, Cartwright KC (1990) Virilization due to Leydig cell tumor diagnosis by magnetic resonance imaging. Clin Pediatr (Phila) 29:414–417
Kay R (1993) Prepubertal testicular tumor registry. J Urol 150:671–674
Kolon TF, Hochman HI (1997) Malignant Sertoli cell tumor in a prepubescent boy. J Urol 158:608–609
Langer JE, Ramchandani P, Siegelman ES, Banner MP (1999) Epidermoid cysts of the testicle: sonographic and MR imaging features. Am J Roentgenol 173:1295–1299
Levy D, Kay R, Elder J (1994) Neonatal testis tumors: a review of the prepubertal testis tumor registry. J Urol 151:715–717
Li FP, Fraumeni JF Jr (1972) Testicular cancers in children. Epidemiologic characteristics. J Natl Cancer Inst 48:1575–1581
Luker GD, Siegel MJ (1994) Pediatric testicular tumors: evaluation with gray-scale and color Doppler US. Radiology 191:561–564
Metcalfe PD, Farivar-Mohseni J, Farhat W, Mclorie G, Khoury A, Bägli DJ (2003) Pediatric testicular tumors: contemporary incidence and efficacy of testicular preserving surgery. J Urol 170:2412–2416
Mirilas P, De Almeida M (1999) Absence of antisperm surface antibodies in prepubertal boys with cryptorchidism and other anomalies of the inguinoscrotal region before and after surgery. J Urol 162:177–181
Mostofi FK, Sesterhenn IA, Davis CJ Jr (1987) Immunopathology of germ cell tumors of the testis. Semin Diagn Pathol 4:320
Nerli RB, Ajay G, Shivangouda P, Pravin P, Reddy M, Pujar VC (2010) Prepubertal testicular tumors: our 10 year experience. Indian J Cancer 47:292–295
Nonomura K, Koyama T, Kakizaki H, Murakumo M, Shinohara N, Koyanagi T (2001) Testicular sparing surgery for the prepubertal testicular tumor. Eur Urol 40:699–704
Pizzocaro G, Zanoni F, Salvioni R, Milani A, Piva L, Pilotti S (1987) Difficulties of a surveillance study omitting retroperitoneal lymphadenectomy in clinical stage I nonseminomatous germ cell tumors of the testis. J Urol 138:1393–1396
Pohl HG, Shukla AR, Metcalf PD, Cilento BG, Retik AB, Bagli DJ, Huff DS, Rushton HG (2004) Prepubertal testis tumors: actual prevalence rate of histological types. J Urol 172:2370–2372
Ross JH, Kay R (2004) Prepubertal testis tumor. Rev Urol 6:11–18
Ross JH, Rybicki L, Kay R (2002) Clinical behavior and a contemporary management algorithm for pre pubertal testis tumors: a summary of the prepubertal testis tumor registry. J Urol 164:1678–1679
Rushton G, Belman BA (1993) Testis sparing surgery for benign lesions of the prepubertal testis. Urol Clin North Am 20:27–37
Rushton G, Belman AB, Sesterhenn I, Patterson K, Mostofi FK (1990) Testicular sparing surgery for prepubertal teratoma of the testis: a clinical and pathological study. J Urol 144:726–730
Shukla AR, Woodard C, Carr MC, Huff DS, Canning DA, Zderic SA, Kolon TF, Snyder HM 3rd (2004) Experience with testis sparing surgery for testicular teratoma. J Urol 171:161–163
Thomas JC, Ross JH, Kay R (2001) Stromal testis tumors in children: a report from the prepubertal testis tumor registry. J Urol 166:2338–2340
Valla JS (2001) Testis sparing surgery for benign testicular tumors in children. J Urol 165:2280–2283
Weiner ES, Lawrence W, Hays D, Lobe TE, Andrassy R, Donaldson S, Crist W, Newton W, Johnson J, Gehan E (1994) Retroperitoneal node biopsy in childhood paratesticular rhabdomyosarcoma. J Pediatr Surg 29:171–178
Weissbach L, Altwein JE, Stiens R (1984) Germinal testicular tumors in childhood. Eur Urol 10:73–85
Young RH, Lawrence WD, Scully RE (1985) Juvenile granulosa cell tumor—another neoplasm associated with abnormal chromosomes and ambiguous genitalia, a report of three cases. Am J Surg Pathol 9:737–743
Young JL Jr, Ries LG, Silverberg E, Horm JW, Miller RW (1986) Cancer incidence, survival and mortality for children younger than 15 years. Cancer 58:598–602

Index

M.A. Hayat (ed.), *Pediatric Cancer, Volume 3: Diagnosis, Therapy, and Prognosis*, Pediatric Cancer 3,
DOI 10.1007/978-94-007-4528-5, © Springer Science+Business Media Dordrecht 2012

N

O

Printed by Publishers' Graphics LLC